ALTHEA HAYTON is a womb twin  in that order. She began her writing care addiction to food. Then, after several ye sociated with the loss of a baby before bi mourning, she discovered in 2002 that she ⸺ ⸺ that time there was no information or psychological support available for womb twin survivors, so she began work at once to put this right. She started recruiting hundreds of womb twin survivors by means of a web site. In 2007 she founded a non-profit organisation, WombTwin.com, to provide information, help and support for womb twin survivors around the world. She has edited two anthologies, *Untwinned* and *A Silent Cry*. Her womb twin research project continues with the help of an online questionnaire. She gives talks and seminars around the world about the psychological effect on the survivor when a co-twin dies before birth. She also facilitates group workshops for womb twin survivors to help them to heal. Althea was educated at Oxford University and is a qualified social worker and counsellor. She is married with two sons and lives in Hertfordshire, England.

The Womb Twin series

Other works by Althea Hayton

Womb Twin Survivors

The lost twin in the Dream of the Womb

Womb Twin Survivors

The lost twin in the Dream of the Womb

Althea Hayton

Wren Publications

First published in 2011
by Wren Publications, P.O. Box 396, St Albans, Herts, AL3 6NE
England

www.wrenpublications.co.uk

ISBN 978-0-9557808-2-0

Printed and bound in UK and USA by
Lightning Source:

Lightning Source Inc. (US)
1246 Heil Quaker Blvd., La Vergne, TN, USA 37086

Lightning Source UK Ltd.
Chapter House, Pitfield, Kiln Farm, Milton Keynes, MK11 3LW, UK

Two in a pod, two in a hold, two in a teacup,
commas curled together, Yin & Yang tumbling end over end.
Yet one grows fatter as one thins. One drinks in
as one seeps away. One's shape sharpens
as the other's lines blur. One grows fingers and toes;
for the other, at the wrists and ankles, clumps,
then knots, then fraying threads,
as cells flake off, migrate across the black waters.

From "Chimera" by Frances Ruhlen McConnel

*This book is dedicated to all the womb twin survivors
who did not win their lifelong battle against despair.
No one explained why they wanted so much to die.*

They are the inspiration for this book, so they did not die in vain.

CONTENTS

PART FIVE : The Healing Path

APPENDICES

LIST OF ILLUSTRATIONS AND TABLES

ILLUSTRATIONS

ACKNOWLEDGEMENTS

This book would not have been possible to write without the help of a huge number of people. First and foremost, my husband John, who has patiently endured my eight-year quest for understanding of this difficult subject, the subsequent years of research and writing, not to mention the hard work of preparing this book for publication. I owe everything to him.

Rose Powell allowed me to use her beautiful image for the cover, for which I am very grateful. Many thanks also to Lindsey Kevan and Neil Spencer of the University of Hertfordshire, who produced the statistical report which underpins this book.

Dr. Louis Keith, Elizabeth Noble and David Chamberlain have been my champions from the beginning of this project and I thank them for boosting my confidence during my lonely quest for understanding.

Because I believe that people deserve their privacy, I will mention my many other helpers by their first name only: Andrew and John were my loyal and honest mentors as I made my first uncertain attempts to create these chapters. Shirley, Monica and Barbara gave support when times got tough. Jean struggled through the early draft and gave an honest and helpful opinion. Tracey proof-read the final manuscript with true professionalism. Thomas and Natalie gave advice on the cover.

The hundreds of people who sent me their stories by email and agreed to their stories being used are too numerous to mention here. Words cannot express my gratitude for the trust and honesty they have shown in sharing their story with me. This whole book is my tribute to them, for their stories have greatly illuminated what may have otherwise been a rather dry discussion of a lengthy research project.

Editor's note:
To preserve the authenticity of the stories, which have been sent from various countries of the world, the original spelling is retained.

Introduction

At the start of this century, I suddenly came to the conclusion that I once had a twin but my twin died before I was born. Almost at once, I began to research this unusual phenomenon. I quickly came across the concept of the "vanishing" twin and discovered that this was more common than I could ever have realized. I named the survivors of twin or multiple conceptions "womb twin" survivors. As I made my own pathway towards healing, I embarked on a journey of discovery that has lasted until this day and will no doubt continue.

I now know that on average just one percent of births in the world are twin births. Research has revealed that for every pair of twins born there are at least ten babies born whose twin died in the womb, their "womb twin." So we now know that there are more than 600 million womb twin survivors in the world. It is astonishing that society has somehow managed not to notice or correctly identify such an enormous group of millions of people. This is probably because, until the 1980s, the loss of a twin in the womb was not fully recognized or acknowledged. People can hardly be expected to pay any heed to the needs of the sole survivors if the lost twins remain hidden from view.

Research using ultrasound scans has repeatedly shown us how many twins are lost in the first few weeks of life. These are called "vanishing twins" but they don't really vanish - they die. Their tiny bodies may be miscarried, disintegrate or gradually fade away, leaving tiny traces that an expert may be able to identify but that many people would not even notice. Since that amazing day when I realized that I am a womb twin survivor, I have been looking for the others. One by one, womb twin survivors have come to me by means of my web site. With their help, I have learned how to identify them and help them heal. I know that womb twin survivors have a need to understand why they feel as they do and in order to help them, I intend to bring these little lost twins out of the darkness and into the light: this book is their story.

We will begin by exploring the big idea of human reproduction and some seemingly trivial events occurring in the womb which are actually of vital importance. Bit by bit, we will explore the development the Womb Twin hypothesis that underlies this work. We will discover the intricacies of twinning - an extraordinary but common anomaly of human reproduction that has far-reaching consequences for the survivor when a co-twin dies. We will uncover the implications of zygosity and the different physical consequences of losing your twin at different stages of development.

We will then consider the psychological effect of such a personal loss on the sole survivor and examine closely the pre-birth experiences that lie in your Dream of the Womb. We will take a look at the science of prenatal psychology, which lies on the fringes of general psychology but at the very heart of this book. Next, we will carefully scrutinize what was learned during my seven-year Womb Twin research project, which I carried out with the help of many hundreds of womb twin survivors.

On almost every page you will hear the voices of womb twin survivors from all over the world, telling a story rarely told in public. There is plenty of room for interested observers who are not womb twin survivors but with important questions to ask. Some of those questions and their answers will be scattered along the way. By the end of this stage you will hopefully have a clearer idea of how it feels to be a womb twin survivor.

The final stage sets out a pathway to healing. This is a step-by-step progress through five stages of healing that may take you three years or three weeks to do, depending on your level of engagement and desperation. The rewards will make all the difficulty and pain worthwhile. You will end up with a new way of seeing the world. On almost every page, dozens of inspirational stories, sent to me from womb twin survivors across the world, will give you hope as you make your own journey to autonomy as a womb twin survivor who has awakened from the Dream of the Womb.

Althea Hayton
St Albans, England

PART ONE

The death of a twin before or around birth

There Should Have Been Two

I am born alone.
I push into the world
One, not two.

You were expelled: a bloody mess.
Mucus mixed with foetus
disintegrating to slip and slide
your bloody lumpy way out.

Your heart used to beat in time with mine.
We were joined until separation.
One egg into two: my other half.

Your unbirth was messy.
You gave your life, so mine could begin.
You were pulled from me -
into the dead abyss.

We were content together.
Curled around each other
in a two-fold foetal position,
thumbs in our mouths, feeding from one source.

You left me in that cavity.
Ripped from you –
my sister, my mirror image,
who I had starved to save my own soul.

I greedily took from you.
You happily gave to me.
My embryonic soul sister.
I couldn't stop you. I couldn't help you.
Like you'd helped me.

As I pushed through
into this bright, noisy world alone
there should have been two
there should have been you...
I miss you.

Julie Rae

1
The making of you

Yes – the history of man for the nine months preceding his birth would, probably, be far more interesting, and contain events of greater moment, than all the three-score and ten years that follow it. [a]

Whoever you are reading this, when you were no more than a twinkle in your father's eye, the making of you had already begun. You came into being as a separate, unique, brand-new little person at the moment of your conception. Now conception requires two tiny single-cell gametes to meet, one from Mum and one from Dad. Mum's gamete is called an *ovum* - sometimes called a human egg - and Dad's gamete is called a *spermatozoon* - usually known as a sperm.

Sexual reproduction - and this is after all what we are talking about - has been going for a very long time. Largely by a process of trial and error, this extremely complex and delicate process, operating at a microscopic level, has been honed to a nicety over the generations.

Your Mum and Dad played their biological part to perfection, as they negotiated themselves into position to enable conception to occur. It may have been carefully planned, impulsive, entirely inappropriate or even morally wrong, but once Dad's sperm and Mum's egg were in exactly the right position and in precisely the right environment, they made that impossible, crucial connection and merged. That created you. Whatever else you may say about yourself, you are a miracle. We all are.

As we will discover later on, all those years of evolution have not eliminated the hundreds of mishaps that prevent conception or the successful development of the embryo. Over time, intricate and elaborate means have been developed to ensure the survival of our species. Today, if conception and development simply won't work, despite Mum's and Dad's best efforts, we now have artificial means to try and ensure that

---

a. That was how Samuel Taylor Coleridge (1772-1834) marked a passage in his own copy of Sir Thomas Browne's *Religio Medici*.

they can have a baby. They may be still uncertain, but the various new fertility treatments have helped us to understand a little more of how we all came into being, because these pregnancies are so carefully monitored at the very earliest stage of embryo development. [b]

DNA - the stuff that genes are made of

You probably already know that you have half your mother's genes and half your father's genes. Your body is made out of many millions of cells, which for the whole of your life have been constantly dividing in half. In each cell is a genetic code that decides what kind of cell is made and how it functions. We are beginning to understand just a little of what these genes may do, but there is a lot that we don't know. The whole science of genetics is very mysterious indeed. We do know that genes are laid out along chromosomes, which are long strings of a protein called DNA.[c] The chromosomes are always grouped in pairs. Human DNA is arranged in a set of 46 chromosomes in 23 pairs. Pair number 23 decides your gender. In males the two strands of pair 23 do not look alike: one is like a letter X and the other looks a bit stunted and is known as the "Y" chromosome.

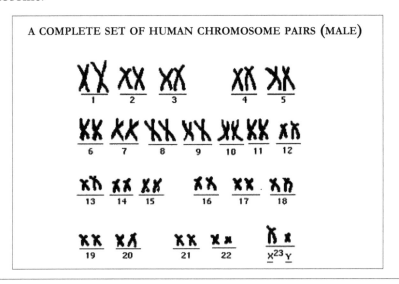

A COMPLETE SET OF HUMAN CHROMOSOME PAIRS (MALE)

---

b. The various fertility treatments now available are collectively known as Assisted Reproductive Technology, or ART.

c. Deoxyribonucleic acid.

In females both chromosomes in pair 23 are complete, so in simple terms females are described as "XX." Also in simple terms, males are described as "XY."

The most important thing to remember about a gamete is that it is specially created with half the usual number of chromosomes. If two gametes of opposite genders fuse together, they make up a whole new organism. That is exactly what gametes are designed to do. So each *ovum* (egg) in your mother and each *spermatozoon* (sperm cell) in your father had only a single chromosome in each pair. Mum's tiny egg was a spherical single cell, just about the same diameter as a human hair. In the nucleus of the egg was half of the DNA needed to create you, the new zygote.

Each one of Dad's sperm cells had a head about as big as a flake of pepper with a thin tail ten times as long as its head, which contained the half package of Dad's DNA. Scientists at Bath University are discovering that there is far more to a sperm cell than its genetic payload of DNA. Each one carries other proteins that have a direct influence on the processes of fertilization and embryo development. Even the proteins in the tail may be crucial in some way.[1]

Apart from the half set of chromosomes, your mother's egg carried mitochondria, tiny powerhouses of energy that keep every cell alive. These same little packages are now found in every cell of your body, and the mitochondria you now carry came from your mother's egg, which was made in the ovary of your grandmother and contained mitochondria from her mother, and so forth back through the generations. This aspect of inheritance has been the focus of extensive research in recent years and the Mitochondria Research Society, founded in the USA in 2000, is leading the field. The debate includes the notion that Dad's mitochondria also made it into Mum's egg, so had some part to play.

The merger

The Grand Plan of Reproduction requires a continuous supply of high quality eggs and sperm. To guarantee this, a simple rule applies: the weak go to the wall and the superior organisms survive. As a womb twin survivor you are already a superior organism because you survived. Remember that next time you are feeling inadequate.

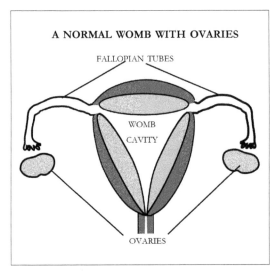

A NORMAL WOMB WITH OVARIES

FALLOPIAN TUBES

WOMB
CAVITY

OVARIES

In the womb, a female *foetus* (unborn baby) has about seven million oocytes (immature eggs) in her tiny ovaries. Some of these never mature and others die off so that at birth she only has about two million.[2] Approximately 500 times in her life (i.e. once a month from the age of about 14 to 55) about 15 eggs matured in your mother's ovaries. One of these same 15 eggs, sometimes more than one, were shed from one or both ovaries. The egg floated off away from the ovary and down the fallopian tube, ready and willing to meet with a sperm.

If a mature egg is not fertilized within a day of its ejection from the ovary, it dies. Therefore the sperm have got to swim all the way up the fallopian tube. This is a journey of about eight inches which, if you are a microscopic organism, is a very long way. Sperm may reach the fallopian tube within 20 minutes of ejaculation. This is very fast swimming indeed, made in a spiral rotating movement which propels the sperm forward. To increase the probability of one sperm achieving a successful meeting with an egg, the normal sperm count is 20 million sperm in every ejaculation. Only about half of the sperm are normally developed and able to swim. If the concentration is less than that it may impair fertility, unless there are some excellent swimmers involved. The whole arrangement acts as a quality control system, so that sexual reproduction is a risky and wasteful business.

Meanwhile, the egg that was about to be fertilized was making its slow and gentle way into the fallopian tube, turning slowly as it moved towards the womb. The next step was one of the most mysterious of all. Surrounding Mum's egg was an area called the *zona pellucida* that acted like an impenetrable barrier to sperm. Only the sperm with the right chemical "signature" was allowed through. The few sperm that survived as far as this had been primed and prepared during their long, hard swim in a process known as "capacitation." Only capacitated sperm can attempt to penetrate the *zona pellucida*. Capacitation re-energizes these selected Alpha sperm after their long swim. They start to lash their tails back and forth in a huge effort that latches them onto the welcoming surface of the *zona pellucida* that surrounds the egg. There they are bound to the surface of the egg by an irresistible mix of organic chemicals. Right at the tip of every sperm's head is a little package of zone-digesting enzymes.

You owe your very existence to the strength and endurance of a certain Alpha sperm cell which faced the final challenge. This particular sperm made it because it had both the strongest tail and the most efficient zone-digesting enzymes. It was able to thrust and digest its way through the *zona pellucida* like a microscopic drill and about 20 minutes of frantic effort later, it was through. When the two sets of DNA met, they fused into one enormous zygote. The zygote was you, with a whole new set of chromosome pairs and therefore a brand new mix of genes never seen before - half from Mum and half from Dad. That was the moment when your life began.

Morula to blastocyst (1-4 days)

A series of rapid chemical changes then took place in the *zona pellucida* that made it quite impenetrable so that no further sperm could get through. It took about 24 hours, but in the end the new zygote was complete and that was the very beginning of you. Your zygote began to divide in half almost immediately, creating a series of cells called "blastomeres." Research is beginning to suggest that the first division of the

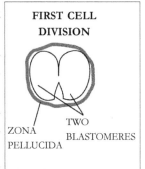

FIRST CELL
DIVISION

ZONA
PELLUCIDA

TWO
BLASTOMERES

zygote sets the trend for how the subsequent cells from each of the two halves will be employed in the developing body of the blastocyst.[3] We will see in the next chapter how twins may form if the zygote divides in half and separates into two individuals. For now, we will concentrate on the development of a single embryo, so we can trace the developmental stages of the embryo that apply to everyone.

Each cell division takes about a day to happen. After two or three days you consisted of about 16 blastomeres held together in a bundle, called a *morula*. Your ball of blastomeres surrounded by the *zona pellucida* floated gently down the fallopian tube. After three or four days, as your little bundle of blastomeres moved along, you formed into a blastocyst, which had a hollow within it.

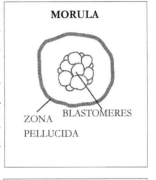

Your blastocyst moved into the vast space of your mother's womb. Your bundle of blastomeres had differentiated themselves into two groups - an outer layer and an inner layer. The outer layer was designed eventually to keep you fixed onto the wall of the womb and nurture you as you grew. The inner mass of cells was designed to develop into your body. Within a day or two, your blastocyst eventually found a place to rest, somewhere on the wall of your mother's womb.

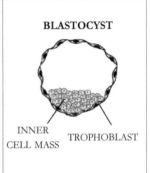

Implantation (4-7 days)

It takes two people to enable implantation. You had to get there, stay there and go on growing but your mother's womb had to welcome you. Your mother's ovaries went on producing progesterone and this thickened the wall of her womb making it receptive for your arrival and implantation. The outside of your *zona pellucida* became thinner and your blastocyst "hatched out" and broke loose. The outer layer (now known as the trophoblast) came into contact with the womb wall and began to excrete an enzyme that broke down the outer membrane and dug a little hollow. The outer cells of your blastocyst also began to produce human chorionic gonadotropin (HCG) that stimulated the blood supply in the walls of the womb. The edges of your new "nest" space became swollen with new capillaries.

We have already emphasized that you were a brand-new being never seen before. However, as far as your mother's body was concerned, you were a "foreign body" trying to "invade" the womb lining. In the same way as when a splinter enters the skin, your mother's immune system should have been triggered at once to expel you. This does not happen in pregnancy. There appears to be a special quality to the lining of the trophoblast cells that conceals the in-built genetic "otherness" that would otherwise have triggered your mother's immune system and cause rejection. If you had been rejected by your mother's immune system you would have never implanted but would have floated away and passed out of the vagina, too small to be noticed. Once the pregnancy hormones begin to flow, there also seems to be a special quality to the membrane that lines the womb that also helps to prevent rejection of a pregnancy. The crucial aspect of implantation for our consideration here, is that the lining of the womb is capable of supporting several pregnancies at once. However, where one trophoblast may make a good contact with the mother's blood supply and continue to develop, another may do less well and so fail to develop. An unknown number of fertilized eggs are lost because they fail to implant adequately, if at all.

Bonding (7-12 days)

Your trophoblast had to make a good enough hollow but not create a hole in the womb wall. It had to make direct contact with your mother's blood supply. Your mother's womb produced substances designed to slow this process down, but your trophoblast eventually got through to be alongside the tiny capillaries of your mother's blood supply. The capillaries gradually altered and became more stable, so as to provide a good blood supply to the developing pregnancy. At this time there may have been be a small amount of vaginal bleeding - known as implantation bleeding - if maternal blood leaked into the womb. The amount of HGC being produced gradually increased. As your trophoblast began to implant your Mum may have started to feel queasy in the mornings.

The placenta (12-14 days)

Your trophoblast was gradually developing into a little placenta, rooted to your implantation site in the womb wall. Your placenta was a vital part of you and was your life support system for your whole time in the womb. It was made of the same tissue as yourself, with the same genes.

It was amputated shortly after birth when your cord was cut. Meanwhile, your inner cell mass grew into a ball of many thousands of cells that were dividing constantly every day. By the time you were 13 days old, your mother would have been expecting her monthly period and would have found it was delayed. The hormones of pregnancy inhibit menstruation. A pregnancy test, designed to detect the level of HGC hormone in the urine, would be positive. From this day forward you were considered an "embryo" but so far you were just a blob of cells, growing very rapidly. Some significant changes occurred, beginning about the 13th day.

Your life as an embryo begins - (13-14 days [d])

By this time a streak (known as the "primitive streak") had begun to appear across the mass of developing cells which would one day become your body. The streak was the first sign of some kind of noticeable organisation in the ball of cells that was you. You were no bigger than a grain of sand but you were growing larger every day. The process of organisation within the ball of cells that was you had been going on since the very beginning. For a start, there had to be a decision about what was "up" and what was "down"; what

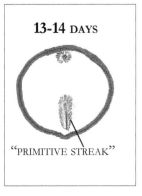

13-14 DAYS

"PRIMITIVE STREAK"

was "left" and what was "right." It has been suggested that the usual trigger point for this decision may be the original site where the sperm entered the egg.[4] Your limbic system was the first area of your brain to develop as a separate system of neurons which can be detected from the 15th day by using special microscopic chemical analysis.[5] The limbic system it is the most primitive part of your brain in the evolutionary sense, but it is still, even today, the regulator of all brain activity. It is involved in emotions and motivations to do with survival, including fear, anger and feelings of pleasure.

Three-layered development - (16-21 days)

According to your genetic blueprint, your body began to develop into three layers of cells.

---

d. All diagrams of the development of the embryo published in this chapter are adapted from photographs of the Kyoto embryo collection.

- *The outer layer* became your skin, nails, hair, the lenses of your eyes, the lining of your ear, your nose, mouth, anus, tooth enamel and your nervous system.
- *The middle layer* made your muscles, bones, and internal organs, such as your blood cells, heart, lungs, kidneys and reproductive organs.
- *The inner layer* formed your bladder and digestive tract.

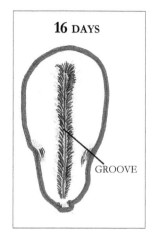

16 DAYS

GROOVE

A groove had formed along the line of your body. This would become your neural tube. Your body was pear-shaped. The wider part would eventually become your head and the narrower part your hips and legs. You had a very simple blood circulation system, which was just a tube.

New shapes and ridges - (21-23 days)

By now your mother had probably begun to wonder if she was pregnant or not, because her menstrual flow would now be a week overdue. Your body was now elongated, with all kinds of bumps and ridges along it. Every ridge was there for a purpose and everything was developing according to the genetic blueprint that was laid down at fertilization. Your neural tube was beginning to develop: this was the start of your spinal cord. The tubes containing blood began to develop muscles. As the days went by, your body gradually began to curve into a C-shape. You were developing so fast that every day made a difference.

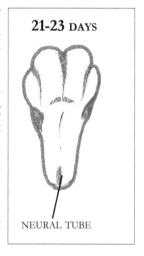

21-23 DAYS

NEURAL TUBE

A beating heart - (23-25 days)

The first ultrasound scan may be made at this time. No bigger than a grain of rice, you would just be visible. Your spinal cord was still an open tube and did not form an enclosed tube for a few more days. The buds for your eyes and ears were in place. The tube that contained your blood began to grow into an S-shape. The cardiac muscles that lined the tube begin to flutter and this set all the fluids moving through your body. Your shape was determined by your neural tube, which ran along your back. Your nervous system was the most developed system of all and you had a very primitive, simple brain. You had a bulb-like tail and a connecting stalk joining you to the placenta. The stalk would gradually grow longer and become your umbilical cord. Your yolk sac contained nutrients to sustain you while your placenta was still forming and developing.

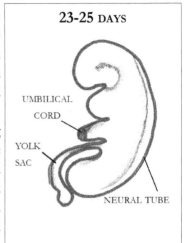

23-25 DAYS

UMBILICAL CORD

YOLK SAC

NEURAL TUBE

Developing eyes and ears - (26-30 days)

By now, you were about the size of a lentil. Your neural tube had closed and your eyes and ears had begun to form. Your brain and spinal cord were by now clearly differentiated. Your placenta was providing a good blood supply. Your tiny little heart was developing valves. There were signs of the future locations of your liver, lung, stomach and pancreas. Little buds were appearing that would soon form your arms and legs. On the ultrasound scan there would have been clear early signs that you were alive, for from six weeks of pregnancy the fluttering foetal heart can clearly be seen. [e]

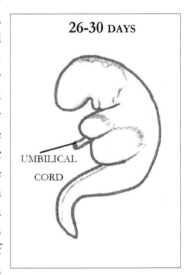

26-30 DAYS

UMBILICAL CORD

Enclosed in skin - (28-32 days)

This week showed astonishing progress, and your mother became

---

e.   Please note that the length of a pregnancy is calculated from the date of the start of the last menstruation and so does not accord with the number of days given in this chapter, which describes the age of the embryo in days from conception.

more and more convinced that she was pregnant. Your forebrain began to fold over your mid-brain into the position it now occupies - at the front of your head. All the time new neural networks were being developed to serve your organs as they developed. You had the beginnings of a lens for your eyes. Your tongue, heart and liver were all developing well and connected to your brain. Your liver received blood from your placenta via your umbilical cord. Your placenta was functioning properly. Limb buds were forming. A thin surface layer of skin covered your developing body.

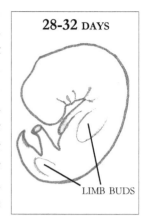

28-32 DAYS

LIMB BUDS

Big head - (31-37 days)

Your brain and head were growing rapidly and your head was enormous compared with the rest of you, which was about the size of an apple pip. The lenses of your eyes were on the surface. Your arms were little cylinders with nerves spreading along them. Your legs were just beginning to appear. Your brain was developing rapidly. Your hindbrain, which is responsible for heart regulation, breathing and muscle movements, was beginning to develop. Your legs were divided into three sections and were supplied with nerves.

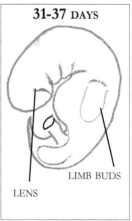

31-37 DAYS

LIMB BUDS

LENS

Developing rapidly - (38-41 days)

You were the size of a pea, and most of it was your brain and your head. Your mother had missed a second period and there was no doubt: she was expecting a baby. Your arms were now divided into three sections and one of them would become your hand, but it was not yet served with nerves. Your legs were just little cylinders. Your heart had four chambers and you had a sense of

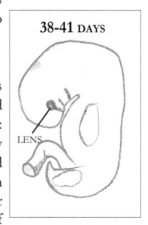

38-41 DAYS

LENS

13

smell. Your intestines began to develop in your umbilical cord. Primitive germ cells arrived in your genital area - they were the only cells in your body capable of dividing in half to form gametes for the next generation.

Beginning of a skeleton - (42-46 days)
You were about the size of a kidney bean and cartilage was beginning to form in your limbs and spine. Your eyes were pigmented and your eyelids had begun to develop. You had nipples on your chest and your kidneys began to produce urine for the first time. Your arms were in the proper place and your hands showed the beginnings of fingers. You were beginning to twitch a little as your limbs moved.

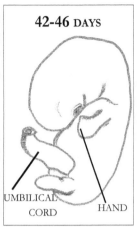

42-46 DAYS

UMBILICAL CORD   HAND

Brain waves and muscles - (47-50 days)
By now, you had grown to the size of a quail's egg. Your brain was giving out the first detectable brain waves. Your head was more erect and your inner ear was developing. If you are male, you had testes and if you are female, you had ovaries. Your legs were now almost complete, down to the toenails. Your skeleton was becoming more solid and your muscles were growing stronger as you swam about in the amniotic sac.

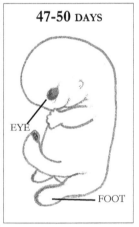

47-50 DAYS

EYE

FOOT

Intestines move inside - (51-56 days)

Your intestines began to migrate into your abdomen from the umbilical cord. Your body had by then grown big enough to accommodate them. Your fingers and toes were still webbed but your fingers were lengthening and your hands could now meet across your chest. Your eyes were well-developed. Your heart was fully formed. The cartilage in your skeleton was beginning to harden into bones. You had proper fingers, well-defined toes and a little

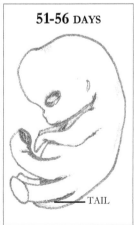

51-56 DAYS

TAIL

14

tail that would soon disappear. Your sexual organs were now visible. You were about the size of a walnut.

Development completed - (57-60 days)

By eight weeks of pregnancy you looked quite recognisably human and you were much larger than your own front door key. You had completely developed ears, fully-pigmented eyes, taste buds on your tongue and the beginnings of primary teeth. Your arms and legs were well-formed, your fingers were longer and your toes no longer webbed. A new surface layer of skin was forming. Your tail had disappeared. You measured nearly three inches (7.5 cm) long from head to rump. You looked fully human.

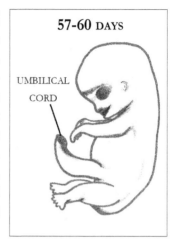

57-60 DAYS

UMBILICAL CORD

A tiny human

In 1970, Dr. Rockwell, Director of Anaesthesiology, Leonard Hospital, New York wrote a compelling description of a 57-day-old embryo he had seen in 1959, which was still enclosed in its amniotic sac. It had been an ectopic pregnancy.

> *Eleven years ago while administering an anaesthetic for ruptured ectopic pregnancy (at two months' gestation) I was handed what I believe is the smallest living human being ever seen. The embryo sac was intact and transparent. Within the sac was a tiny (approx.1 cm) human male swimming extremely vigorously in the amniotic fluid, while attached to the wall by the umbilical cord. This tiny human was perfectly developed, with long tapering fingers, feet and toes. It was almost transparent, as regards the skin, and the delicate arteries and veins were prominent to the ends of the fingers. The baby was extremely alive and swam about the sac approximately one time per second, with a natural swimmer's stroke. This tiny human did not look at all like the photos and drawings and models of 'embryos' which I have seen, nor did it look like the few embryos I have been able to observe since then, obviously because this one was alive. When the sac was opened, the tiny human immediately lost its life and took on the appearance of what is accepted as the appearance of an embryo at*

this age. Six months later, at a lecture in embryology at Harvard University, I had occasion to ask the approximately 150 physicians present whether any had witnessed such a phenomenon. All were amazed and none had seen nor heard of such an event. [6]

We have come a long way since 1959. These days we can watch moving, swimming embryos by means of ultrasound. The womb is no longer the dark and mysterious place it once was and the embryo is no longer a stranger.

By the time you were 12 weeks old, doctors called you a "foetus" and they continued to call you that until the day you were born. Life as a foetus spans approximately six months, from the twelfth week until birth. During that time you had an intricately-formed, finely-balanced hormone system which was regulated by that all-important limbic system in your brain. This enabled you to stay alive in the ever-changing womb environment.

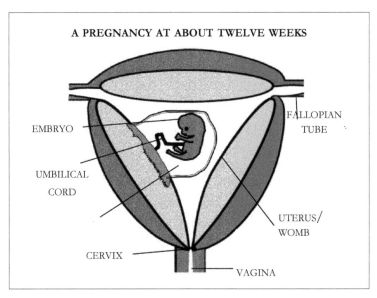

A PREGNANCY AT ABOUT TWELVE WEEKS

EMBRYO

FALLOPIAN TUBE

UMBILICAL CORD

UTERUS/ WOMB

CERVIX

VAGINA

Your developing senses

Your main sense organ was your skin. It was served by neurons that could detect temperature and texture. Everything in the womb was soft and warm to the touch as you floated in a bath of warm amniotic fluid, twitching slightly as your body learned to move. Your sense of taste and smell had developed very early on, at about four weeks. You had muscles and could react physically. You were tiny but there was a lot going on. A few days meant enormous changes in your body.

Beginning to move

Your autonomic system had from the very start taken care of your fluid balance and circulation, as it still does today. Your placenta took care of nutrition and waste disposal without any effort from you at all. Your mother's blood kept you warm and her hormones circulated in your body. Then somewhere between the 6th and 10th week your tiny body burst into motion. You twitched and wiggled about in frantic bursts with only a few minutes of rest between them. [7]

Exploration

By the time you had been alive for about a hundred days, the number of neurones in your brain was almost as many as you have now. They were reaching outwards towards each other, touching one another and making contact and reacting to stimuli from various parts of your body. Then the feedback began. As your body moved in the amniotic fluid it came into contact with Something Else - but that is another story.

Not alone

If you are a womb twin survivor, your pre-birth development was unusual in many ways. At some stage in the womb you were not alone. In the next chapter we will take a look at twin or multiple pregnancies and consider some of the mishaps that can lead to the death of one twin, leaving a sole survivor.

2

The making of twins and more

Once a twin, always a twin
Raymond Brandt (1929-2001) [a]

In the last chapter we explored how a single baby is conceived and begins to develop in the womb. Sometimes, two or more embryos begin to develop in the same menstrual cycle and the result is a twin or multiple pregnancy. In this chapter we will consider what happens in a twin or triplet pregnancy. We will begin with twins. There are two very different kinds of twin pregnancy. In one kind, two eggs are produced in the same menstrual cycle, each is fertilized by one sperm and more than one zygote is produced. The two zygotes develop into fraternal twins. In the other kind, the original zygote splits into two individuals, which creates identical twins.

THE MAKING OF FRATERNAL TWINS

Fraternal twins develop from two eggs. As a result of the conception of both eggs, two zygotes are created. This is why fraternal twins are also called dizygotic (DZ) twins. If you are the sole survivor of a fraternal twin pair, you can call yourself a DZ womb twin survivor, which is the term we will use from now on. In the case of DZ twinning, two eggs are produced in the same menstrual cycle. Each egg is fertilized by a different sperm. They become two separate zygotes, which in turn develop into two foetuses, sharing the womb.

Ovulation

Ovulation in a fertile woman is the production of mature eggs, each ripe and ready for fertilization. The production of an egg is a complex hormonal process - so complex in fact, that every single conception is a miracle, as we have seen. Within the ovary, special cells with just one set of chromosomes are developed. These are called oocytes (immature eggs).

---

a. Founder of Twinless Twins Support Group International.

It is common knowledge that, at a certain time each month, one egg matures and is released from one of the ovaries. The egg passes down the fallopian tube and may - or may not - encounter some sperm. This sounds simple enough but, like so much else in the delicate business of sexual reproduction, a whole orchestra of hormones, specific proteins, genes and microscopic processes are required for an immature egg to mature, be released and begin its journey down the fallopian tube.

One of the necessary hormones for this process is FSH (Follicle Stimulating Hormone) which, as the name implies, stimulates the follicles to help the eggs mature. Follicles are balloon-shaped structures in the ovary each containing an immature egg. If the FSH hormone levels are high, then several follicles may be stimulated and several immature eggs ripened. Next, as part of a woman's the menstrual cycle, Luteinising Hormone is released, which develops the follicles even more and triggers the release of the eggs. Her monthly surge of Luteinizing Hormone makes a women particularly fertile and is known to increase the chances at that time that sexual intercourse will occur.[1] This is of course most convenient for the survival of the human species.

Double ovulation

It can happen that two mature eggs are released from either or both ovaries and pass down the fallopian tube, heading towards the womb. This is a double ovulation. The eggs may meet with some sperm, perhaps not at exactly the same time, but certainly within hours or days of each other. Once a sperm enters one of the eggs the two sets of chromosomes come together within the egg and cell division begins as usual. It can also happen that the other egg is fertilized. Should that occur, then two zygotes begin their journey towards the womb: these are DZ twins.

The necessary support for a successful DZ twin pregnancy

From conception to birth, a twin pregnancy is a risky and uncertain business, since the human womb is designed to carry only one baby at a time. To guarantee the conception and birth of a pair of DZ twins, that particular menstrual cycle must be well able to support a twin pregnancy, but unfortunately that is not always the case. Several criteria must be met if twins are to be conceived: it has to be the right time in the month for the womb to be receptive to sperm, so that plenty of sperm can reach both of the eggs. There must be enough mucus for the transport of two eggs down the fallopian tube. There must be at least two viable eggs, capable of being fertilized by the partner's sperm. There must be enough sperm released around the time of ovulation, within a window of six days, so that one sperm can successfully fertilize each of two eggs. The womb must be well-supplied with blood vessels so that both of the fertilized eggs can implant successfully in the uterine wall.[2]

Different life journeys

DZ twin zygotes are very different individuals. They do not have the same genes and their life journeys diverge from the start. Each zygote takes a separate route as they develop into blastocysts. The two blastocysts may travel close together or far apart. They might be in the same fallopian tube or in separate tubes. As implantation begins one trophoblast may embed in a more advantageous position than the other. If they both come to rest on a good site on the womb wall, one DZ twin may manage to implant more successfully than the other. After implantation one DZ twin may develop faster than the other. The two placentas may develop on opposite sides of the womb wall or close together and side by side. If the two placentas develop close together, they fuse into one placental mass.

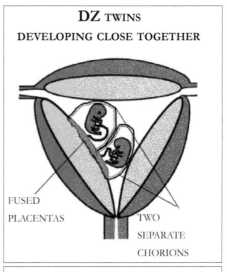

DZ TWINS
DEVELOPING CLOSE TOGETHER

FUSED PLACENTAS

TWO SEPARATE CHORIONS

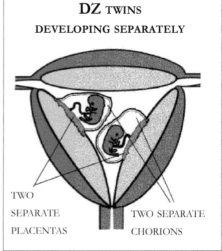

DZ TWINS
DEVELOPING SEPARATELY

TWO SEPARATE PLACENTAS

TWO SEPARATE CHORIONS

Unusual situations creating DZ twins

Superfetation

Usually, when one egg is fertilized and begins to implant, hormones are produced by the other to inhibit further ovulation. However, if there is another egg already mature enough and ready for release, this may be fertilized at a later stage and still be able to implant eventually. It has been known for DZ twins to be born several weeks or even months apart. [3]

Different fathers

If two eggs are fertilized by two different fathers who are racially not the same, then this will create a pair of mixed-race twins. Mixed race twins can be very different from each other - a black boy and a white girl for example. For this to happen, the woman must have engaged in sexual intercourse with two different men within the space of a few days and before the first implanted zygote triggers the hormones that inhibit ovulation. It may be assumed that conceiving DZ twins naturally by two different fathers occurs only rarely, but during IVF *(in vitro* fertilization) the possibilities of a mix-up are greatly increased. Sperm is produced by the would-be father (or a sperm donor) and added to the eggs of the would-be mother (or an egg donor) for fertilization in the laboratory, but they may be wrongly matched. There are mixed-race twins in existence today who were conceived in this mixed-up way. [4]

THE MAKING OF IDENTICAL TWINS

Identical twinning starts with a single zygote. This single cell has within it a blend of genetic material that has never been seen before - a unique genetic individual. But when identical twins are formed, at some early stage of development the zygote splits into two halves. Each half develops into a separate individual with a separate life history. If you are the sole survivor of an identical twin pair, then you and your twin developed from one zygote. The medical term for identical twins is monozygotic, or MZ. That is the term we will now use to indicate identical twins.

How many MZ twins are there?

The rate of MZ twinning across the world is about three MZ twins per thousand live births. The MZ twinning rate does not seem to vary very much over time, or across the continents of the world. [5] The causes of

MZ twinning remain unknown, despite many decades of research into early human development. It has been suggested by experts that MZ twinning is an anomaly[6] and a random event.[7] However, it remains remarkably consistent, widespread and independent of historical, social or geographical factors.

MZ twinning and ART (Assisted Reproductive Technology)

In the last thirty years, doctors have become aware there is a noticeable increase of MZ twinning among pregnancies helped along with ART such as hyper-ovulation drugs or IVF.[8] One study found the rate of MZ twinning to be as much as 12 times higher in pregnancies created by ART than in natural conceptions.[9] Researchers are not sure why this happens. Some have said that it may be caused by the stimulation of the mother's ovaries with fertility drugs.[10] During the process of IVF, sperm and eggs are mixed together in a Petri dish.[b] Eventually, conception takes place and several tiny balls of cells begin to form. These are nurtured for a few days and then carefully placed in the womb of the mother-to-be. The mystery is, why would these transplanted embryos be more likely to split into MZ twins than embryos created in a natural conception? We do not know why, but if you were conceived by IVF there may have been some MZ twinning involved after you were conceived in that Petri dish.

If you were once an MZ twin, this was your story:

At some stage during the first fourteen days from your conception, the single bundle of cells that were produced from the original single zygote divided into two halves and created MZ twins. The outcome for each twin, one of which was you, depended on the stage of development that had been reached before the single cell mass divided into two. We will now consider the various stages of development and what can happen when the split occurs at each stage. If you were once an MZ twin, you may discover your own story described in one of these stages.

Splitting of the morula - days 1-4
The division may happen in the first four days after fertilization, when the *morula* (the bundle of blastomeres) has developed. Within each bundle, every individual blastomere divides into two every day or so, and as a

---

b. A shallow glass cylindrical dish with a lid.

result the bundle rapidly begins to expand. The entire bundle divides into two separate bundles of blastomeres, each contained within their own *zona pellucida*. Within a few days the bundles have both developed into two separate blastocysts, which float gently together down the fallopian tube to implant in the wall of the womb. The two blastocysts may implant so close together that the placentas meet and overlap, or they may end up some distance away from each other. [c] Each DZ twin has its own enclosing membrane (chorion) and amniotic sac. About one third of born MZ

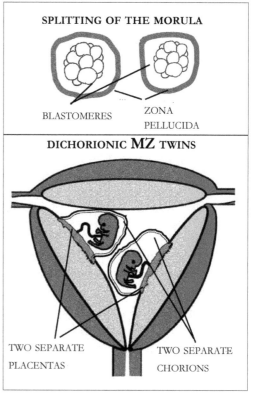

SPLITTING OF THE MORULA

BLASTOMERES   ZONA PELLUCIDA

DICHORIONIC MZ TWINS

TWO SEPARATE PLACENTAS   TWO SEPARATE CHORIONS

twins are dichorionic - i.e. they have their own separate chorion, amniotic sac and placenta. [11] If your original zygote split into two in the first 48 hours, you would have spent the first two days of your existence merged with your twin as a single entity. Then you split apart from your twin and developed in a separate space with your own food supply.

Sharing the same chorion - days 4-8

By the fourth day, the zygote has become a blastocyst. If the split is delayed until now it happens inside the blastocyst where the cells have already differentiated into the three layers. Under a microscope we can watch a blastocyst "hatching" and the tiny single trophoblast reaching out, seeking the womb wall, ready for implantation. Once the whole mass of cells has hatched, we can see how the inner mass of cells has divided

---

c.   It can also happen that one of the twin blastocysts does not implant at all and is lost from the womb altogether, leaving the other to develop alone.

into two cell masses, which in time will form into two tiny developing embryos, joined by separate cords to a single placenta. These twins are "monochorionic" that is, they share the same chorion and placenta, but they are also diamniotic, which means they both have their own amniotic sac in which they continue to develop, close together and side by side. Research with pairs of twins after delivery has found that about three quarters of MZ twins are mono-chorionic and diamniotic, which means that they share a placenta but each has a personal amniotic sac. [12] If the split between you and your MZ twin happened between four and eight days after conception, you would have spent the first week or so of your life as a single entity, merged with your twin. You split apart in such a way that each of you had a personal link to a shared source of nourishment but an individual personal space.

Sharing the same amniotic sac
- days 8-12

If the mass of cells within the blastocyst divides into two a little later, then even more of the original ball of cells is shared between the twins. Twins developing within the same chorion are sustained by the same placenta and share the same

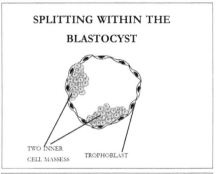

SPLITTING WITHIN THE BLASTOCYST

TWO INNER CELL MASSES   TROPHOBLAST

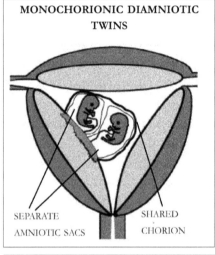

MONOCHORIONIC DIAMNIOTIC TWINS

SEPARATE AMNIOTIC SACS   SHARED CHORION

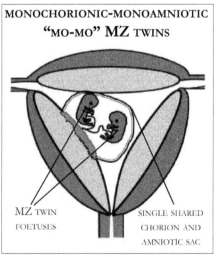

MONOCHORIONIC-MONOAMNIOTIC "MO-MO" MZ TWINS

MZ TWIN FOETUSES   SINGLE SHARED CHORION AND AMNIOTIC SAC

amniotic sac. They are known as monochorionic-monoamniotic, or "Mo-Mo" MZ twins. As they develop, Mo-Mo MZ twins live entwined lives in the same space, to the extent that their cords can sometimes become entangled. They spent more than a week as one mass of cells before splitting apart., so they share everything. This is a very rare form of twinning, for research has shown that only about 1% of twins once shared a chorion, placenta and sac. [13] If the split between you and your twin occurred between eight and twelve days after conception, you spent more than week merged with your twin. Then the mass of cells split into two and you were twins, intimately sharing space and nourishment.

Splitting on days 12-14
The later the split occurs, the more is shared between the twins, and if splitting occurs anytime after the twelfth day, they will be conjoined and share a body. This is extremely rare and usually fatal. A considerable amount of effort has gone into the surgical separation of conjoined twins. They might be quite separate with just a little skin between them, as in the case of Chang and Eng, the famous Siamese twins of the nineteenth century. [14] With today's surgical expertise, Chang and Eng could have lived separate lives if they had been given the chance. There are some cases today of conjoined twins who still survive, joined at the head or abdomen or sharing entire parts of the original single body. [d]

Diagnosing zygosity

During the mother's pregnancy, MZ twins are usually diagnosed as such because they seem to be sharing the same placenta or sac. However, as we have seen, they may have separated in the first two days and found separate implantation sites with separate placentas. This means they can look exactly like DZ twins, both on the ultrasound scan and after birth. After a twin delivery, the midwife or obstetrician can carefully examine the afterbirth and check how many sacs there were, but this is an uncertain way to establish zygosity. The membranes may be broken or totally destroyed by the process of delivery. For example, two amniotic sacs may become joined if the dividing membrane splits when the twins interact in later pregnancy. When the babies are newborn, they may look

---

d. We will discuss this form of twinning in more detail in Chapter 6

vaguely alike, but whether they are identical or not can remain a mystery.

MZ twins are not identical

Monozygotic may seem to be a complex and unnecessarily scientific term for an identical twin but in fact it is more accurate, for MZ twins are far from identical.[15] For example, despite having the same genes, MZ twins do not have the same fingerprints. They are very similar in many ways, but not identical. Even DNA can vary between MZ twins, if only slightly. Scientists have found that MZ twin embryos can differ considerably in their genetic makeup because of slight differences in the arrangement of the chromosomes as the two separate balls of cells continue to divide in the first few days of life. This asymmetry may produce an obvious physical difference between the twins that could be fatal for one of them. It may be that a critical number of the original germ cells is required for normal development, and if one twin lacks a few of these critical germ cells, then some organs may develop abnormally or not at all - such as one kidney or even the heart.[16]

Mirror-image twinning

It is thought that, when split in the conceptus is delayed to eight or more days after conception, a different kind of splitting occurs and the result is mirror-imaging between the twins. Although it is not yet clear exactly why this occurs, mirror-imaging has been found in about one in four MZ twin pairs.[17] MZ mirror-image twins have the same genes but they are not identical for they are complete opposites. They look like mirror images of each other and have opposite features, such as one twin being right-handed and one being left-handed.[18] They may have opposite hair whorl patterns or may each have a facial mole on the opposite side to the other. They may have uneven facial features that mirror each other. Double organs, such as their kidneys, may be of unequal size and the difference may be mirrored between the twins. In some cases, single internal organs such as the heart may be on the reverse side from the normal in one twin.

Epigenetics make a difference

However equal or unequal the original split, each MZ twin has a separate and individual experience of being alive and is even subject to subtly different environmental influences from the other. MZ twins are known to become less alike as they grow older, and part of that individuality is genetic. As cells continue to divide, variations begin to occur in how the genes on each chromosome are copied. [19]

The science of epigenetics is the study of the way that genes can be "switched" on and off in response to changes in the environment, diet, blood supply, etc. Epigeneticists are now exploring the subtle but crucial ways in which our genes begin to change as our cells divide after conception. It is because of this gradual change that identical twins can begin to vary genetically from each other, even from the first moments of conception. From the earliest days of embryo development, every day brings a fresh cell division. Any slight differences between the genes in each twin embryo will become fixed as a new cell line is created. Each cell line will then be slightly different in each twin. [20] As the weeks pass, there can be other genetic changes over time in response to the changing uterine environment, in a process known as epigenetic drift. [21] From the very beginning of life, epigenetic influences may be brought to bear differently on each member of an MZ twin pair. Their individual genes, development and capacity for life may end up being very disparate indeed. A fatal defect in one embryo may not be present at all in the other, who may go on developing normally and be born alone

Same zygote, different sexes

It has happened in rare cases that, during the split of a male zygote, one twin lost a Y chromosome and thus became a girl with just one X chromosome. This has been named as "Turner's syndrome" after the doctor who in 1995 first identified a specific syndrome caused by having only one X chromosome. Meanwhile, the other male twin remains truly male and develops normally. [22]

Rejection and dissimilar genes

The concept of rejection has been used as an explanation for identical twinning: the idea is that the very first cell division may produce two cells with such genetic difference that they reject one another and develop each into a distinct cell line. Paradoxically, according to this theory, so-called "identical" twinning may be caused precisely by the non-identical nature of these early cell masses. When an MZ twin offers their co-twin an organ for transplant, it may still be rejected. [23]

THE MAKING OF TRIPLETS AND MORE

Twin pregnancies are high-risk pregnancies and triplet pregnancies even more so. The human womb, unlike that of a cat or a dog, is not designed to carry a litter. One baby is quite enough and singleton pregnancies are best for both mother and baby. It requires a healthy, well-fed mother over the age of thirty if there is to be a good chance that she will carry three babies for long enough for them all to be born alive. In the advanced stages of pregnancy, a woman carrying triplets is disabled by the size of her enormous womb. The three babies also take their toll on the woman's body. It takes a long time to recover physically while she is exhausted by the need to care for three babies at once. Multiple pregnancies can kill: some triplets may die before or at birth simply because the pregnancy is insufficient to keep them all alive. A high level of medical care is required to keep the pregnancy going, keep all the babies alive, ensure the safe delivery of the babies and assist the mother's recovery. Triplets are 12 times more likely to die in very early life than singletons. [24]

Triplets are now far more common than they were thirty years ago and the increase is almost entirely due to the use of ART. [25] Louis Keith, an identical twin himself and the director of the Centre for the Study of Multiple Birth in Chicago, USA, has become so concerned about this epidemic of triplet births, that he and his colleague Isaac Blickstein gathered together 48 contributions by experts on triplets from all over the world and in 2002 they created the first book on the subject, *Triplet Pregnancies and Their Consequences*. [26] Because of the large number of triplet pregnancies in the USA, research workers at Matria Healthcare of Marietta in Georgia have been able to gather data on 3000 triplet pregnancies and the book contains an analysis of them. Thanks to this data set, we are beginning to understand some of the unique biological circumstances associated with triplets.

In 1998 in the USA only 20% of triplets were conceived naturally. The rest were conceived with ART. [27] If your parents used ART, you may be the survivor of a triplet set - or more. Even if you were born as one of a living twin pair there may have been the pre-birth loss of a triplet or more, so any twin pair born alive could be two womb triplet survivors. This means that twin pairs may not be what they seem - particularly if they were conceived with the help of IVF or fertility drugs.

28

Various combinations of triplet embryos

In order to clarify how triplets are made, here are some of the various combinations of embryos.

One zygote splits three times
The triplets may be monozygotic if the zygote egg splits twice and then one of the halves splits again. This creates a pair of monochorionic-monoamniotic MZ twins, plus an extra embryo enclosed in the same chorion. The timing of the split may be early or late, and one split may be at a different stage than another. This can also produce MZ quadruplets, if both "halves" again each split in half.

MZ twins plus one other
There may be just two zygotes to start with but one of them splits into two, to create a pair of MZ twins with an additional embryo alongside. This is the most common kind of triplet pregnancy to result in three live babies and is known affectionately as a "Pair and a Spare."[28] When the babies are born, it can be clearly seen that two of the triplet set are identical twins.

Trizygotic
As we have seen, some women have a natural tendency to ovulate more than once in a month. They are more likely to conceive twins or more. The triplets (or more) created by hyperovulation develop in the same way as a DZ twin pregnancy, with every zygote separate.

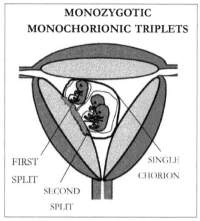

MONOZYGOTIC
MONOCHORIONIC TRIPLETS

FIRST SPLIT
SECOND SPLIT
SINGLE CHORION

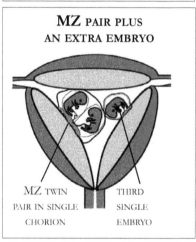

MZ PAIR PLUS
AN EXTRA EMBRYO

MZ TWIN PAIR IN SINGLE CHORION
THIRD SINGLE EMBRYO

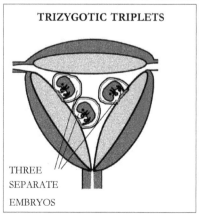

TRIZYGOTIC TRIPLETS

THREE SEPARATE EMBRYOS

29

There can be any combination of boys and girls in this kind of triplet set and they may also look quite different from each other. Women with fertility issues also hyperovulate, because of the drugs they are given. Hyperovulation drugs may work exceedingly effectively and in a single month large numbers of eggs may be stimulated into production. After IVF it is normal practice to place several embryos in the womb of the mother-to-be. As a result, more than two embryos may implant and begin to grow. Trizygotic triplet pregnancies are common after IVF if three embryos implant successfully and begin to develop.

Multiple birth: a risky business

Many more babies are conceived than are born, particularly in a twin or a multiple pregnancy, which is a risky business. The existing published research on multiple birth has concentrated on analysing the twin pairs and triplet sets that develop as far as birth.

> *I'm the sole survivor of the four womb mates that I shared the womb with. My three womb mate brothers died as babies and my womb mate sister died the night before our fifth birthday. It's not easy, as with early loss twins, we aren't considered twins at all if our twins died early. It feels like my womb mates are following me everywhere I go. That bond I feel with them grows stronger over the years instead of weaker. Although I only have life memories with my sister, I still miss our womb mate brothers equally so.*
> *Iris, USA* [e]

Alpha twin or Beta twin?

Studies have shown that in every twin pair there is one twin who is more dominant than the other. The difference may be very slight, but it is always there. Research has shown that even before birth this difference is noticeable. When twins are observed by ultrasound interacting in the womb, it can be seen that, after a period of rest, the dominant twin is seen to start moving first, which triggers the less lively twin into action. We will call the more dominant twin the "Alpha" twin and the more compliant twin the "Beta" twin. Italian psychoanalyst Allesandra Piontelli, who studied twins interacting in the womb and observed them for five years

---

e. In the remaining chapters of this book you will find many other such stories from womb twin survivors from around the world, in their own words.

after they were born, showed that the Alpha/Beta difference in pairs of twins tended to persist long after birth.[29] Usually it is the stronger Alpha twin who survives and the weaker Beta twin who dies. If you are a womb twin survivor, the chances are that you were the stronger of the two – the Alpha twin.

The lone twin

Sadly, not every twin pregnancy results in two living healthy babies and one twin may die. The next chapter will explore some of the reasons why one twin may die in the final trimester of pregnancy or shortly after birth.

3
When a twin dies close to birth

*My sister was stillborn. From childhood, I've felt that
part of myself was "missing".*
Lyn, UK [a]

This chapter will focus on the various ways in which a twin may die immediately after birth, at birth or in the last three months before birth. After many months of expecting twins, with all that this entails - the excitement, the anxiety and two sets of everything to buy - it is very painful indeed for parents to find that after all, there is to be only one baby.

Alexa Stevenson wrote her book: *Half Baked, The Story of My Nerves, My Newborn, and How We Both Learned to Breathe,* about the premature birth at 25 weeks of her daughter Simone, whose twin died at 22 weeks of pregnancy. The book describes the scene after the ultrasound had revealed the death of Ames, one of her DZ twins: "Simone is flipping around, indecently enjoying the extra space. Ames is still and crooked at the edge of the screen, but Simone is waving, showing us her eyeball and tiny chin." [1]

Audrey Sandbank, a psychotherapist working with the Twin and Multiple Births Association in Guildford, UK, completes her book *Twins and the Family* with a chapter entitled *...And then there was one.* She points out that the loss of one twin is a tragedy, not just for the parents, but also for the surviving twin for whom their missing co-twin is "an ever-present reality." [2] If you are a womb twin survivor, I am sure you would agree with that.

I was born breech and two months premature. My twin was stillborn. I have her birth certificate. Almost every day I wonder what life would have been like if she had lived.

Diana, USA [a]

---

a. All stories in this book are written by womb twin survivors, in their own words.

Multiple pregnancy is dangerous

A multiple pregnancy is by definition a dangerous and risky pregnancy for both the mother and her babies. The problems continue for the mother after delivery and for the children after birth.

A mother carrying twins or more will probably experience some problems throughout her pregnancy. She may quickly grow large, even in the early weeks. She will require more rest and nourishment than in any other previous singleton pregnancies, which may make it difficult for her to continue to work or care for any existing children. As she enters into the third trimester she is more likely to suffer toxaemia of pregnancy, pre-eclampsia and gestational diabetes. The doctors may require that the babies be delivered early by induction or caesarean section to preserve her life and save her babies.

After her babies are born she will have the double work of caring for two newborns at once and she may find it totally exhausting. This experience has been described as "twin shock." [3] Twins are more at risk of abuse and accidental injury than singleton born children. Twin birth is considered in some countries to be a risk factor for abuse and neglect. [4]

> *I was born a fraternal twin; my twin sister died shortly after birth. I don't remember when my parents told me about her; I must have been fairly young. It wasn't really a topic for further discussion, although they did take me to see her grave at one point. I was always very curious about my twin, but I definitely got the message that it wasn't something my parents felt comfortable talking about.*
>
> *Sally, USA*

Sudden infant death of one twin

Sudden infant death syndrome (SIDS) is a form of neonatal death that has caused a great deal of anxiety to parents. There is occasionally a slight suspicion of foul play on the part of the carers, which makes the situation much worse. It can happen that apparently healthy babies die suddenly while sleeping, or even in a doctor's surgery. Twins are at a greater risk of SIDS than singleton babies. Furthermore, twins are occasionally, but rarely, found dead together. [5] Sole surviving twins, particularly same-sex twins, are at greater risk of SIDS than singleton babies. [6]

Here is what one SIDS survivor had to say about her twin loss experience:

Our conception was the result of a violent rape of a young woman. We were born - a few medical difficulties, plastic bins and isolation and all that medical stuff - spent six weeks in a foster home and then home to our new loving family. At eight months my twin sister died of something similar to SIDS - stopped breathing in the doctor's office, of all places.
Judith, USA

Stillbirth of one twin

When labour begins, even after careful examination of the mother it is not always obvious that there are twins. These days, a twin birth is often induced early or at least monitored with extreme care. However, before ultrasound scans were available, a second baby was sometimes delivered who took everyone by surprise. This can happen even today in less well-equipped hospitals. Under those circumstances things can go very badly for the second twin, especially if he or she is in a breech presentation (head uppermost.) With these unexpected twin deliveries, the second baby is often stillborn or lives only for a very short time. Many do not survive the trauma of birth. The stillbirth rate in twins is double the rate for single births.[7]

The doctor had no idea my mother was expecting twins until she went into labour. I was born first with forceps. Then my twin was delivered in a breech position but was stillborn. I was told I had a twin at about the age of five, but it was not considered to be very important.
Lynette, UK

Accidental death of one twin

Even shortly before birth, a trauma to the womb or the mother may cause the death of one twin by precipitating a sudden labour when insufficient medical attention is available to prevent disaster. Sometimes one baby is born dead as a direct result of the trauma.

Two weeks before my identical twin brother and I were due to be born, my mother was in a car accident. The limited technology of the day left my mother's doctor unaware that she was indeed carrying twins, and assured her after hearing my heartbeat following the accident, that "the baby" was all right. Only when

34

we were born did they learn that my mother was right, and she had indeed been
carrying identical twin boys.
Fred, USA

Umbilical cord complications causing the death of one twin

The average umbilical cord is about 55cm long. If the cord is much longer it can twist into a knot. In that case, the blood supply can no longer reach the baby. The baby dies of asphyxiation. If the cord is too short, then when labour begins the placenta may be torn from the wall of the womb causing a fatal haemorrhage. When MZ twins share an amniotic sac, the two cords may become entangled and the blood supply to one or both babies may be interrupted, with fatal consequences. During delivery, a longer cord can become wrapped around the neck of one of the babies, who is at risk of asphyxiation. As prenatal ultrasound is becoming increasingly sophisticated, many of these difficulties can be diagnosed before birth. However, some of these problems are not apparent before delivery, even with the use of ultrasound.

Where the placentas of DZ twins overlap, this may badly affect the position of the cord of one twin. Meanwhile, the other twin has a centrally-attached cord and will thrive and grow rapidly. The twin whose cord is poorly attached to the placenta will have little access to nourishment and may not survive.

My twin died five days before I was born. I knew of this as a child, but would
recount it with about as much emotion as telling what we had for dinner -
although I had an inner fascination with it. The loss of my twin was devastating
to my mother. The doctors told my family that I had killed my twin, that I had
taken too much of the resources.
Eleanor, USA

Infection causing the death of one twin

Bacteria entering the vagina can cause an infection and inflammation of the amnion and chorion (the membranes surrounding the baby.) If an infection develops in the third trimester of an MZ twin pregnancy the inflammation of the shared membranes can trigger premature labour, as a result of which one or both twins may be born dead or die at birth.

I was born at 27 weeks pregnant. My Mom went to the doctor, and they thought my placenta was infected so they induced labor. I weighed 1 lb 10 oz when born. I don't know how much my twin brother weighed. The doctor said that if they could have kept him in the womb, he would have lived. I have always wondered why I lived? What was so special about me?
Greta, USA

Increased chance of premature birth of both twins

The presence of twins in the womb tends to shorten the usual 40 weeks of pregnancy. Spontaneous delivery may begin several weeks early. When dealing with a twin or multiple pregnancy it is common practice in hospital maternity units to induce an early labour with hormones. The twins may be delivered by Caesarean section particularly if the babies are large or if one baby is in the breech position.

Delivery before 40 weeks of pregnancy may mean that the twins are not properly developed. A baby is described as premature if he or she is born less than 37 weeks of pregnancy.[8] The definition used to be based on weight, in that any baby weighing less than five pounds and five ounces, even at full term, was once described as premature.[9] Today, the sole criterion for premature birth is the length of gestation, but this criterion is still under review.[10]

Premature delivery can mean developmental and health problems for the babies. If the babies differ greatly in size and development, one twin may be ready to be born while the other is not yet sufficiently grown. In the last three months of a twin pregnancy, even after weeks of hospital bed rest for the mother, labour may begin and cannot be stopped. Consequently, neonatal death is common in premature birth, and this is also the case when twins are delivered many weeks early.

We were born two and a half months premature, identical twin sisters. My parents didn't know we were twins until a few days before our birth. I'm visually impaired as a result of my prematurity. My diagnosis is retinopathy of prematurity or ROP for short. It is generally thought that ROP is caused by giving babies too much oxygen at birth. In my case, this was done to keep me alive. I have no vision in my left eye and am partially sighted in my right eye. It was traumatic losing my sister and my vision too, at such a young age.
Brenda, USA

36

The prematurity dilemma

Because of the advances in special care for tiny babies, twins may be delivered as early as nine weeks premature. This is at the very margins of viability. These tiny babies bring with them an ethical dilemma. With the new technology now available in special care baby units, very premature babies can be kept alive, even against the wishes of the parents.

For instance, Vicki Forman describes in her book *This Lovely Life* how she gave birth to twin boys at 23 weeks. [11] She and her husband did not want their babies resuscitated, because they knew that the extreme prematurity of their twins would create major health problems for them, if they managed to survive at all. However, the medical staff, according to their professional code of practice, did their best to keep their two babies alive. One twin died shortly after birth and they were left with the sole survivor, who had severe developmental difficulties, seizures, cerebral palsy, mental retardation, a congenital heart defect and blindness. Vicky Forman wrote, "Being the parent of a medically fragile child or a very premature child or disabled child is possibly the loneliest and most devastating experience a person can have. Nothing in life prepares you." Sadly, her son died suddenly when he was eight years old from intestinal complications, apparently related to having been tube-fed at birth.

The abnormal development of one twin

If one twin develops some kind of lethal abnormality, it does not necessarily follow that the other twin will have the same problem. It may be possible for the affected twin to survive in the womb for many months or even the entire pregnancy, only to die close to birth. If the abnormality is caused by a faulty gene, DZ twins usually do not share it, for they develop separately from each other in separate sacs and do not share genes. MZ twins on the other hand do share genes, but even so it is possible for only one MZ twin to develop a fatal abnormality. [12]

I learned at an early age that I had a twin that "died at birth." I have never been given details about how she died but my Mom did tell me one time that if my twin sister had lived, she would have been severely disabled. I thought I was the only person in the world who felt a loss like this. I thought there is no one on the planet who can understand this emptiness inside.
Katie, USA

Missing organs in one twin

If one or more major organs do not develop in the body of one twin, that baby cannot survive outside the womb. For example, a twin with no kidneys may be lively and grow well in the womb where the placenta is taking care of excreting bodily toxins. After birth however, the body quickly becomes fatally toxic. An acardiac twin (with no heart) may be felt moving in the womb but be dead at birth. Sometimes one twin is born without a brain, which is almost always fatal within hours of birth. Meanwhile, their co-twin develops normally and is born alive and well.

Twin-twin transfusion and monochorionic MZ twins

When MZ twins share a placenta, this can cause problems for them both. A transfusion of fluid and blood between the twins can take place via the placenta. Left untreated, this can lead to death or disability in one or both twins. This can also happen in a triplet pregnancy, but only if there is a monochorionic MZ twin pair within the triplet set.

The first sign of twin-twin transfusion is a different amount of fluid in each of the amniotic sacs. Amniotic fluid is constantly being swallowed by the twins who both urinate the fluid out again, but when a twin-twin transfusion begins, the amniotic fluid increases in volume in one sac because one twin starts to urinate excessively. Meanwhile, the other twin stops urinating and their amniotic fluid is reduced to such a very low level that movement is no longer possible.

Removal of fluid

An excessive amount of fluid in one of the amniotic sacs can trigger premature labour, which could mean a poor outcome for the babies. The cure for this problem is to remove fluid from the distended sac by inserting a hollow needle into the uterus via the mother's abdomen. Mo-Mo MZ twins, who share an amniotic sac, do not have this problem.[b] Therefore, where there are dichorionic MZ twins, in separate sacs, the fluid levels between the two sacs can be regulated by puncturing the membrane that divides the two sacs. This causes a sudden readjustment to a normal amount of amniotic fluid around the immobilized twin. For many years this was the only treatment for

---

b.   Monochorionic-monoamniotic twins - i.e. sharing a placenta and amniotic sac

twin-twin transfusion. Sadly, the eventual outcome in some cases was the death of one or both twins, so why did some twins die and some survive? It seemed that there was much more to this imbalance between twins than just the level of amniotic fluid.

A fatal blood transfusion

It has become clear over the last twenty years that twin-twin transfusion is of blood, not amniotic fluid. In the placenta some blood vessels are shared between the twins and it is between these shared blood vessels that the transfusion of blood occurs. However, it is important to stress that twin-twin transfusion does not always happen. Everything depends on the timing of that original split into MZ twins.

As we have seen, if the original zygote splits within the first three or four days, then the two MZ twins develop separately, each with its own placenta, chorion and amniotic sac. For these twins there is no problem with twin-twin transfusion. If the original zygote split after eight days or so, then the MZ twins share a placenta and a sac. The transfusion doesn't happen in this case either.

When the original zygote splits between five and eight days, the MZ twins share a placenta but do not share a sac. In the shared placenta the blood vessels from each baby may become connected at some stage of the pregnancy. When the vessels become connected, there is a sudden and dramatic shift in the blood supply between the two babies as a transfusion of blood begins between them. Whether a transfusion occurs or not between the twins depends on the specific nature of the connected blood vessels.

Artery-to-artery connection

Where Mo-Mo MZ twins share a single amniotic sac, the blood vessels that are connected are both arteries because of the way their placenta is configured. In that case, the sharing of blood is equal and is not fatal for either twin.

Artery-to-vein connection

The risk of fatal transfusion comes when the MZ twins each have an amniotic sac but share a single placenta. Within the single placenta, arteries or veins may become randomly connected. Arteries carry bright red, oxygenated blood, pumped by the heart at considerable pressure into the body via the lungs. Veins carry the darker red blood passively back towards the heart so there is very little, if any, pressure in the veins. It is possible for various connections to be created: artery-to artery, vein-to-vein or artery-to-vein. It is only the artery-to-vein connection that is potentially fatal for one or both twins. If that happens, blood under pressure in an artery from one twin (the "pump" twin) comes into direct contact with a vein from the other "recipient" twin. The effect is that the pump twin's blood is pumped along the vein into the body of the other twin. The increased blood pressure in the recipient twin puts the heart under stress, which means there is a risk of heart failure for the recipient twin.

Resolution of the problem

Twin-twin transfusion is usually diagnosed when there is a visible difference in size between monochorionic MZ twins. If the two babies are sufficiently developed, they can be delivered by Caesarean section to save their lives. This may not be necessary however, for the situation can resolve naturally if the "pump" twin dies in the womb. This reduces the blood volume in the body of the recipient twin. The excess blood flows back via the vein into the body of the dead pump twin and naturally resolves the problem. [13] It is a different matter if the recipient twin dies. In that case, some rapid medical intervention is needed to help the surviving "pump" twin, for in this case the blood transfusion continues but there is no pumping heart in the dead recipient twin to send the blood out again. The blood pools in the body of the dead recipient twin, leaving the survivor severely anaemic and bloodless. Even when the two babies are delivered the surviving pump twin may soon die of severe anaemia. Methods have recently been developed to give the pump twin some extra blood before birth. After carefully taking a sample of foetal blood to get a good match, a blood transfusion can be given to the foetus while in the womb. This is fast becoming a standard procedure for restoring blood levels in a sole surviving "pump" twin. [14]

The loss of a twin or more: the tragic cost of ART

Since the onset of Assisted Reproductive Technology (ART), multiple birth - of twins, triplets and higher order multiples - has been on the increase in the Western world. It was reported in the New York Times in 2008 that, since the onset of IVF treatment in 1980, the rate of twins in all births has climbed by 70%.[15] Multiple births as a result of IVF have been described as having reached epidemic proportions.[16] The toll on mother and baby when a multiple pregnancy is created by ART can be enormous. This is reflected in costs of another kind: multiple pregnancies require a huge investment in health care costs, social care for families with multiples and lifetime support for any disabled children of the family. A good example of this high cost was reported in October 2009 in the New York Times: the Mastera family live in Colorado, USA and their twins were conceived by IVF after two years of fertility treatment. In that same period they spent more than 23% of their income on these treatments. The two boys (DZ twins) were born nine weeks early, each weighing barely more than three pounds. After many weeks of special care, the babies returned home at last and are both thriving. The medical bills for everyone involved over the whole exercise was over a million dollars. A leading expert in all matters relating to multiple birth has made it clear that the press and media coverage of successful IVF pregnancies has carefully omitted the tragic stories of twins born so premature that they are left permanently handicapped. The risks increase with the number of foetuses in the womb and the number of babies delivered. Where the foetuses arise out of a single egg (MZ) they do less well than where several eggs have been fertilized.[17]

A conflict of interest

As a result of the increase in multiple births caused by ART, some fertility centres are beginning to change their tactics. In the UK and Europe, new regulations have been put in place to try and reduce the number of multiple births. In some fertility clinics it is already common practice to replace only two embryos or blastocysts after IVF, or to select the two that seem to be of the highest quality. That means leaving the cells to divide to the blastocyst stage and seeing how well the various blastocysts are developing. The ones that develop the fastest are isolated and just two of them are chosen and replaced into the womb. An interesting by-product of this practice is that a greater proportion of the babies that result are boys.[18] This is because from the very start of life males grow more rapidly than females.[19]

41

Deaf ears

There is a certain conflict in the minds of both fertility specialists and the would-be parents. On the one hand there is the desire to see a happy outcome: the so-called, "Take-home-baby" rate. On the other hand, there is the desire to ensure the health and welfare of the babies. In gathering material for her book *One and the Same*, which is about the life of MZ twins, Abigail Progrebin, who is one of a pair of MZ twins herself, interviewed several fertility specialists about their work. They claimed that they do make it a practice to point out the many risks of multiple pregnancy and birth to their clients, but this tends to fall on deaf ears.[20] After a series of failed fertility treatments, increasing age and perhaps also a rising level of debt as a result of the fees involved, the parents' desire for a baby of their own seemingly eclipses any other thought. Indeed, to these parents, two babies for the price of one may seem to be a favourable outcome. The conflict of interest between doctors and fertility clients is likely to continue for a long time and the use of ART will doubtless continue. Increasingly desperate couples, rapidly running out of time and funds, will take the risk of having twins or triplets sooner than remain childless.

Death on the increase, more sole survivors

As the incidence of multiple births increases, there will be a greater number of cases where one twin dies in the third trimester or close to birth, leaving a sole survivor. In the next chapter, we will take a closer look at the death of one twin in the second trimester of pregnancy, which is a dangerous time for all concerned.

4

The death of a twin in the second trimester

My mother has told me that I had a twin in the womb but it died when we
were at six months into the pregnancy. I just always wondered what things
would have been like if she or he were to survive. I would probably not be so
sad at times when my life is going wonderfully.

Jenny, USA

Pregnancy is usually divided into three trimesters, each being a period of
three months. This chapter will take a close look at what can happen when
one twin dies in the second trimester. This is the middle three months
of pregnancy (13-27 weeks). The second trimester of a twin pregnancy
encompasses the period when the developing foetuses are completely
formed and are growing rapidly. The lungs and digestive system are
developing in this period, but only when the lungs are developed
sufficiently to enable the baby to breathe air will that baby be able to live
outside the womb. This is known as the "limit of viability" which in most
countries is defined as 23-25 weeks of development. [1] The prognosis for
babies born at this early stage is very poor, but some babies are safely
delivered at the very margins of the second trimester. Despite efforts by
medical staff to prolong the pregnancy, labour may start naturally, causing
premature delivery. A delivery at this stage often leads to the loss of both
twins. Occasionally one of them will be just strong enough to survive
but will probably have to spend several weeks in a hospital neonatal care
unit.

Premature delivery

In a healthy twin pregnancy, the pregnant mother sees her abdomen
swell rapidly as she enters the second trimester. The kicks and surges
of activity of the babies in her womb are sometimes quite pronounced.
However, at this stage of her pregnancy her physical state is being
carefully monitored. If her blood pressure increases, if there is protein in
her urine or she notices her hands and feet starting to swell with retained

fluid, then she may be in a state known as "pre-eclampsia." Pre-eclampsia is more common in twin pregnancies and even more common in multiple pregnancies.[2] Pre-eclampsia is potentially very serious for the mother and can be fatal for both the mother and the babies. If a medical emergency of this kind happens to arise, it may be necessary to hasten delivery for the sake of the mother. Both twins may be delivered at the very margins of viability by Caesarean section. If at the time one twin is poorly developed, then the stronger one (the Alpha twin) may just manage to survive, but the other (the Beta twin) will almost certainly die.

> *I have asked my Mum about my birth and as far as she knows I am an only child, but I still feel I had a twin sister. Back then there was no ultra-sound and my Mum was unconscious for a couple of days. I was born by Caesarean section after she developed pre-eclampsia.*
> Adam, UK

One twin stillborn

One twin may be stillborn in the second trimester while the other one just manages to survive. The definition of a "stillbirth" varies around the world: in the UK a stillbirth is defined as a baby delivered without breath at 24 weeks or later.[a] In the USA there is no federal law on stillbirth, but the Wisconsin Stillbirth Service Program considers a baby to be stillborn if he or she is delivered without breath at 20 weeks of gestation or later.

Asynchronous delivery

It can happen that one twin is delivered in the second trimester, too early to survive, while the other twin remains in the womb until birth. Several cases of the asynchronous delivery of twins have been reported. In one such case, a DZ twin pregnancy was diagnosed but it looked as if the premature delivery of both twins was likely. Yet despite the birth of a stillborn girl at just 20 weeks of pregnancy, the pregnancy continued for another 110 days and eventually a healthy baby boy was delivered

---

a. In the UK the Stillbirth (Definition) Act 1992 changed the definition of stillbirth to a baby born dead after 24 weeks completed gestation (previously it had been 28 weeks). A baby who is stillborn is now recognized in law as an individual and so the death of the baby must be registered and the baby buried or cremated. In the USA there is no general formal definition of the term "stillbirth".

at 35 weeks.[3] The way to maintain this kind of pregnancy is to cut the cord of the delivered child as close to the cervix as possible and leave the placenta of the dead twin in the womb. At birth, the placenta of the dead twin is either delivered separately or is fused to the surviving twin's placenta.

> *My mother told me when I was almost a teenager that she delivered a perfectly formed little girl, dead, when she was pregnant with me. She explained that my twin died before I was born and I was really large. So large, that I broke her tail-bone. I was not delivered until a couple of months later.*
> Lara, USA

Miscarriage of one twin

In the second trimester of pregnancy the foetus is perfectly formed but is usually too tiny and undeveloped to survive outside the womb. If labour begins too soon and the twins are miscarried (i.e. delivered before 20 weeks) then they will certainly both die during delivery or after birth. Sometimes one twin dies in the womb while the other survives. The death of one twin in the womb at less than 20 weeks is emotionally very hard for the mother. She has carried twins for so long but after all only one baby will be born alive. In addition, the loss of one's co-twin at this stage is traumatic for the survivor.

> *I always felt a sense of separation from others, and that I was incomplete. From a young age I had the perception that my friends and others were whole individuals, complete, while I was not. There was always this sense of something missing, something "out there" that I was somehow bound and connected to and they were not there. I remember questioning if I was adopted, and at the age of twelve my mother, through some questioning regarding this, told me that she had a miscarriage around four months of pregnancy, and recalled seeing the hand of a foetus. I believe that she must have endured some emotional state during and following this episode. She does not recall if my twin was male or female and this topic is rarely spoken of. This revelation allowed many pieces of the puzzle to fall in place.*
> Geoff, S. Africa

When the body remains in the womb

Twin pregnancies are not just dangerous for the mother. The babies can easily be adversely affected by having to share the space and available resources. Abnormal development, twin-twin transfusion and other pregnancy complications can cost the life of one twin around birth and these same conditions can arise in the second trimester of pregnancy. In this case, the adverse conditions in the womb may not allow both twins to live until birth. As always in a competitive environment, only the strongest will survive. The difference at this earlier stage in pregnancy is that if the surviving twin has not yet reached the age of viability (about 24 weeks or so) then delivering the survivor as soon as possible is not an option. The dead twin must remain in the womb alongside the survivor until delivery. The adverse conditions that cause the death of one twin may be the mother's severe illness or some kind of trauma to the womb such as an accident or being kicked in the stomach.

> *I was born as a single, my Mom was kicked in the stomach early in her pregnancy. I dream of my brother and I, communicating in the womb before a great force comes and we spin and fall, then he disappears after the spinning quits. I have always felt I had a twin, asked my Mom about it when I was three and continually after that.*
> Michela, USA

Only one chorion: when one MZ twin dies

In a twin pregnancy where there is only one chorion surrounding the entire pregnancy and there is only one shared placenta, the twins are always MZ. A recent study has established that the risks of one twin dying in the second trimester are six times greater if the twins share a chorion and placenta. All twins of this kind are MZ.[4] Monochorionic MZ twins share a blood supply and consequently there is a strong possibility that connections will develop between the major blood vessels. As we have seen, where there are shared blood vessels and after the death of one of the twins, blood may be transfused from the living twin into the dead body of the other.[b] When this happens in the second trimester it cannot be resolved by an emergency Caesarean delivery, for at this early stage

---

b.   For more about twin-twin transfusion, see page 38

neither of the babies can survive outside the womb. Instead, an attempt at laser ablation may be made which severs the blood vessels connecting the twins, in order to rescue at least one baby while they are both still alive in the womb.

Laser ablation in twin-twin transfusion has been under development since the early 1990s and is now regarded as a feasible solution for foetuses that would not be viable if delivered.[5] Directed by ultrasound, a laser is used to cut off and seal the connected blood vessels at the earliest possible moment before the recipient twin dies. Where possible, the operation takes place between 20 and 28 weeks of pregnancy, by which time any transfusion of blood between the twins can be verified and the blood vessels are large enough to see.[6] Laser therapy is now the standard procedure in the case of twin-twin transfusion and has been found to be more effective than the removal of amniotic fluid as a solution to the problem.[7] Sadly however, in some cases it is necessary to sacrifice one of the twins in order for the other to survive.[8]

Twin embolization syndrome
If a dead monochorionic MZ twin remains in the womb alongside their living co-twin, this can put the co-twin's life at risk. Monochorionic twins share a placenta so if there are connected blood vessels twin embolization syndrome may occur. This syndrome develops as the dead twin's blood begins to clot soon after death. The clots may be passed through the shared blood vessels into the body of the living twin, causing major damage to the brain and other organs. Sadly, in the second trimester of pregnancy it is too early to deliver the survivor and there is every chance that both twins will die.

The various complications of shared blood supply found in MZ twin pregnancies are known collectively as "twin disruption sequence." One rare study of 18 sole survivors of twin disruption sequence revealed that the prognosis is poor for them all.[9] Before the introduction of laser surgery for twin-twin transfusion in the 1980s, there was nothing that could be done to prevent these problems. The survivors, such as there were, died close to birth or survived with major disabilities.[10] Laser surgery does provide hope that at least one twin will survive, as long as the surgery itself does not trigger a miscarriage of the whole pregnancy.

47

It can be supposed that there is a small but increasing number of MZ womb twin survivors in the population as a direct result of this new development in surgery.

Fatal abnormality in one twin

There are certain abnormalities of development that may prove fatal in the second trimester and they may arise in only one twin of the pair. One or more essential organs may fail to develop normally, such as a missing brain (Anencephaly) or both kidneys missing, (Bilateral renal agenesis,) or no heart (Acardia).[11] Developmental abnormalities of this kind have many and various manifestations and causes. For instance, some may be related to the fertilization of an abnormal ovum.[13] Fatal abnormalities are more common among monochorionic pregnancies, which are almost invariably MZ.[12]

> *I didn't find out I was a twin until I was about 14 when I mentioned to my Mum how I'd loved to have been a twin, when she casually said, "You were." She only really said my twin didn't form properly in the womb, and at the time I was a bit shocked and didn't probe it any further. From time to time I would think about it, especially if someone mentioned twins, but I didn't really dwell on it, only to think that I too might have twins one day.*
> *Nikki, UK*

Two separate chorions – DZ and MZ twins

In about a quarter of MZ pregnancies and all DZ twin pregnancies the twin babies develop quite separately. Each placenta and amniotic sac is surrounded by an outer membrane - the chorion. The placentas may fuse into one, but rarely is the blood supply shared. Twins who do not share a chorion, be they MZ or DZ, stand a much better chance of surviving with no problems if their co-twin dies in the second trimester. If you were an MZ twin whose twin died in the second trimester and you have no problems, then you probably did not share a chorion and placenta with your twin.[14]

> *It seems that my mother took medicine to induce contractions and abort the pregnancy. My twin died at between four and five months but the pregnancy continued. I survived and held myself still in the womb next to my dead twin, afraid to move. I get into relationships where I recreate myself as being "the*

dying twin" - subconsciously of course. I try to push myself out of the "womb space" I've created with this person or other, and leave the relationship. Then when the other person does fine without me and is successful in "living" I have a weird thing of getting suicidal. It's as if one of us has to metaphorically "die". I want to live and not feel guilty about it. I have this deep subconscious "unwritten law" that if I live, someone close has to die.
Linda, USA

Problems with the placenta

If during a twin or multiple pregnancy the mother suffers an infection such as influenza, measles or polio, this can compromise the development of one or both twins. It is not so much the infection that causes the problem but the subsequent damage to the placental blood supply.[15] The placenta of one twin may suffer more damage than the other and may die, leaving a sole survivor.

My mother contracted polio and was expected to die. Mum recovered but I was left with a huge aching hole in me that seemed to get bigger as I got older culminating in a breakdown at the age of sixteen.
Joan, UK

A common infection in pregnancy is Cytomegalovirus, which in a twin pregnancy may spread to both MZ twins where the blood supply through the placenta is shared. However in the case of dichorionic pregnancies one twin may have the virus and die, while the other remains healthy and survives.[16]

Poor implantation

The death of one twin in the womb and the delivery of a healthy survivor can be the result of the poor implantation of the affected twin. In a dichorionic twin pregnancy one twin may implant first and the second twin may attempt to implant in the same place, upon the placenta of the other twin. When one twin implants upon the placenta of the other, it can be fatal for the second twin who, unable to obtain enough oxygen or nourishment, asphyxiates and starves to death while the other one continues to thrive. When this has happened, the placenta of the dead twin can be seen at birth as a patch of different placental tissue, embedded in the surviving twin's placenta. After birth and when tested

49

for DNA, the cells of this embedded patch are found to be belonging to the dead twin. This is known as a "mosaic placenta," for a mosaic is any tissue containing two sets of DNA.

Intrauterine growth restriction (IUGR)

Intrauterine growth restriction (IUGR) means that in the womb the normal growth of a foetus is in some way compromised. Sometimes, in a twin pregnancy where the twins each have their own separate chorion (DZ or MZ), one twin grows very slowly while the other one thrives. This can lead eventually to a great difference between them in both size and vitality. IUGR is caused by a general restriction in nourishment and oxygen via the placenta. In a twin pregnancy IUGR favours one baby over the other. The restriction in growth in one twin is caused by reduced access to nourishment and oxygen, which is related to the different functioning of the two placentas. The increasing difference between the two babies is visible on the ultrasound scan. The difference between the twins may persist, even after birth. In MZ twins this can create a life-long disadvantage for the growth-restricted twin. A study of MZ twins, where one twin of each pair was smaller than the other, showed that in each case the twin who weighed less at birth had a lower IQ than the larger twin. [17]

The foetus papyraceous - a "papery" foetus

If one twin stops growing but both of are sufficiently developed to be able to survive outside the womb, then may be appropriate to hasten delivery and risk the complications of a premature birth. However if at least one twin is not sufficiently developed, the pregnancy is allowed to continue. The smaller twin must remain in the womb, slowly dying. After death, the body remains intact inside its own sac and attached to the placenta by the umbilical cord. The body of the foetus is compressed as the tissues begin to deteriorate. It may become embedded in the other twin's placenta. Once exposed to the air after delivery, the skin of the dead foetus may become papery and white. This papery appearance gave rise to the term *foetus papyraceous*, which is Latin for "papery foetus".

This Latin name has been given to the body of a second trimester twin because science has known about these tiny dead twins for more than five hundred years. This papery creature, born alongside a healthy baby, was described in 1497 by an Italian doctor named Michele Savonarola in his book *Practica Major.* This book contained all the knowledge of medicine at the time, some of which dated back to the ancient Greeks. Under the section on obstetrics there is a short piece on what he called "*De Mola.*" This was his term for the strange objects that formed in the womb of women and were born with their babies. Savonarola wrote, "The women call them *fera*, which means "a wild animal." [18] According to how squashed and misshapen the tiny twin's dead body may have become by the time of delivery, with a little imagination and a great deal of ignorance, they could be taken to resemble the young of a wild animal. This notion gave rise to some speculation, including the assumption was that this strange object might have been conceived in a separate sexual encounter by a process of superfetation. Furthermore, the nature and status of the "wild animal" that was seemingly delivered alongside the newborn baby would be assumed to vary with the social standing of the putative father. If the *fera* seemed to look like a hawk, then that was considered much better than a lizard!

Today, the *foetus papyraceous* is properly understood to be the dead body of a twin that has developed as far as the second trimester before death ensued. The tiny body may become so compressed that it is easily overlooked or ignored, so it is hard to know how often this occurs. However, the presence of a papery foetus at birth can be anticipated when a dichorionic twin pregnancy is interrupted by selective foeticide.

Selective foeticide

In the last 20 years, the use of ultrasound as a diagnostic tool has become increasingly sophisticated, as have pre-birth tests for foetal abnormality. At around 16 weeks of pregnancy, the pregnant woman is subjected to a battery of tests to establish whether her developing foetuses show any signs of abnormal development. In a dichorionic pregnancy where the placentas are not shared and one twin has some kind of abnormality it is relatively safe for the survivor if their co-twin dies. Therefore, it is now common practice for the anomalous twin to be aborted by lethal injection and delivered as a papery foetus along with the sole survivor.[19]

Multi-foetal pregnancy reduction (MFPR)

Foeticide can be carried out on healthy foetuses in the second trimester of a multiple pregnancy if there are too many foetuses developing.

51

In that case there is a risk that they will all be lost if the numbers are not somehow reduced. There is usually some natural loss of one or more foetuses in the very early stages of a multiple pregnancy. If this does not occur, by the second trimester there may still be too many foetuses, so a multi-foetal pregnancy reduction may be made. Through the 1980s and 1990s, various forms of selective foeticide were developed. These were based on an earlier system developed in the 1970s, of puncturing the heart of the selected foetus and injecting air into the circulation.[20] The selection of foetuses for MFPR is usually made in the first trimester, but where possible it is considered helpful to wait until the second trimester, when the foetuses are a little more developed and any abnormalities can be more easily diagnosed.[21] The method of choice today for selective foeticide is potassium chloride injected directly into the heart of one or more of the selected foetuses. This causes cardiac arrest.

Concern about MFPR

The policy now adopted by some assisted reproduction clinics is to transfer only one or two embryos during IVF. Also, some steps are being taken to limit the irresponsible use of fertility drugs. As a result the number of pregnancies with triplets and more is gradually reducing. However, the focus now is on twins. Because the reduction procedure is now available, some parents are asking for twins to be "reduced" to a single baby in order to guarantee delivery of one healthy baby. One study in Denmark of 44 multiple pregnancies reduced to two foetuses included 16 pregnancies reduced from twins to a singleton. In this study the good effects of reduction from twins to one were clear in terms of the size of the babies and the length of the pregnancy.[22] In the light of positive reports such as this, the practice of selective foeticide is

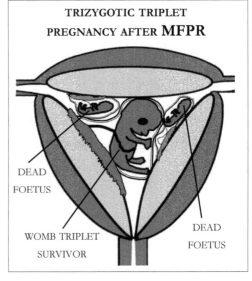

TRIZYGOTIC TRIPLET PREGNANCY AFTER **MFPR**

DEAD FOETUS

WOMB TRIPLET SURVIVOR

DEAD FOETUS

likely to continue despite the misgivings of some professionals. An article entitled *"Do reduced multiples do better?"* published in 2005 stated clearly that they do. [23] The same article reports that women over 40 carrying twins benefited from a relative lack of pregnancy problems when their twin pregnancy was reduced to a single womb twin survivor. The emotional problems experienced by the parents, who have the option of watching while a selected few of their multiples are destroyed, are only now being addressed. It is known that the parents find MFPR very difficult, in particular the arbitrary nature of the selection. [24] Some professionals have been voicing their concern about the emotional difficulties associated with MFPR, because no details are available about the possible effect on the survivors or how the parents should tell them. [24]

The survivors of MFPR

In published articles about MFPR there is little mention of any health and disability problems caused to the surviving babies. We know that dichorionic DZ and MZ twins suffer fewer problems when their co-twin dies, so it is to be assumed that most successful pregnancy reductions take place among foetuses who are developing in their own a separate chorion. Held safe in their own private life-support system, dichorionic twins presumably suffer no physical ill-effects as a result of the sudden heart failure of one or more of their fellow womb-mates. MFPR is a recent development, so the survivors are still young at the time of writing. It seems to suits the interests of both parents and professionals not to emphasize the physical effects on the survivor when a co-twin dies, let alone a larger number of fellow foetuses. This is understandable, as no one would want to cause unnecessary anxiety to a pregnant woman. However, more and more large-scale studies are being carried out and it is becoming clear that there are definite physical effects on the survivors, particularly if their MZ co-twin dies. [26]

Death in early pregancy

In the next chapter will discuss how a twin may die in the first trimester of pregnancy. There are many survivors of this eventuality and we will be hearing some of their extraordinary stories.

5

The death of a twin in the first trimester

I lost one of my twins at about two months pregnant. I had some bleeding.
We went to the doctor and my remaining baby was doing great. Oddly, when
I delivered my baby there was a second little placenta.

Jenny, USA

The first trimester spans the first three months of pregnancy. For the
first 57 days of pregnancy, (i.e. the first eight weeks) the unborn baby is
described as an "embryo." When all the major organs are in place and the
skeleton is beginning to form, the name is changed to "foetus." Using the
two names for the same unborn baby may be a bit confusing, but for the
sake of accuracy both terms will be used in this chapter. The two terms
signify the stage of development and that is all.

By the end of the twelfth week, a mother carrying twin foetuses
is already aware that her womb is larger than would be expected in a
singleton pregnancy at such an early stage. Her family may have already
remarked on how quickly she is expanding. She is probably finding her
normal clothes a little tight around the waist. She will be considering
maternity clothes and wondering if it is a little early for such things.
We saw in the last chapter that as the pregnancy proceeds there may be
dangers ahead, but for the moment all seems well. After some weeks of
wondering she may be prepared to announce her pregnancy to her family
and friends.

Miscarriage of one twin

It is usual among pregnant women to keep their pregnancy a secret until
three months or so have passed, for it is in the first trimester that there
is the greatest risk of miscarriage. In a twin or multiple pregnancy the
risk is even higher. This early pregnancy loss is described in the medical
literature as "natural wastage," which may sound cruel and random at
first hearing. It is certainly a hard truth for pregnant mothers to face if
they have invested a great deal in their pregnancy, only to see their hopes
dashed in a miscarriage.

I was told at about eight or nine years old that my mum miscarried my twin. This news was at the time devastating yet somehow a relief because I always felt different. Having learnt of my twin, new fears and worries began - was it my fault my twin had died? Did I harm or kill it? These thoughts would go round and round, even to this present day.

Laura, UK

Conversely, an early miscarriage of the whole pregnancy is a bittersweet experience for women who are afraid of rearing twins or who have an unwanted pregnancy. The loss of one twin can be a great relief to many mothers. If we stand back a little and see the global picture, the womb is where evolution starts. The ruthless eugenics of Nature are at work to ensure the health and strength of the next generation by a process of Alpha-Beta pruning. Only the strongest survive. This is a point that will be made again and again as we explore the lives of womb twin survivors.

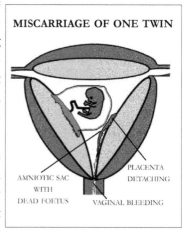

MISCARRIAGE OF ONE TWIN

AMNIOTIC SAC WITH DEAD FOETUS

PLACENTA DETACHING

VAGINAL BLEEDING

When my Mom became pregnant with me, she had just married my father and couldn't be happier. Then she had a miscarriage at around nine weeks. She went to see the doctor in the middle of the night and he proceeded to console her, stating that he was deeply sorry for her loss. At the time my parents were clearing trees and brush to build a new house, so after my Mom lost the baby, she got to work. All day she worked hard so that she wouldn't think of the child she lost. A few weeks later she couldn't shake the feeling that she was still pregnant, for the signs were still there. She went back to the doctor and to his amazement he saw that she was still carrying a baby that was just as far along as her previous one should have been. She had been carrying twins and I was the survivor.

Anne, USA

Why did my twin die?

There are many reasons why one twin may die in the first trimester: we will now consider just a few.

55

A "blighted ovum"- developmental failure

If at the start of pregnancy a gestational sac appears but there is nothing in the sac, it is known as a "blighted ovum." This is a zygote that implants in the uterus, begins to develop a gestational sac which can be seen on the ultrasound scan but no embryo develops in the sac. The embryo may begin to form but development does not get very far before it fails to survive. Until the 1970s little was known about the abnormalities that can occur in the first trimester of a

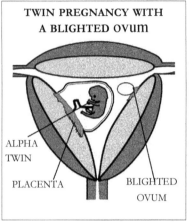

twin pregnancy. However, when ultrasound came into regular use in pregnancy in the 1970s, this opened a window on the early weeks of foetal development. In 1979 it was reported that 41 cases of an abnormal multiple pregnancy had been diagnosed by means of ultrasound and the most frequent occurrence was a normal pregnancy with a blighted ovum for a twin. [1]

Developmental abnormalities

If development goes badly wrong for one DZ twin in the first trimester of a twin pregnancy, the affected twin will probably not survive longer than a few weeks. A failure to develop major organs, in particular the heart, the kidneys, the intestines or brain, means an early death for the twin concerned, who is the weaker, Beta twin. As the weeks pass, the Beta twin gradually disappears from view on the ultrasound screen. When a twin pregnancy is diagnosed at the time of the first scan but one twin has gone by the next scan,

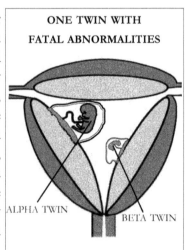

this is known as a "vanishing twin" pregnancy. As the DZ survivor has a separate life support system intact, there will be no ill-effects.

Congenital abnormalities

In a twin pregnancy, there may be one twin with defective or missing genes or chromosomes while the other has a set of normal chromosomes. Otherwise one or more chromosomes in one of the twins may be normal to start with, but become damaged. This may compromise the development of the affected twin to the extent that survival is impossible beyond a few days or weeks. Meanwhile, the other twin will have no development problems at all.

Problems with the placenta

In the first three months of a twin pregnancy the placentas are still developing. One twin's placenta may not have implanted very well and could easily be dislodged if the mother falls or sustains an abdominal injury. A very stressful and traumatic episode such as a disaster, an accident, or the death of a loved one can reduce the blood supply to the placenta because of the adrenaline produced. The consequent loss of oxygen and nutrients could prove fatal for an already-weakened or disadvantaged twin. It is not known exactly how stress affects pregnancy in humans, but we know that stress can induce a miscarriage. [2] However, animal studies have found that a period of psychological distress can create hormonal changes that may affect implantation and development. [3]

> *Mom's partner was very violent and he told her that he would prevent any child being born. So she looked for another man, my father, to get pregnant secretly. When the abusive guy found out he treated her in a very violent and abusive way. Mom got a singular size around the waist, so one of her coworkers told her, "I think you are carrying twins." But before three months had passed she started to bleed, so she thought she had had a miscarriage, but the pregnancy continued. The ninth month arrived and there were not any signs of birth, but the doctor told her that they could wait, so the tenth month arrived and nothing happened, so the doctor said it was time for a Caesarean. I was lying horizontally inside Mom's womb. They pulled me out but there was no breathing, no crying, nothing. The doctors put me in an artificial respirator for a day and a half, and then I started breathing by myself.*
> *Martin, USA*

Vaginal bleeding

Various studies suggest that vaginal bleeding complicates a quarter of all pregnancies. The nature of that bleeding has been subjected to careful analysis. The term "light spotting" is used to describe the situation when a woman discovers bleeding by wiping but does not require use of sanitary protection. "Heavy bleeding" soaks underwear or requires a pad. In one study, three quarters of women who experienced bleeding reported "a single episode of light spotting" in the first trimester.[4]

Spotting or slight vaginal bleeding, at a stage when one is still unsure of a pregnancy, is a private matter. For most women it is too embarrassing to discuss at all. Furthermore, according to several studies, most women with vaginal bleeding in the early weeks of pregnancy go on to achieve a live birth, so an episode of light spotting could easily be overlooked or ignored.[5] Until the advent of ultrasound and its use in early pregnancy, vaginal bleeding was an unexplored area. It is now generally assumed that significant vaginal bleeding in early pregnancy probably signals the foetal death of one twin.[6] One study of first trimester bleeding revealed a "blighted" ovum in every case.[7]

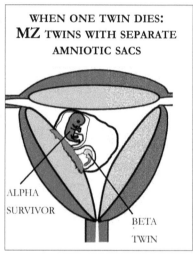

WHEN ONE TWIN DIES: MZ TWINS WITH SEPARATE AMNIOTIC SACS

ALPHA SURVIVOR

BETA TWIN

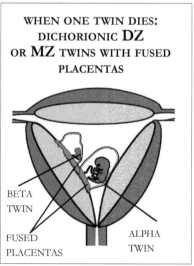

WHEN ONE TWIN DIES: DICHORIONIC DZ OR MZ TWINS WITH FUSED PLACENTAS

BETA TWIN

FUSED PLACENTAS

ALPHA TWIN

Changes in the placenta

When one MZ twin dies in a mono-chorionic twin pair (i.e. sharing a chorion) the placental blood supply shifts and changes as a result of the changed demands made upon it. There may be some leakage of blood from around the placenta. The pregnant woman may notice this as a show of blood. In a dichorionic twin pregnancy (i.e. with separate chorions) the twins may be DZ or MZ and two placentas develop. If the two separate placentas are fused together, then the placenta of the dead twin remains in the womb, attached to the surviving twin's placenta. Even so, the changes in the placenta when one twin dies may cause some bleeding.

Vaginal bleeding misinterpreted
When a mother notices some vaginal bleeding, depending on the stage of pregnancy that has been reached, she may assume that this is her menstrual flow back again and she is not pregnant after all. If she knows she certainly is pregnant, she has no idea she is carrying twins and no ultrasound scan is made to check, then she may assume that the bleeding signals the end of her pregnancy and that her baby is lost. Later on, experiencing all the symptoms of pregnancy, she may take a test and be surprised to find she is still pregnant. After an incomplete miscarriage, that is, where there has been bleeding but no sign of a foetus or placenta, a doctor may recommend a dilatation and curettage procedure (D&C) to clear all remaining detritus of the pregnancy out of the womb. This is to prevent a major bleeding episode or an infection, which can happen if parts of the placenta are left behind. For many years it has been common practice to carry out a D&C after a miscarriage. It is probable that many sole surviving twins have been surgically removed in this way after the miscarriage of their twin.

> *My mother always told me her pregnancy with me was extremely difficult. She had a severe bleeding episode and her doctor suggested she come in for a scraping. I just feel incomplete, always have. I had a very bad dream when I was about three or four years old of a dead baby chasing me, and I was running away but I felt like I could not run. I remember that dream even today.*
> Matt, USA

Abortion of one twin
When a woman goes for an abortion but is unknowingly pregnant with twins, she may remain pregnant afterwards if both babies have not been removed. Some women in this situation may attempt a claim for compensation to cover the cost of bringing up the remaining unexpected child. One such claim was successful: Kim Nicholls, from Staffordshire

in England, successfully claimed £10,000 compensation when she was given an injection to abort her pregnancy yet remained pregnant and delivered a healthy daughter some months later. [8] As a result of successful claims such as these, doctors are now advised to take particular care to check that only one foetus is present before every abortion procedure.

Ectopic pregnancy

In an ectopic pregnancy, the developing embryo does not implant in the womb but instead attaches to some other surface. In most ectopic pregnancies the embryo begins to develop in one of the fallopian tubes. This is also known as a tubal pregnancy. An ectopic pregnancy can occur alongside a normal pregnancy in a version of twinning or as part of a twin pregnancy as a kind of triplet set. If an ectopic pregnancy is left to develop and no intervention is made the results are potentially fatal for both the mother and the other twin. Either the embryo must be stopped from growing or it must be removed from the tube where it has implanted. When there is a twin pregnancy with an ectopic embryo and another embryo developing in the womb, the ectopic embryo can be stopped from growing with drugs or surgically removed from the fallopian tube. The other twin is at risk from the effects of this treatment but may survive unharmed. Ectopic pregnancy has been associated with IVF, especially among older patients with some existing damage to the fallopian tubes. In one reported case only two embryos were transferred during IVF treatment but an additional ectopic pregnancy resulted nonetheless. [9]

PROBLEMS SPECIFIC TO DZ TWINS

If you are a DZ womb twin survivor, how genetically different you were from both your parents and your twin may have been a matter of life and death from conception. According to research it looks as if humans may avoid prospective mates who are too similar in the genes that drive the immune system. This set of genes is called the human leukocyte antigen system, or the "HLA system" for short. It is found on chromosome number six. [10] In a DZ twin pregnancy the twins have different sets of genes. One twin's HLA gene set may vary more from the mother's genes than the other twin. This genetic difference has an effect on how well the womb will tolerate the presence of one particular twin. It may decide which twin is to be rejected by the mother's immune system in the first trimester and cast out of the womb in a miscarriage.

It has been suggested that one role of the HLA gene set in the immune system is to differentiate "self" from "non-self" and reject any tissue that is not an exact match. This "foreignness" would presumably spell trouble for the twin with the most different genes from the mother's, but not so, in fact. Exactly the opposite is true and for a very good reason. Several studies have found that a miscarriage is more likely when a man and a woman with similar HLA gene sets conceive. If the fittest individuals are to survive then the best kind of immune system to have is one able to produce a wide variety of antibodies to various diseases. The reasons are not clear but it may be assumed that, because pregnancy is in fact an invasion of foreign tissue, the HLA gene set is involved in miscarriage. The HLA gene set may simply provide protection against a wider range of diseases, both in the womb and in later life. In other words, having a wide variety of combinations in your HLA gene set means that you will have a stronger immune system. [11] If you are a DZ womb twin survivor, the nature of your HLA gene set may have been the deciding factor in why you were the only twin to survive.

PROBLEMS SPECIFIC TO MZ TWINS

As MZ twins develop from the same zygote they share the same genes. This means that if there is an inherited genetic defect that proves to be fatal it will affect both twins and neither will survive. In the first trimester the most likely defect specific to MZ twins is an asymmetrical splitting of the original cell mass. That would prove fatal to the Beta twin but leave the Alpha twin developing normally. It could also leave the Beta twin alive but with a fatal condition, such as a cardiac defect or *spina bifida*. [a]

Monochorionic MZ twins - a shared placental blood supply

If you are a womb twin survivor, began life as an MZ twin and shared a chorion and placenta with your twin, you may have also shared a placental blood supply. Twin-twin transfusion via a shared placenta, which we discussed in the last chapter, is not such a problem in the first

---

a. The neural tube does not fully close. See Glossary.

trimester as it is later on in pregnancy. [12] This is probably because the connections between the two blood supplies are not sufficiently developed to create a shared blood supply. Where a blood supply is shared between twins, that share may have been unequal. If that is your story, this fact alone may be enough to explain why you made it to birth but your Beta twin had died by the end of the first trimester. In this case your Beta twin had an insufficient share of the placenta, managed for a while to adapt to "famine conditions" but eventually starved to

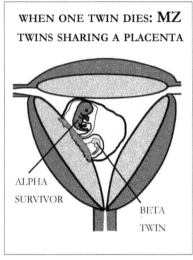

WHEN ONE TWIN DIES: MZ TWINS SHARING A PLACENTA

ALPHA SURVIVOR

BETA TWIN

death. Exactly where the two cords are joined to a shared placenta is very important regardless of how the blood vessels are connected, if at all. The shared placental blood supply is connected to the mother's blood supply. In the early weeks of pregnancy her blood volume increases to meet the demands of her growing babies. At this early stage there is more than enough food and oxygen to go round but it may be that one twin gets a little bit less nourishment and oxygen than the other. If your twin's cord was joined to your shared placenta away from the major source of blood but your cord was more centrally placed, this may have held back your twin's growth and development. Starved of both food and oxygen, your twin may have struggled to survive until their major organs begin to fail. This would have been a slow but inevitable death.

Twin-twin transfusion resolved naturally

We saw in the last chapter how untreated twin-twin transfusion can cause the death of one MZ twin and leave any survivor at risk of multiple abnormalities and disabilities, if there is a survivor at all. [b] When twin-twin transfusion begins as early as the first trimester it may resolve naturally. Even so, in the process it may cause some problems for the survivor. After a transfusion of blood between twins in the first trimester, the body of the recipient twin embryo becomes over-hydrated.

---

b.   For more about twin-twin transfusion, see pages 38 & 46

When the recipient twin dies

If the recipient twin dies, even more blood drains through the connected vessels and pools in the body of the dead twin. The dead recipient twin's heart has stopped pumping it back into the shared circulation. Meanwhile, the once-donor twin has lost a lot of blood and may be severely anaemic. Acute anaemia and the neurological damage that this can bring may be a cause of cerebral palsy (CP).[c] A statistical study carried out by Peter Pharoah at Liverpool University in England has revealed that, if you are a twin or it is known that you lost an MZ twin before birth, you are many times more likely to have CP than if you never had a twin.[13] Pharoah maintains, along with his fellow workers, that the cause is probably connected to twin-twin transfusion in an MZ twin pregnancy with a shared blood supply that has resolved naturally after the death of the recipient twin.[14] Connected blood vessels in a shared placenta might also lead to abnormalities of development in the surviving donor twin. This may be because in the first few weeks of life the major organs are developing. A shortage of circulating oxygenated blood in the donor twin may hold back development of some major organs, such as the lungs or nervous system. Pharoah has also found, as part of his study of the causes of CP, that people with CP also have an increased chance of cerebral impairment. He also suggests that singleton babies born with CP may have lost a twin early in pregnancy.[15]

When the donor twin dies

Meanwhile, if the donor twin dies it is the recipient twin's chance of life. The donor twin may pump out a bit too much blood and die of acute anaemia because of a fatal lack of oxygen to their brain. In that case twin-twin transfusion simply ceases. The donor's arterial blood is no longer being pumped into the veins of the recipient twin, who urinates out any excess fluid. Following this bonus gift of oxygen and nourishment, the once-recipient twin settles down to a more normal rate of growth.

Mo-Mo twins

When MZ twins share a sac and a placenta they also share a blood supply. Twin-twin transfusion can occur between the twins but it is less common

---

c. Spastic paralysis and/or other disabilities. (See Glossary.)

than in a diamniotic twin pregnancy. Connections between Mo-Mo twins[d] are usually artery-to-artery. In this configuration twin-twin transfusion does not occur.[e] After the death of a Mo-Mo twin in the first trimester the body of the dead twin remains in the shared sac but soon disintegrates and is resorbed. This is how the Beta twin briefly lives alongside the Alpha twin and dies, leaving no evidence that they had ever existed

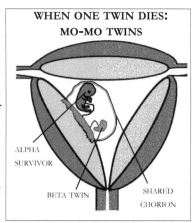

WHEN ONE TWIN DIES: MO-MO TWINS

ALPHA SURVIVOR

BETA TWIN

SHARED CHORION

THE BETA TWIN'S BODY

There many different outcomes for the body of a Beta DZ or MZ twin after death in the first trimester, depending on whether or not the Beta twin is enclosed in a separate chorion.

Twins developing in two separate chorions (dichorionic)

In later chapters we will discover the importance of working out what happened to the body of a Beta twin who died in the first trimester, for if you are a womb twin survivor that will be part of your womb story.

Expelled from the womb

In the first case, cramps and contractions begin. The body of the dead embryo twin, the placenta and the surrounding membranes gradually part company with the wall of the womb. The cervix opens slightly and the body sac and placenta and are eventually expelled from the womb. There is bleeding, sometimes severe, but the surviving twin's placenta remains anchored in place. The survivor continues to develop until birth.

The body remains intact

The second case arises when the twins have developed for more than ten weeks and their skeletons have begun to form. One twin dies but the body is not expelled, for it is too solid to pass through the cervix and remains in the womb alongside the surviving co-twin. The amniotic sac

---

d.   Monochorionic-monoamniotic twins - i.e. sharing a placenta and amniotic sac

e.   For more about this aspect of twin-twin transfusion see page 39

of the dead twin shrinks as the amniotic fluid drains away. The squashed little foetus, pushed to one side by the expanding amniotic sac of the surviving twin, lies embedded in the surface of the placenta. This is an early example of the *foetus papyraceous* ("papery" foetus.) A close histological examination of the placenta after delivery would be needed to establish whether or not there had been a second foetus developing, just for

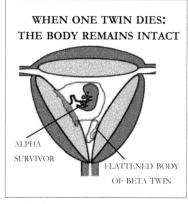

WHEN ONE TWIN DIES: THE BODY REMAINS INTACT

ALPHA SURVIVOR

FLATTENED BODY OF BETA TWIN

a few weeks. This facility is not normally available, so we do not know how often this happens.

The embryo body disintegrates

The third case arises during the first ten weeks when only the soft tissues of the twin's body have formed. Some pregnancies, especially those created by ART, are monitored from the first week. There is nothing to be seen until just over four weeks from conception, when one or more gestational sacs are visible. If inside the gestational sac there is a yolk sac that means there is a conception. From five to six weeks the foetal pole can be seen. It is generally from six weeks onward that the foetal heartbeat is detected. From this stage foetal viability can be assessed in either twin, according to whether or not the foetal heart is beating. The first sign of death is that one of the foetal hearts is not longer beating and the tiny body begins to disintegrate. After this there are three more eventualities:

A sac and cord are left: The disintegrated tissues of the twin's body are gradually absorbed into the placenta. The twin's placenta may remain intact and be delivered later with a second cord and empty amniotic sac attached, either as a separate placenta or integrated into the placenta of the surviving twin.

Only a placenta remains: The body, the cord and the sac all disintegrate and the dead twin's placenta remains embedded into the survivor's placenta.

Everything disappears: The body of the twin, the placenta, the cord, the sac and all the membranes disintegrate entirely and gradually disappear.

Sometimes there is vaginal bleeding but often there are no symptoms at all. Without the tiny images on the ultrasound scan – if a scan was made early enough to catch a glimpse of it – there would be no indication at all that the Beta womb twin ever existed.

> *Although there is no medical reason I should think so (although I have never asked my mother about my actual birth), I have always felt horrifically lonely and as if I was missing something vital to myself. Someone suggested perhaps I was a womb twin survivor, which when I read more about the subject really struck a deep chord with me.*
> Leila, UK

MZ twins developing in a shared chorion (mono-chorionic)

Where there have been MZ twins sharing a chorion, after the Beta twin dies the body is held within the chorion. It cannot be expelled from the womb and remains alongside in the womb until birth. After 10-12 weeks, the skeleton is sufficiently developed to form a "papery foetus." If death occurs in the first eight weeks the embryonic tissues are still very soft and will disintegrate. The dissolved tissues are gradually and totally resorbed into the placenta, which is now supporting a lone Alpha survivor. Within a few more weeks all visible traces of the dead twin will have disappeared. There may be another sac, some thickening or nodules to be seen on the single placenta after birth which would be the only evidence of the lost twin.

The twin within

As we continue to explore the various pre-birth experiences that womb twin survivors may encounter, we will next consider the situation when the lost Beta womb twin becomes merged into the body of the Alpha survivor.

6

When twins unite

I was a twin in the womb, and I believe that I "absorbed" my other half.
Melly, USA

It seems to be axiomatic that DZ[a] twins can never merge to become one person and MZ[b] twins are split apart for life, but this chapter will show you how this can happen. Under very particular circumstances both DZ and MZ twins can unite and mingle with one another. The various forms of merging take place along a spectrum, from conjoined twins to the merging of two sets of DNA. In this chapter we will follow the same spectrum as we explore the merging of twins.

Conjoined twins

If separation of the original zygote does not happen for 14 days or more, the two parts cannot separate completely. The result is MZ twins whose bodies are physically joined together. They share body parts with their twin. The phenomenon of conjoined twins, sometimes called "Siamese" twins, reveals a failure of the zygote to split completely apart. Today, the general assumption is that conjoined twins are better off surgically separated, if that is medically possible. Conjoined twins are separated as babies, or when very young, depending on how and to what degree they are connected. The possibility of a successful outcome of surgery - defined as where one or both twins survive - depends upon where the twins are connected. There are medical terms for each area of connection, based on the Greek word *pagus,* which means fixed, stuck or fastened.

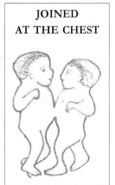

JOINED AT THE CHEST

One heart
The commonest situation is *thoraopagus* twins, who share part of the chest wall and sometimes share a heart. This means that if they are separated one twin must be

---

a. Dizygotic - formed from two separate zygotes
b. Monozygotic - formed from one zygote

sacrificed for the sake of the other. Very few operations of this kind have been carried out and any survivor of such an operation rarely survives beyond infancy. [1]

Joined at the chest (Omphalopagus)

When twins are united from the waist to the lower breastbone, they may share a liver but each has a heart. If both twins are strong and equally developed, then separation can be successful. If one twin is weak, then the organs of the other must work harder to support the co-twin. The tragic case of Gracie and Rosie Attard, whose family came from Gozo, made headlines in the UK in 2001. [2] Gracie had a fully-functioning heart, lungs and brain but Rosie had an enlarged heart, her lungs did not inflate and she showed some signs of serious brain damage. If the twins had remained connected it was unlikely that they would both survive, but separation meant certain death for Rosie. Gracie's heart and lungs were keeping them both alive. It led to legal action and a court hearing, after which it was decided that separation would take place. [3] Rosie died during the operation but Gracie is well and thriving. [4]

Back to back (Pygopagus)

Twins joined in this way are very rare. They are connected back-to-back, usually at the rump. They may share internal organs such as part of the digestive tract, which can cause great difficulty to surgeons if they attempt a separation operation.

Bottom of the spine (Ischiopagus)

The connection between the twins is at the very bottom of the spine this is rare, but there have been successful separation operations. Success depends on how connected the limbs and skeleton happen to be and to what extent other internal organs, such as the bladder, are joined. Most conjoined twins who make it to birth are female, so after separation of twins joined in this way there is invariably a need for further surgery and on-going treatment, particularly

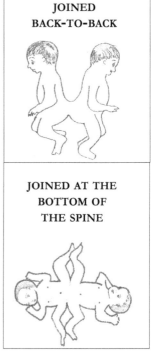

JOINED BACK-TO-BACK

JOINED AT THE BOTTOM OF THE SPINE

with regard to defecation and urination.[5]

Two heads, one body (Dicephalus)

These twins have two heads but share one body. One outstanding case of a happy, healthy twin pair of this type has been widely reported. The dicephalus Henshel twins, who live in a small town in the USA, seem to be happily living "lives unpunctuated by solitude."[6]

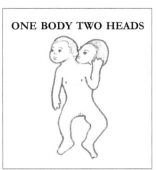

ONE BODY TWO HEADS

Being the survivor of conjoined twins

At one time the birth of conjoined twins came as a terrible shock. Today, the fact that twins are conjoined can be visible on ultrasound scans as early as ten weeks of pregnancy. In this case it is usual for the mother to be offered an abortion. In one case a woman was diagnosed at ten weeks of pregnancy with "twins" but it quickly became clear that the second "twin" was in fact a pair of conjoined twins so this was in fact a triplet pregnancy.[7] The conjoined twins were aborted by lethal injection and over the next few weeks they slowly disintegrated and disappeared, leaving a surviving womb triplet. If conjoined twins are surgically separated but only one survives, it is very difficult for the sole survivor. One such twin, following the death of her twin after they were separated aged three, was reported to have experienced "an initial period of grief" and was in need of on-going family support for many years afterwards.[8] You may be the sole survivor of a conjoined twin pair. If you are this fact will be very visible to you, for the scars left by the surgical separation are extensive and lifelong.

A parasitic twin

A parasitic twin is a variant of a conjoined twin, where one twin has not developed fully.[9] In this case the Beta twin develops abnormally and vital organs are missing. There is no heart (*acardiac*) and little or no brain (*anencephalic*). Connected to the other twin by shared blood vessels and nervous system, the Beta twin may develop arms and legs and even a head. If there is a rudimentary nervous system, there may be some slight movement. However the body does not develop enough to survive as a separate individual. After birth, the Alpha twin may carry one or two extra legs, or an extra arm, attached to their body as a parasite, usually in the abdomen but sometimes along the spine. There are some rare cases of an acardiac twin consisting only of a head, such as one case where the head of the twin was embedded in the check of the survivor and extensive plastic surgery was needed to repair the face.[10] With today's technology and surgical techniques, it may be possible to surgically remove the additional limbs from the body of the host twin, but in places remote from sophisticated medical treatment, the surviving twin is forced to carry their co-twin as a burden, everywhere they go.

A parasitic tumour

A parasitic twin may not develop into anything recognisably human, but just be a mass of tissue, joined to the body of the twin and sharing a blood supply. In one case a mass of tissue attached to the sacrum of a newborn baby was found to contain imperfectly-formed limbs and a backbone.[11]

The twin within: three different forms

In a twin pregnancy, very soon after conception, the embryonic stem cells of the Beta twin may become enclosed within the body of the Alpha twin. The body of the Beta twin develops within the Alpha twin. The Beta twin takes on a variety of different forms depending on what level of organisation is reached in the developing tissues.

Foetus in Foetu: a "Twin-in-a-twin"

A parasitic twin can be completely enclosed within the body of the survivor, connected to the blood supply and therefore able to develop to a certain extent, usually in the abdominal cavity. This is known as a *foetus in foetu*, or a "twin-in-a-twin."[c] This condition is thought to result from the formation of MZ twins, when there is an unequal division of the cell mass in the blastocyst

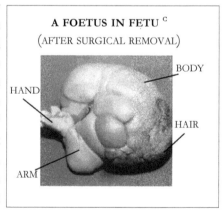

A FOETUS IN FETU [c]

(AFTER SURGICAL REMOVAL)

BODY

HAND

HAIR

ARM

c.   Image from Khalifa, N.M, et al. (2008) Foetus in foetu: a case report, *Journal of Medical Case Reports*. Vol 2. p.2

and the twins merge together at a very early stage. The tiny Beta twin embryo continues to slowly develop inside the body of the Alpha twin, connected to the Alpha twin's blood supply. Typically, the Alpha twin develops a lump somewhere in the abdomen that slowly increases in size and may even be felt to move. When ultrasound scanning in pregnancy is not used, a "twin-in-a-twin" can remain undetected for many years. As a result there are several reported cases of adults who have unknowingly carried their twin around within their abdominal cavity for decades. This has been described as being "pregnant with your own twin." [12]

I feel abandoned and a failure. I think others will think that I am weird and not normal. I have a history of "vanishing" twins in my family, with the evidence being the partially-absorbed body of the other foetus joining with the living one. Grandfather had extra toes on one foot and his brother had part of a head on his back.

Jen, USA

Until forty years ago, the origins of the *foetus in foetu* remained a rarity and a mystery. In the 1970s ways were found to examine the tissues after removal and it became clear from the arrangement of chromosomes that the "twin-in-a-twin" is an MZ twin.[13] Today, with sophisticated DNA tests available, it is now possible to check the DNA of both the excised foetus and the Alpha survivor. Invariably they have identical genes. [14]

Teratoma [d]

When a non-cancerous lump is found and surgically excised, it can be hard for doctors to decide exactly what it is. At first glance, it looks like a mass of cells with no particular form. On closer examination the tissues show signs of a rudimentary but disorganized foetal development. This is a *teratoma*. Some reports suggest that a teratoma is a less developed form of a "twin-in-a-twin." [15]

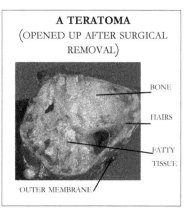

A TERATOMA
(OPENED UP AFTER SURGICAL REMOVAL)

BONE

HAIRS

FATTY TISSUE

OUTER MEMBRANE

Or conversely, a "twin-in-a-twin" can be considered to be a more

---

d. Teratoma image from Wikipedia.org (public domain image)

developed and differentiated teratoma. [16] Like the *foetus in foetu*, a teratoma is a completely enclosed Beta twin. It seems that some teratomas are comprised of cells with slightly different chromosomes from the Alpha twin. As a result they can trigger an immune response and may even become malignant. [17]

> *I started feeling like I was pregnant when I was young, which is interesting in as much as I'm a male. As a child I had an undescended testis that turned to cancer as an adult. Part of the cancer was in the form of a small teratoma. CAT scans showed a very large mass in my mid-section which turned out to be a huge unrelated teratoma. I had surgery and when I woke up after surgery my wife said I was speaking of "losing my baby" or "my baby died." All I can tell you is that I was happy I survived the surgery but had this profound feeling of loss. I was empty inside, having lost something.*
> David, USA

A teratoma can grow to the size of a grapefruit and may contain any kind of tissue, sometimes organized into a recognizable form such as hair, tiny hands or feet. Otherwise there may be a mass of specific cells that would form a specific organ, such as brain, liver or lung cells. In one rare case, a tumour developing externally at the base of a baby's spine was opened during surgery to reveal a rudimentary organ resembling a heart, which pulsated with a different rhythm to the baby's own heart. [18]

Dermoid cysts

There has been some dispute among experts about the nature of dermoid cysts. [e] They are known to be derived from embryonic cells, but there are few people who would be prepared to describe a dermoid cyst as a "twin." Womb twin survivors are quite prepared to think of a dermoid cyst as an absorbed twin but most medical professionals are more circumspect. Dermoid cysts are usually smaller than teratomas but they can grow very large. The difference between a dermoid cyst and a teratoma is not their

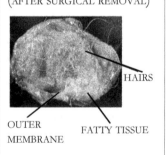

A DERMOID CYST
(AFTER SURGICAL REMOVAL)

HAIRS

OUTER MEMBRANE

FATTY TISSUE

---

e. Dermoid cyst image courtesy of TheOvarianCystCure.com

relative size but the recognisable tissues to be found within them and how organized the tissues have become. Usually, dermoid cysts contain hair and a few teeth, for the cells are derived from the outer layer of cells in the embryo known as the ectoderm that forms into skin, teeth, nails and hair. Dermoid cysts are often found on the ovary, in which case they are known as ovarian cysts, but they still contain hair and fatty tissue.

I had a dermoid ovarian cyst which twisted and ruptured. I had surgery when I was sixteen. Another tumor developed on the other ovary, which was removed age eighteen. I had a vivid imaginary friend until I was five or six. I always felt weird, lonely and different. I'm not sure why I'm here on this planet.
Dee, USA

Two different sets of DNA

When two twins merge into one it can happen very early indeed, within days of conception. One DZ zygote becomes swallowed up in another DZ zygote and the resulting individual contains two sets of DNA. [f] The sole survivor of this merger is truly two individuals in one with a body made of two types of tissue, one from each individual.

I continue to see one sac with two embryos drifting in my mind. I feel early on we began splitting into two, then her side stopped, and mine didn't. She didn't die, but became part of me - or rather, we became one - I engulfed her. I feel as though she is a part of me, part of my DNA.
Katie, USA

Inside every cell there is a nucleus, a small dark patch which can be seen under a microscope. In the nucleus of every cell of your body is a complete set of your personal chromosomes (23 pairs in all.) Each chromosome is made out of two twisted strands of DNA molecules. As we saw in Chapter One, each egg in your mother and each sperm cell in your father contained only a single chromosome from each pair. The two sets of single chromosomes met and merged to make a fresh set of chromosome pairs, in a combination never seen before.

When DZ zygotes unite

When two DZ zygotes merge this creates a chimera, which is an individual with cells derived from two genetically distinct sources.

---

f. Deoxyribonucleic acid - see Glossary

73

A chimera may be formed as a result of transplantation, tissue grafts or the embryonic fusion of DZ twins. As they merge, the cells of the absorbed twin migrate to various parts of the body of the host twin under the instructions of the genetic code in each cell. The cells of the absorbed twin end up creating different tissues, such as parts of the skin or the ovaries, in the host twin. This means that the body of a chimera may contain one or more patches of tissue made up of their twin's DNA. We can detect a DZ chimera by testing the DNA of different tissues.

When MZ zygotes unite
Sometimes a single zygote splits to form MZ twins but for some reason the cells in each twin, although they have exactly the same DNA to start with, lose chromosomes or individual genes. That means that the DNA in each MZ twin is slightly different.[g] Two slightly different cell lines develop in each MZ twin but at a very early stage the two balls of cells recombine to form a new individual - a mosaic. [19]

Being a chimera
A chimera is hard to detect without DNA evidence, but there can be visual clues. Experts believe that there may be many undetected chimeric womb twin survivors walking the streets and completely unaware that right at the beginning of their lives they once had a twin and their twin's DNA is still within them.[20]

> *I have always felt that I have "missed" someone, like a twin. I feel I am not complete without my other half, so to speak. I try to find my other half in other people, but can't. Maybe I am too keen to make new friends - that I put them off. I have missing organs, eg. one ovary, one kidney and a divided womb.*
> *Annabel, UK*

Life can get very complicated for a chimeric womb twin survivor if the organs of their twin replace their own as fully-functioning organs. This is a particular difficulty for a woman if the organ in question is her ovaries.

> *I began menstruating at age thirteen and hemorrhaged about every second month from then on. Around age twenty-two I began telling doctors that I "knew" my left ovary was the source of the problem and that I knew I was not ovulating from it either. They ignored me, probably thought I was a bit crazy. Then by*

---

g. For more about how MZ twins are not identical see page 26

age thirty-five (after twenty-two years of hemorrhaging) I nearly bled to death. Luckily, my brand new gynecologist (who performed the emergency surgery) decided to investigate my "theory." I was stunned when he told me he had discovered that my left ovary was in fact my twin: (hair, teeth and bones) and it was never an ovary. So my diagnosis about not ovulating was also correct!
Barbara, USA

If you are a DZ chimera your two sets of DNA may be circulating all around your body in your blood or lymph system. If you have your DZ twin's DNA in one of your organs, that organ may consist solely of your twin's DNA. For instance you may have your twin's DNA in your hair, but not in the skin cells of your cheek, which is where experts usually take cell samples for testing. We generally only find out about chimeras when DNA is analysed - it can certainly make crime-solving difficult!

An odd side-effect of this is that sometimes in a female chimera, any eggs produced by the ovary do not contain the mother's DNA, but rather the DNA of the merged twin. The legal ramifications can be complex. For example, Jane, a kidney patient, needed a transplant, and so her family underwent blood tests to see if any of them would make a suitable donor. As a result, she was told that two of her three sons could not be hers because they did not have any of her DNA. After much investigation they worked out that Jane is a chimera of DZ sisters. Some parts of her body are her own, but some parts, including her ovaries, belong to her twin sister. [21]

Blood chimera

Blood chimeras can arise when developing DZ twins share a blood supply. This can happen if DZ twins have fused placentas. The stem cells that form the blood are tiny enough to pass through from one placenta to another. If you have a blood test and the doctors check what blood type you are they may discover that you have two types of blood. If so, your twin's blood is mixed with yours but the DNA in your other tissues is your own. There are many people who remain unaware of being a blood chimera until they have a blood test. [22]

Visible signs of a chimera

Without the benefit of DNA testing it is possible to see DZ chimerism in yourself or the people around you.

Eye colour. DZ Chimeras may have eyes of completely different colours or have patches in the iris of a different colour.

Patchy skin colour. Another common problem with DZ chimerism is to have patches of different-coloured skin on various parts of your body. This condition is called vitiligo and can be very embarrassing if the patches are on the face or hands. This condition is found in people of both light and dark skin but is particularly noticeable in very dark-skinned people.

> *The left side of my body looks completely different from the right. I'm African-American and have "marble-cake" swirls of pigment (light brown swirled with a darker brown) on the left side of my torso. Thank goodness, the color is consistent on my face, hands, and feet. My pigment issues have plagued me my entire life. I'm ashamed to expose a lot of skin, as doing so would force me to answer a lot of questions that I don't know the answer to. I'm sure that my twin was a male. I switch often from my male-dominated personality to that of a female. I have an extremely muscular body, though I don't exercise and eat junk at times. I lose weight very easily, like my Dad, and follow dietary guidelines for men.*
> *Melly, USA*

Hermaphrodites

If you are a chimera who merged with your DZ twin and they were the same sex as you, then in the absence of any skin or eye colour anomalies, there would be little proof unless you happened to take a DNA test. However, if you merged with your DZ twin and they were the opposite sex to you, chimerism would be more easily identified because you would have both male and female chromosomes in your body and they can be easily detected. This is because the formation of each chromosome in pair number 23 varies according to whether the individual is male or female. Once the chromosomes are visible under a microscope the different shapes can be clearly seen. The male chromosome pairs look like

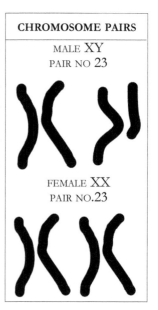

CHROMOSOME PAIRS
MALE XY
PAIR NO 23
FEMALE XX
PAIR NO.23

the letters "XY" and the female chromosome pairs look like the letters "XX." Chimeras with both male and female DNA are called "XX/XY." Another word for people with mixed-sex DNA is "hermaphrodite." They are both male and female. If you are a hermaphrodite you have XX/XY chromosomes but that doesn't say you will also have physical characteristics of the opposite sex.

A spectrum

Hermaphrodites can be grouped on a spectrum, depending on the degree to which the opposite sex DNA is expressed physically. At the "male" end of the spectrum we have hermaphrodites who are normal, fertile males and have all their sexual equipment present and intact. At the opposite "female" end, we have hermaphrodites who look like normal, fertile females, also with their sexual organs present. [23,24,25] In the middle of this spectrum there are people with the sexual characteristics of the opposite sex. They are described as "inter-sex" if their bodies express both sexes, such as having both sets of genitalia. They are "trans-sexual" if they begin life as one sex but have an overwhelming desire to change to the opposite sex. In the medical literature there is so much emphasis on people with sexual ambiguity that the "normal" male/female chimeras remain unnoticed, simply because they look and act normal.

I am often mistaken for a eunuch, and my friends frequently tell me I am very masculine at times, or very androgynous. Even I, while looking in the mirror, sometimes question my own gender, especially since my mother has confided in me that I am a hermaphrodite, and to save my dignity she had it removed from my medical information.
Alice, USA

Being a mosaic

When two MZ twins and made and then merge almost immediately after conception, this forms a mosaic. An MZ mosaic may have one side of the body smaller than the other. Another indication that someone may have once been an MZ twin are divided, missing or duplicated internal organs. The organs involved may be the uterus, the kidney or the digestive system. For example, some womb twin survivors have an additional kidney. Having additional organs is one of the signs of being a womb twin survivor. There has been one reported case in Scotland of a woman who had a double womb. She conceived a baby in each womb in the same month and delivered fraternal twins as a result.[26]

> I had never heard of a chimera until I was called one. I was told that I most probably started out as a mirror twin and that the egg didn't completely split. Externally, my left side is smaller and weaker than the right. I have very little feeling in that side and it is a few shades lighter than my right side. Internally, the organs on my left side are healthier and larger than on the right side. I have two extra ribs, my heart is backwards, I only have four lumbar vertebra and discs, my reproductive organs were very small and I had a tooth in my sinus.
> Angela, Canada

It may be that there are many millions of people in the world who are chimeras or mosaics but never realize that they are womb twin survivors. For those people, a strange, vague feeling of something missing will be the only evidence that, at the very start of life, they once had a twin.

7

Womb companions

As a child and young adult, I often spent a lot of time searching crowds looking for my twin. My mother told me that when I was born, another sac had come out but it had been empty.
Manda, USA

In the womb we were never alone, whether we are womb twin survivors or not. This chapter will take a closer look at the various objects that surrounded you during those vital months of development before you were born. You were held within your mother's body in the world of the womb and surrounded by objects of various kinds: they were your womb companions. The theory behind this book is that all the experiences you had in the womb are hard-wired into your brain as a vague but profound impression. In the back of your mind are all your companions in the womb and how their presence affected you as you developed. As we describe each one of your many possible womb companions, we will also consider how you may have experienced them.

Your mother's womb

First of all, we will consider the space where you spent those early formative months. The womb is a small, muscular space about the size of a pear. It was nestling between your mother's hip-bones and designed to be the perfect growing space for you. To begin with it was much larger than you. Gradually, as you grew and took up more and more space, it became very cramped and you had to fold yourself in half.

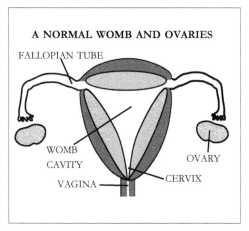

A NORMAL WOMB AND OVARIES

FALLOPIAN TUBE

WOMB CAVITY

VAGINA

OVARY

CERVIX

A double womb

The normal womb, also known as the uterus, is an inverted triangle with the two points at the top connected with the ovaries by means of the fallopian tubes. A double womb can be T-shaped or divided into two uterine cavities, in either or both of which a baby may be carried. Some women

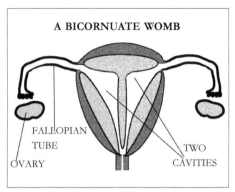

A BICORNUATE WOMB

FALLOPIAN TUBE

OVARY

TWO CAVITIES

with a double womb, known as a bicornuate womb, can be pregnant in both uterine cavities at the same time. There was one case of a woman with a double womb who had a triplet pregnancy, with twins in one womb and a singleton in the other.[1]

The uterine blood supply

Right from the start of your development and until you were finally born, you depended on your mother's blood supply. In her blood and therefore in yours, there were toxins and stress hormones which you shared with her. If she was afraid, so were you. If she was shocked or traumatized, so were you. Through her blood supply you shared in the inner workings of her body and some of the events in her life. Your mother was your constant companion and she shared her blood with you. Not only that, but you shared your blood with your mother. When you first implanted, your trophoblast excavated a little hollow in the side of the womb wall and you made direct contact with your mother's blood supply. Some of your tiny blood stem cells made their way across into your mother's blood supply. This is called "micro-chimerism," which is chimerism on a microscopic scale. A few of your mother's cells also crossed the placental barrier into your blood supply and gathered in your lymph nodes, where they became part of your immune system. They are probably still there.[2]

A foreign body

For your mother to have a few of your cells in her body was an excellent idea in terms of your survival. In your mother's womb you were a "foreign body" as far as her immune system was concerned. Without some mechanism to enable her body to tolerate your presence, you would have been ejected from the womb in a miscarriage. Micro-chimerism is that mechanism. Your mother's cells, now residing in your own lymph system, have "taught" you how to balance the need for self-defence on the one hand and the requirement for tolerance on the other. You had to tolerate the presence of your mother's cells in your own body or else your body would have turned against itself in some kind of autoimmune disease. [3] That early lesson in the womb may well have become a life lesson in tolerance. Your mother's womb was far more than a mere vessel, it was a place where you were prepared, in a hundred different ways, for your life after birth.

The cervix

The cervix - the entrance to the womb - was of little account to you until the day you were born, when it gradually dilated and opened as your mother's contractions came and went during labour and birth. After a long struggle for both you and your mother, the cervix widened enough to let you to pass down the vagina and into the world. Usually, the cervix closes tight as soon as a pregnancy begins and remains tightly closed for the whole nine months of pregnancy. However, if you are a womb twin survivor and your mother experienced bleeding or your twin was miscarried, then it may be worth considering how your mother's cervix behaved at that time.

A "complete" miscarriage meant the cervix opened enough for your twin and all associated tissues, including the placenta, to pass out of the womb.

An "incomplete" miscarriage meant the cervix opened and your twin was delivered but the placenta remained attached to the womb wall.

A "threatened" miscarriage describes bleeding in early pregnancy where the cervix remained tightly closed so nothing was lost.

A "delayed" or "missed" miscarriage meant that although your twin had stopped growing and died, the cervix remained closed and there was just a small amount of dark-brown blood loss.

During your mother's pregnancy with you, her cervix may have never been closed tightly enough and she may have had difficulty retaining the pregnancy. Her cervix may have been stitched together in a surgical procedure called a "cervical cerclage."

81

Your life support system in the womb

In the womb you had a chorion, amnion, placenta and cord for a "life support system." Your relationship with this system could hardly have been more personal, since it was created out of the original zygote and was the same human tissue as yourself.

The chorion

Your chorion was the first thing to develop from the mixing of DNA from your father and your mother. The chorion was formed from the trophoblast layer, which met with your mother's womb wall and enabled you to implant. Throughout pregnancy, until the breaking of the waters during labour, your chorion contained all your growth and development. If you were once a DZ twin or a monochorionic MZ twin, your chorion contained all that was personally yours in the womb. You did not share it with your twin. There was no one else there and the space inside the chorion was all yours. On the other hand, if you were an MZ twin and shared your chorion with your twin, then from the very start your twin was there alongside - your constant companion. The shared chorion was the container within which you and your twin developed together.
It was the limit of your shared world.

The amniotic sac

The amnion is a thin membrane made out of your own human tissue which surrounded a bubble of amniotic fluid in which you first learned to swim - the amniotic sac. At first, the amniotic fluid consisted mainly of water taken out of your mother's blood. Then after about 12 weeks of pregnancy, your own urine made up most of the fluid. When you were in the womb, your amniotic membrane would have felt shiny and smooth to the touch. The upper surface of your placenta had a shiny surface, because of the amniotic membrane that covered it. The umbilical cord also had a shiny covering of amniotic membrane. Everything was soft, smooth and warm. The little puddle of amniotic fluid inside the sac was once your whole world. The fluid played a crucial role in your ability to develop normally. It cushioned and protected you. It also provided you with fluids as you constantly drank it and urinated it out again. As your lungs developed, you breathed in the amniotic fluid but you did not drown, for the placenta provided you with oxygen through the umbilical cord. If you find yourself feeling relaxed and sleepy in a bath of water at blood heat, this is because it is the closest you will ever come in born life to how it felt to be in the womb surrounded by warm amniotic fluid. Finally, the first sign of your mother's labour starting was probably "the breaking of the waters" when your amniotic sac split, the amniotic fluid dribbled out and it was time to be born.

The umbilical cord

Your umbilical cord was the vital link between you and your placenta, but as it grew, it changed. It began as a little stalk at about 20 days or so and contained your digestive tract, for at that time there was not enough room in your abdomen. By the time you had been alive for 50 days or so, you were big enough for your digestive tract to migrate into your abdomen. After that, your cord grew thinner and longer until all that remained were three blood vessels: two arteries to bring blood in and one vein to send blood out. By then, as a fully-functioning human being growing very fast, you needed more and more room to grow and move about under your own volition. The cord became progressively longer until about 28 weeks of pregnancy, reaching a final length of about 22 inches (50cms.)[4] It was not smooth like a water pipe, it was corded like the trunk of a tree. As it grew, it twisted around itself and became coiled. It pulsed with the flow of blood and it had knots on it at various points. It floated about with you as you moved, moving with you and tethering you to the placenta. The cord was as much a part of your life as the amniotic fluid you swam in. If the cord was long enough, it may have coiled around you and been in your way as you swam about, exercising your developing muscles.

The cord may have been be a source of danger: some foetuses dance about so violently that they tie their umbilical cord in knots, a practice that can be fatal because it interferes with the flow of blood along the cord. They may grab hold of the cord and hold it so tightly that the blood supply is temporarily reduced. The cord may grow so long and the foetus may move about so much that the cord can become wrapped around their neck: that eventuality may have strangled your twin or nearly strangled you. After birth, your cord was cut and the small, knobbly scar that you now carry in your navel is all that remains of your life support system.

The placenta

Your placenta was joined to the womb wall in a convoluted series of minute projections that provided a large surface area in direct contact with the minute blood capillaries of your mother's blood supply.[5] The surface area, including all the tiny projections, increased from about one and a half square metres at 100 days gestation to about 14 square metres in the later months of pregnancy.[6] As the quality of ultrasound images improves, we can observe with increasing clarity the way that unborn babies use their own placenta like a trampoline as they dance and swim about. After delivery, it can be seen that the placenta is red, thick and circular, the size of a large dinner plate and covered with a soft, smooth surface. By means of your placenta, you had a direct link with your mother but you also had a relationship with your placenta as a separate object in your life. It provided a good supply of nutrients and oxygen but was also a source of toxins if your mother smoked or took drugs. In the last few weeks of pregnancy you were feeling very cramped. To make matters worse, you were beginning to outgrow the ability of your placenta to feed you, provide you with oxygen and clean your blood of carbon dioxide and waste. The placenta not only stopped growing during this period but it became less efficient. The increased toxicity of the womb would be an important factor in your being born: it was time to go, for the sake of your own health.

After birth, your umbilical cord and placenta were discarded as waste. The disposal of a placenta is a vexed question, for some people become very attached to the concept of their own placenta. In some traditions, the mother buries it under a fruit tree so that it will feed the tree that feeds those who eat the fruit. The most usual fate for a placenta is to be thrown into a bucket and incinerated. Some people have a problem with that, for in the back of their mind is a nurturing companion who was always there from the beginning but is now gone. You never saw your placenta again, however hard you may have tried to get your mother to deputize for it since. Your relationship with your mother or primary carer is in many ways a straight re-enactment of the relationship you had with your placenta. Your placenta was an organ capable of multi-tasking, much like a busy working mother. Like Mother making mushy meals for you as a baby, it broke down food for you into a form that you could digest. Like Mother, your placenta kept you clean inside and out, removing waste from your body and breaking down any toxins into harmless substances that could be eliminated safely. Mother gave you continuous liquid feeds, only to change your wet nappy six times a day, likewise, your placenta maintained your fluid balance by bringing fluids in and removing them in equal measure.

To be fully born, you had to be separate from everything in the womb. That meant jettisoning your own, self-made, life-support system. From then on, you had to hope that your carers would support you until you built another life support system of your own in born life.

Other objects found in the womb

It may be that other objects were there in your mother's womb while you were developing. If there were other objects there, then you developed a relationship with them, as you did with your own private life support system. The concept of being entangled in fibrous growths, squashed by more rounded shapes or cramped within an amorphous mass of fibrous matter may still be hard-wired into your brain.

Fibroids [a]

The commonest growth to be found in the womb is the fibroid. Fibroids are benign tumours made of muscle fibres. About a quarter of women of reproductive age have fibroids in their womb. As women are having children much later in life, fibroids are becoming more common during pregnancy. If a fibroid were growing in the womb with you, the doctor would have been able to diagnose its presence by feel when making a vaginal examination, and it may have been visible on an ultrasound scan. Fibroids can take different forms: in the wall of the womb they are rounded protrusions. In the womb cavity they vary in consistency from hard and stony to soft and rubbery. They change

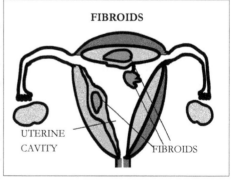

a. Also known as a uterine leiomyoma, or myoma.

in consistency as they degenerate and may become rounded, encysted and hard, stringy, branching or fibrous. About 10-15% of women with fibroids will have complications during pregnancy but in one study only 40% of fibroids diagnosed during pregnancy had been clinically detectable.[7] Some fibroids change the shape of the whole uterine cavity and cause miscarriages to occur. Pregnant women with fibroids may be at a greater risk of experiencing premature labour. Due to the increase in oestrogen levels during pregnancy, uterine fibroids may enlarge and displace the placenta. Large fibroids in the uterine cavity can create a shortage of space for the growing baby.

Sometimes the presence of fibroids in the womb wall makes it a very difficult environment for an embryo to implant. Multiple fibroids located in the lower part of the uterus can even block the vagina during pregnancy, making it necessary to deliver the baby by Caesarean section. In most cases however, the majority of fibroids are small and do not cause any symptoms at all. If a fibroid was present with you, then in the early months of pregnancy your mother would have noticed that her womb was unusually enlarged. At first, the fibroid would have been much bigger than you, leaving you a little cramped. Only later in pregnancy would the fibroid be smaller than you. It may have shrunk or even disappeared completely by the time you were born.

Polyps

Endometrial polyps are growths in the endometrium, the lining of the womb. They are very common and usually benign. They hang on a stalk into the womb cavity like tiny trees or figs, but they can be rather flat. They can obstruct the womb and prevent implantation. They tend to be small but may grow to the size of an orange. It is quite possible for a foetus to implant next to a polyp. If you had a polyp for your womb companion, there would not

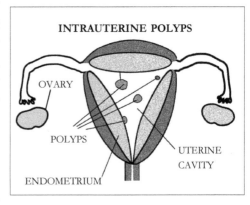

86

have been the same pressure on space as with a fibroid. Depending on the size of the polyp, however, there would have been a time when it was bigger than you - but not for long. Any growths in the womb with you may have changed in size, shape and consistency as the pregnancy advanced. The growths may have occupied the womb space to a greater or lesser extent in those crucial first 57 days. You grew and they got relatively smaller, until they ceased to be of consequence.

IUD's

Intra-uterine contraceptive devices (IUD's) have been in common use now for over 40 years, so if you are under the age of 40 and your mother used an IUD, it is possible that you had for a womb companion one of these devices designed to prevent implantation. IUDs can be T-shaped, rigid and branching, made of metal or

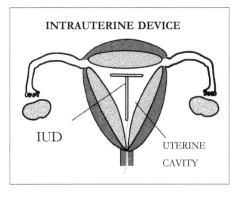

plastic, with a string attached, which extrudes through the cervix and can be used to remove the IUD. If you were conceived alongside an UID it would have stayed there all the time and would have been expelled from the womb along with you at your birth.

A living twin companion

If you are a womb twin survivor, for a certain length of time your living twin shared the womb with you. You may or may not have been able to feel the physical presence of your twin as they moved and twitched, somewhere close by. If you were an MZ twin and shared a single amniotic sac with your twin, then swimming with you in that same bubble of amniotic fluid there would have been another tiny human - the closest womb companion anyone could ever wish to have. How long your twin remained as your companion depends on how long your twin remained alive and what happened to the body of your twin after death. We will explore this in a later chapter.

The twin that wasn't

It may be that your twin never lived as a separate individual from you, or if a separate embryo did briefly exist, that life was almost instantly extinguished. Here are some examples of how that can happen:

A chimera

If you are a chimera, then your twin was hardly a living twin companion at all, but rather a tiny and imperceptible presence within you.

A parasitic twin or teratoma

A twin of this kind would be a constant "inner companion" and part of your own body.

A very early MZ split

If you are an MZ twin and your zygote split in the first day or so, your twin may never have implanted at all.

A blighted ovum

This may have been in an empty sac attached to your placenta at your birth. Apart from a very brief life, this would have been an inert, empty and lifeless presence.

A hydatidiform mole

If two sperm penetrate an empty ovum without any functional maternal DNA, then a molar pregnancy may develop. This is caused by the abnormal development of a zygote, which gets as far as implanting in the wall of the womb but the placenta develops rapidly into a bulky mass with a classical "bunch of grapes" appearance known as a

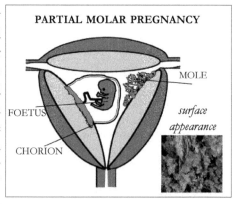

PARTIAL MOLAR PREGNANCY

MOLE

FOETUS

surface appearance

CHORION

hydatidiform mole. There can be an abnormal embryo, with the wrong number of chromosomes, developing within the mole. If this was your story but you still managed to implant and develop, then you are the survivor of what is called a partial molar pregnancy. In this case your twin would have promised something for a brief time but developed into a strangely-formed and silent companion, taking up space but never responsive. If a tiny embryo did develop, then apart from a barely perceptible initial spark of life, your mole companion was totally inert.

Foetus papyraceous: a changeable companion

A "papery' foetus in the womb in the second and third trimester would have not taken up much space as you grew larger and larger. The womb space was now all yours and you would have simply grown into it. Your twin, very much alive in the first trimester, would have become still and silent. Gradually your twin would have shrunk in size, as the tiny body became dehydrated. As you grew, your twin diminished. By the time you were born your twin may have been squashed completely, embedded into the placenta and almost invisible.

Your twin's empty amniotic sac

If your embryo twin died and disintegrated, the empty sac attached to a little umbilical cord may have remained. It would have taken up very little space in the womb as you grew. However, in the very early days of pregnancy your twin was growing in that sac - alive, twitching and bouncing off the placenta. Things changed after your twin died.

> I have vague memories of another "me" – a "she that wasn't me" is how I thought of her. I remember her being so close it was almost as if it was myself, like two of me. Not like another person and not like me exactly, but another me, just like me. I have vague memories of her crying, screaming, blood and death. And then, just emptiness. A huge, empty nothingness.
> Mandy, USA

Secret lives

The use of ultrasound in the last thirty years has given us a window on the womb and has changed our view of twin and multiple pregnancy. We are now able to see two or more tiny embryos develop, even from the very earliest stages. At first there is the dark shadow of a gestational sac. A little later, after about five weeks of pregnancy, a tiny embryo can be seen. Within a short time the fluttering heartbeat is visible, which signals a new life. Sadly however, ultrasound has also revealed that many of these tiny embryos are lost, leaving a sole survivor. But if an ultrasound scan is not carried out early enough and there has been no bleeding or miscarriage, then it would seem that there has always been one baby.

There may be other signs and indications that could suggest a twin or multiple pregnancy, if we only knew where to look. If we were able to discover what these signs and indications were, then we might be able to find out how many supposedly "singleton" pregnancies began as twins or more but ended with a single birth. To bring to light this secret loss, we will gather together what other evidence we can as we try and solve the case of the "vanishing twin." The next part of this book will be dedicated to that task.

PART TWO

Solving the case of the "vanishing" twin

Untwinned

You were left
a slippery wisp of tissue,
flattened ghost of cells,
a bone white filament.

You were wedged against the womb wall
sacrificed, for parts, for me
your sister, sole survivor.

The rest of you tossed at last
into the blood-body mix of origin,
trashed as useless scrap
of miscreation.

You lost your body - I kept your loss.

This bond in the central sac of small beginnings
reproduced as memory,
the loss of which would scream as new
throughout the breath of my existence.

Colleen Werner

8
"Vanishing" twins revealed

*I only heard about womb twins today from a friend, who thought it might be
the answer to my health problems. It struck an immediate chord with me as
my Mum had previously told me that at the time she was pregnant with me,
her doctor thought that she might be carrying twins.*

Mary, USA

The fact that twin pregnancies often result in a singleton birth has been
well-known in obstetric circles for a very long time. A miscarried twin
was first known as a "blighted" twin because it was considered at that
time that most miscarried foetuses were genetically abnormal. The
term "blighted" twin was being used in 1944.[1] In the next few years
the "blighted" twin was made the subject of various other reports, all
of them assuming that the lost twin had died because of some kind of
fatal genetic abnormality.[2,3] By 1958 these lost twins were at last made
visible by X-ray, which was being used to diagnose twin pregnancies at
the time.[4]

The advent of ultrasound

In the late 1950s a team of doctors in Glasgow, Scotland, had been
working on using ultrasound scans for medical diagnosis of various
abdominal cysts and tumours. The first articles on the use of ultrasound
scans for this purpose were being published.[5] It was just a short step
from abdominal cysts to using ultrasound scans to measure the size
of a baby's head in the womb, in order to check on how the baby was
developing. This extraordinary new tool gave doctors a rather fuzzy but
useful window on the womb and they were able to study pregnancy from
beginning to end. By the end of the 1950s, ultrasound scanning took
over from X-rays as the preferred method for investigating pregnancies
as they progressed.

Fibre-optic technology

Fibre-optic technology allowed yet another advance. In 1965, using
special lenses with fibre-optic lights, Lennart Nilsson took photographs

of living foetuses in the womb.[6] He published these images in his book *A Child Is Born.*[7] Nilsson's image of a living 18-week foetus inside the amniotic sac was used as the cover image for Life magazine on April 30th, 1965. Eight million copies were sold over the four days until the entire issue sold out. Clearly, as a result of new technologies the unborn baby was becoming more and more familiar to us.

A new statistic

In the late 1970s the use of ultrasound in pregnancy became more commonplace and an astonishing statistic began to emerge. It had become clear that only a small proportion of the twin pregnancies seen on the ultrasound scan in early pregnancy resulted in the birth of two babies. In a 1976 study of over six thousand pregnancies, 71% of the twin pregnancies diagnosed at ten weeks had naturally reduced to singletons when delivered.[8]

> *I was told by my mother at an early age that a doctor had told her that she had miscarried a twin during the early months of her pregnancy with me. She does not believe me but I have always "known" that I had a twin sister.*
> Tina, UK

An abnormal pregnancy

At the time it was considered an abnormal pregnancy if one of a pair of twins died in the womb. The commonest situation was when a normally-developed foetus was found to be accompanied by a blighted ovum.[9] This was hard to diagnose at first, for there was no way of knowing whether or not the apparently empty gestational sac seen on the scan was a blighted ovum or a healthy embryo at the very earliest stages of development. Only by scanning at a later date would this become clear.[10] Various other forms of twinning were coming to light, such as a normal foetus with an anencephalic (brainless) twin and a normally-developing foetus with a *foetus papyraceous* (the "papery foetus.")[11] Once these abnormal twins were discovered there was concern that the surviving twin may be at risk. It became accepted policy to deliver the remaining baby as early as possible. This policy was short-lived however, for it soon became clear that there was very little health risk to the sole survivor.[12] It was then considered a better policy to let the pregnancy proceed to term than to induce an early labour, for babies born prematurely are also at risk.

A new term for the death of one twin in the womb

At the Third International Congress on Twin Studies, held in Jerusalem in 1980, the term "vanishing twins" was coined. It described the situation when a pregnant woman is scanned by ultrasound and two sacs are seen at the first scan, only to find that one sac has disappeared by the next scan and only one baby is born.[13] The "vanishing twin" quickly became an acceptable medical term. The mystery of the vanishing twin at once caught the imagination of research scientists. In 1982, an article entitled *"The Vanishing Twin"* quoted nine research studies.[14] Another article followed shortly with the same title and quoting even more studies.[15] In April 1986 a new term, "The Disappearing Twin" was coined by the translator of an article in Czech but it never caught on.[16] The term "vanishing twin" was not considered sufficiently scientific for some scientists and in 1992 an effort was made to translate the name into Latin, probably in order to put the whole idea onto a more academic footing.[17] One writer adopted the term *foetus vanescens*, which means "vanishing foetus" but by then the term "vanishing twin" was too familiar to replace with any other term. In 1998 a comprehensive article reviewing the existing literature was published under the title, *"The Vanishing Twin"* and cited over 50 references.[18] The term was by then in common usage, even though it was known that in fact none of the twins "vanished." Their bodies were no longer visible on the ultrasound screen but they did not totally disappear. In many cases there was visible evidence at birth that the twin had once existed, such as an extra placenta, a *foetus papyraceous* ("papery" foetus) or an empty amniotic sac attached to the placenta of the survivor.

In the late 1990s some highly imaginative people took the word "vanished" a little too seriously. They decided that the twins had been abducted by aliens and had been literally removed from the womb. That idea faded along with the century, as report after report on the subject of the intrauterine death of one twin was published in reputable journals.[19] Today, the phenomenon of the "vanishing" twin is widely discussed by obstetricians, gynaecologists and experts in multiple pregnancy. Among the general public some residual scepticism still remains, but not among the pregnant women who witness the disappearance of one of

95

their twins from the ultrasound screen and ask, "Where did it go?"[20]

How many twins die?

Obstetricians and midwives have known for a very long time that more twins are conceived than are born. However, no one knew until the ultrasound studies of the 1980s just how many twins were lost.

> *One day a few years ago, I mentioned to my Mom how I always wished I had a twin and that I felt I should have had one. To my surprise, she told me about her pregnancy with me and that she was in fact pregnant with twins. Her case I believe is the "vanishing twin" kind. She was told by her doctor that she was pregnant with twins. This was discovered at around three months of her pregnancy. It was confirmed by an ultrasound, and there were two heartbeats (not including her own of course.) The doctor also told her it was identical female twins. However, at almost six months she went in again and the ultrasound showed only one baby in the womb, which is me. When she told me about this, I was shocked! I thought I was just weird for the way I've acted or felt, etc. but it makes sense now.*
>
> *Mally, USA*

Once a sufficient number of pregnancies had been monitored to be able to produce some reliable statistics, people began to discuss the "vanishing twin rate" as related to the general twinning rate. Various painstaking ultrasound studies of twin pregnancies were carried out in the USA and England to try and find out how many twins had died before birth. The results in each case were consistent: in about a third of twin pregnancies, one twin died at some stage in the first 12 weeks. Unfortunately for researchers most routine scans on normally-conceived pregnancies are carried out after 12 weeks of pregnancy have passed, by which time many twin embryos have died and disintegrated leaving an apparently "singleton" pregnancy. However, scans are made earlier when the various assisted reproductive technologies (ART) are used to create a pregnancy. As a result, these days we now know much more about the early loss of a twin. In the 1980s, scans of normally-conceived pregnancies were made after a woman had experienced bleeding or if the pregnancy was at risk in some way. As a result, bleeding in the first trimester was soon recognized as a symptom of a "vanished" twin pregnancy. However, some women who have lost a twin early in pregnancy do not bleed. In fact, they have no symptoms at all. These pregnancies had not been considered at risk, so these women had not been included in any of these early studies. For women with normal, symptom-free pregnancies and no ultrasound evidence, the possibility of a "vanishing" twin pregnancy would never have been considered. In 1986 it was calculated that more than 20% of twin pregnancies result in a live singleton birth.[21] For every twin birth resulting from a diagnosed twin pregnancy, it was said that there are at least five babies born alone who were once twins. As approximately 1% of births in the world are twin births, that 1986 statistic implied that an astonishing 5% of the world population were the sole survivors of a twin pregnancy. Research continued as many thousands more pregnant women were scanned. In every group, a certain proportion of these women were found to have conceived twins but gave birth to only one baby.

When I was about six years old I overheard my mother telling a friend of hers that I was a twin but the other embryo just disappeared. So I've known about it forever, but I never really thought about it until last year, mainly because a friend of mine was suddenly extremely interested in twins. When I talked to her about it I remembered what I overheard about nine years before and this time I did some research and learned about "vanishing twins." And some things made sense all of sudden. Why I've always had a special interest in twins, why I have always felt different from other people and kind of "incomplete".
Anna, Germany

A definitive statistic

A statistical study of research studies into twin pregnancies produced a definitive statistic in 1990. The study was carried out by Charles Boklage, a geneticist living in the USA. Boklage is the father of twins and has made twins and twinning a favourite area of study over many years. In the 1980s he carried out an extensive statistical survey of twin and multiple conceptions using published articles and research reports. He came to the conclusion that more than 12% of all natural conceptions are multiple. Of those multiple conceptions, 76% are lost completely before birth, about 2% are born alive in a twin pair and about 12% are born as singletons. A report of this study was published in 1995 as a chapter in *Multiple Pregnancy, Epidemiology, Gestation And Perinatal Outcome.*[22]

So far this statistic has not been superseded by any similar calculations. It is widely used when the subject of "vanishing" twins is discussed. A simple approximation derived from this study will be used in this book to simplify calculations: for every twin conception resulting in the live birth of a twin pair, there are approximately ten babies born alone who once had a twin.

Womb twin survivors around the world

The sole survivor of a twin conception is what we now call a "womb twin survivor."[a] For every pair of twins or multiples born together and alive, there are ten womb twin survivors. So to calculate the approximate number of womb twin survivors in the various countries of the world, we will simply multiply the incidence of twins in each country by ten.

The twinning rate

There is a wide variation in twinning across the world. It is known that the twinning rate for identical twins is constant throughout the world at between three and five twin pairs in a thousand deliveries (0.4%) while the twinning rate for fraternal twins varies a great deal and has increased enormously with the advent of ART into developed countries.[23] From various calculations made by statisticians over several decades, it has been estimated that the average figure for the incidence of twinning worldwide is about 1%. Therefore on average, 10% of the world population consists of womb twin survivors. The actual incidence varies with the local twinning rate.

Africa

Africa has the highest incidence of twinning in any continent of the world, especially in South Western Nigeria among the Yoruba. A recent study of twin births in four hospitals in this area found an average of 40.2 twin births per 1000 deliveries (4.02%.)[24] This means that in South Western Nigeria womb twin survivors make up an incredible 40% of the population. The Yoruba who inhabit that area have a well-developed twin cult, which under the circumstances is not surprising.[25]

North America

The incidence of twin and triplet births in North America has increased

---

a. The sole survivor of a triplet or quadruplet conception is called a "womb triplet" or "womb quad" survivor, respectively.

enormously in recent decades, because of the use of ART. Since 2006 in the USA the rate has stabilized to about 3%, varying from 2.7% in New Mexico to 4% in Connecticut. An approximate value for the number of twins in the population would be 1.8%.

Europe

Europe has an incidence of twinning of only about 1.3% but this rate has increased recently due to the use of ART. [26] In Europe twins have been considered a rarity, marked out as worthy of special study. The first twin study in history was carried out in England by Francis Galton, who was the author of the first publication to consider in detail the biological nature of twinning in humans, published in 1883. [27]

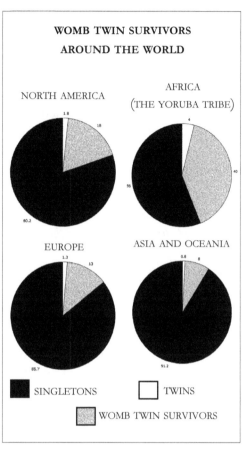

WOMB TWIN SURVIVORS
AROUND THE WORLD

NORTH AMERICA

AFRICA
(THE YORUBA TRIBE)

EUROPE

ASIA AND OCEANIA

■ SINGLETONS   □ TWINS

▨ WOMB TWIN SURVIVORS

Asia and Oceania

In Asia and Oceania (which includes Australasia and the Pacific islands) the twinning rate is much lower, at only 0.8% on average, varying from 1.2% in Australia to 0.4% in China. Most of these are MZ twins. DZ twinning is much rarer in Asia than elsewhere in the world but in developed countries in this region such as Australia, Japan and South Korea, DZ twinning is on the increase with the introduction of ART. For example, the DZ twin rate in South Korea increased almost threefold between 1981 and the period 1991-2002. [28]

IVF and the survivors of a "vanishing" twin pregnancy

In the last 20 years there has been an epidemic of artificially-induced twinning because of the introduction of assisted reproduction techniques including *in vitro* fertilization (IVF) and ovulation-stimulating drugs. The rate of "vanishing" twins varies directly with the rate of twin births. In the USA and Europe in particular, we have recently experienced what has been described as a multiple birth epidemic.[29] Consequently, the number of womb twin survivors in the USA and Europe has risen very rapidly over the last 20 years.

> *I always knew that there were two sacs in my Mom's early ultrasounds, but never thought much of it, until one day we watched a program about vanishing twins and she pointed out that this was me. I had always known, but it hit me at that point. Now that I am in university I have also learned a small amount about chimerism and "vanishing twin" syndrome. While at first I was skeptical, I believe now that there is a possibility that the loss of that tiny object on the ultrasound image did have a profound impact on my life.*
> Naomi, Canada

The first cohort of children to be conceived by IVF are now old enough to be available for researchers to study, so gradually we are learning more and more about them.[30] They are the children born as singletons out of an IVF pregnancy where several embryos were reintroduced into the womb. In each case, more than one embryo may have implanted and a twin or multiple pregnancy may have developed. In the early weeks, the embryos all died except for one - the womb twin survivor. Full details of the early weeks of pregnancy are available for these children, so the womb twin survivors can easily be identified among them. This sub-group has made a useful cohort for researchers to study the effects of the loss of a co-twin before birth. It seems, for example, that this early loss does not adversely affect parenting styles, or the psychosocial development of the child. One study carried out in Italy identified families of 53 singleton births after the loss of a twin or more. They looked for signs of psychological vulnerability in the children. Most of these parents saw their children as strong survivors and not at all vulnerable.[31]

100

A hidden loss revealed

If you have ultrasound images made in your mother's pregnancy showing another tiny gestational sac alongside yours, then that is incontrovertible proof that your twin did once exist. There you will see a real image of your twin. You may be one of the lucky womb twin survivors who has this kind of proof.

When I was thirteen, I found an early ultrasound from my mother's pregnancy with me. It said "twins" on it in the doctor's writing. I asked my mother about it and she said she didn't know what I was talking about and made me stop asking about it. I asked her again four years ago and she said I didn't have a twin. My mother died about two years ago. It was after that I found out about "vanishing twin" syndrome. I feel certain that if I did have a twin she wouldn't have wanted me to know. I've always felt crazy for my feelings of missing my twin. My sister doesn't believe me. I don't know if anyone does and it's frustrating. I feel alone in my sadness about this. I don't know what happened to the ultrasound. I wish with all my heart I still had it, but I'm absolutely certain of what I saw. Even so, I feel I need it to prove to myself that I'm not crazy.

Chrissie, USA

Unfortunately, if you are more than 25 years old it is very unlikely that your mother's pregnancy was scanned early enough to reveal your tiny twin. To know whether you are a womb twin survivor or not is an important piece of personal information. You have a right to know, if anyone is able to confirm it for you. If there is no such confirmation, you may have to search for more clues to help you to find the truth.

Are there problems for the survivor?

When a "vanishing" twin pregnancy is revealed by ultra-sound, it is assumed that the sole survivor will not be adversely effected. Pregnant women, seeing for themselves the disappearance of one of their twins, doubtless find this statement very reassuring. Unfortunately, research revealed some years ago that in some cases there are physical consequences, particularly when a monochorionic MZ twin dies in the womb.

I have always felt like something is missing. I have a very deep-seated fear of being alone. I have panic states and depression. I got very sick in school when

101

we had to view pictures of babies forming. I get panicked if I even see a glimpse of one in a TV advert. I have had dream where I deliver a beautiful well-formed baby girl, only she is made of stone. I am an only child. I was born with a mild form of cerebral palsy. I have managed to graduate with a college degree. I have been married more than 20 years but I have no children. I had never heard of "vanishing" twins until a friend told me about it a year ago.

Vera, USA

The "vanished" monochorionic twin and cerebral palsy (CP)

After years of research, a connection was established in the 1990s between the incidence of "vanishing" twin pregnancies and cerebral palsy (CP). [32] CP was once was attributed to a lack of oxygen at birth, to prematurity and even to the process of twinning itself. Then, in the 1990s, new information came to light. Peter Pharoah, an epidemiologist working in the Department of Public Health in Liverpool University, was studying the fate of twin pairs where one twin was known to have died during pregnancy and closely connected CP to being a sole surviving twin. [33] Monochorionic MZ twins are more at risk of complications following the death of their co-twin. They are also more likely to be born prematurely. Prematurity itself has been found to be a risk factor for CP. [34] In addition, epilepsy and more severe forms of CP appear to be linked. [35] Following another painstaking study of the available statistics, Pharoah came to the conclusion in 2007 that congenital anomalies in children with CP are found much more frequently than would be expected by chance, so CP and various congenital anomalies may be linked to the same basic mechanism. [36] By 2009, the evidence was mounting that the common factor was being the sole survivor of a monochorionic MZ twin pair. [37]

My identical twin sister died at five days old. I have always wished it could have been me who died. I have a very hard time with this. My Mom has always told me about my sister from the beginning. Sometimes I answer for both of us. I see a therapist once a week and have since I was two years old. We were born at 26 wks. I weighed 1lb 8oz and my sister was 1lb 10oz and she was breech. She got a four-degree head bleed from delivery. I have cerebral palsy, seizures and a scoliosis of the spine.

Kyra, USA

Cortical dysgenesis (CD) is abnormal development of the cerebral cortex (the part of your brain that enables you to think.) Thanks to the latest MRI scanning, it has been found that there is a strong association between CD and epilepsy. CD is associated with monochorionic MZ twinning. The "vanishing" twin might be a contributory factor in this, because of the great risks in a shared blood supply when one twin dies.[38] A link has also been recently established between the incidence of CP and multifoetal pregnancy reduction. This is causing concern among experts, who wish to reduce the number of multiple pregnancies because of the wide range of health problems that accompany them.[39] A new syndrome has now been identified which is linked to the loss of a monochorionic MZ co-twin. The symptoms are CP, congenital abnormalities, epilepsy and CD.[40] If you have any of these signs and symptoms, it is probable that you are a womb twin survivor.

Signs and symptoms

In the next chapter we will continue to explore some of the signs and symptoms of what is now commonly called "Vanishing Twin Syndrome" or "Vanishing Twin Phenomenon." We have seen how researchers have carefully put a collection of tiny clues together to reveal the existence of millions of womb twin survivors throughout the world. To follow their example, we will go in search of more clues.

9

Clues to a "vanishing" twin pregnancy

My mother and myself have been talking about my birth. It came up that not only was I very premature, causing me to have my right lung collapse, but the doctors told her during her first ultrasound that she should be expecting twins. She gained a whopping 45 pounds and had first trimester bleeding. Yet I was the only baby at two pounds. Also the placenta was very large. Twins do run in my family. I wish I had more information myself but I don't. I only have the awareness of my personal feelings along with my mother's story.
Joy, USA

Even though a "vanishing" twin pregnancy can be symptom-free there may be some other signs to indicate the existence of a lost twin. Such associated factors as there are may be elusive and vague, none of them adding up to very much. Your deep feeling of having once had a twin may seem to have no basis in fact and may be dismissed as a fantasy by those who do not understand. Even so do not despair, for there is still more to discover as we search for clues.

If you are a womb twin survivor and your mother is unwilling or unable to discuss this with you, the details of her pregnancy may be lost to history. Medical records may be sketchy or missing and family members may not remember anything. If you were adopted and cannot speak to your birth mother, you have no chance of ever knowing what it was like for your birth mother during her pregnancy with you.

I have always been fascinated with twins and wished I was a twin. I am an only child, my mother miscarried three pregnancies, one before me, the rest after, the final of which was confirmed triplets. She told me when I was older that she thought she was losing me because she began bleeding some time during the first trimester. She went to the doctor and I was still there. I did some research and discovered information on "vanishing" twins and womb twins. I feel like that must be me, I always wanted a twin (still do) and wished for siblings, particularly a big brother. I want to know for sure, was I a twin?
Mary, UK

104

Twins in the family

If there are twins among your blood relations, then perhaps you were once a twin also. But were you a dizygotic (DZ) twin or a monozygotic (MZ) twin?

Dizygotic (DZ) twins

It has been assumed for a long time that DZ twins run in families, for there is a strong genetic basis to this kind of twinning. The exact reason has never been clearly identified but it is probably an inherited tendency to hyper-ovulate (that is, to produce more than one egg per month.) It is also possible that the environment, in particular the everyday diet, may have an effect. We have seen that the people of the Yoruba tribe of South Western Nigeria are the twinning champions of the world. They eat white yams several times a day and, according to a student at Yale, the white yam is rich in a biochemical substance that seems to be linked to hyper-ovulation. This student fed white yams to rats in the laboratory and the size of their litters soon doubled.[1] Meanwhile, in Japan they eat no yams at all but rather eat soya beans in various forms several times a day. Many people believe that soya can adversely affect fertility. Perhaps as a consequence DZ twinning was extremely rare in Japan until the advent of ART.[2] ART has greatly increased the twinning rate. In 1998 the number of DZ twins being born was considered to be at epidemic levels.[3] If you were conceived with the help of ART or if there are fraternal twins in your family, these could be valuable clues.

My grandmother was the oldest of twelve children. Her mother gave birth at least nineteen times. She gave birth to twins many times, but they were always premature and didn't survive. My grandmother had four successful births and my mother was one of them. My mother only had me. My second pregnancy started out with a very early positive test at least four days before my period was due. I had massive morning sickness by week five. At week eight, it all stopped. I went in for a blood test to see if levels were dropping and the doctor suspected a miscarriage. She decided to do an early ultrasound, saw a heartbeat and sent me home. At 20 weeks, I started bleeding, mostly spotting. When the baby was born, my midwife said there was the product of two conceptions when I delivered the placenta.

Jane, USA

Monozygotic (MZ) twins

According to experts, MZ twinning does not seem to be inherited but due to some kind of chance effect, independent of both genetics and environment. It has been said that a pair of MZ twins is created approximately once an hour throughout the world, but no one knows exactly why. High rates of monozygotic twinning are found in clusters, one of which is in Kodinhi, a village in rural Kerala in India. In this small village there are over 200 sets of twins, most of them MZ. Scientists have assumed there is some environmental influence, presumably a very local effect.[4] Another smaller cluster of MZ twins, remarkable but not quite on the same scale as Kodinhi, is to be found in China. Heshan, a village in the Hunan Province of China has earned the nickname, "The Village of Twins" because 98 pairs of MZ twins have been born there since 1954.[5]

> *I have always had a fascination for twins. I always wanted to have a copy of myself, to the extent of naming my daughter after me. When I was pregnant I wished to have twins. I asked both my boyfriends I had in long-term relationships if they had twins in the family.*
> *Veronica, Spain*

There may be MZ twins somewhere in your family, but even if there are no MZ twin pairs to be found that doesn't mean there is no twinning. There may be other unaware womb twin survivors in your family who have never even considered this possibility.

Zygosity and survival

DZ twins have a greater chance of surviving to birth as a complete pair than MZ twins. Complete monochorionic[a] twin pairs are three times more likely to be lost before birth than dichorionic[b] twin pairs. A study of aborted foetuses made in 2005 revealed that 17.5 monochorionic twin embryos or foetuses were lost for each dichorionic twin embryo or foetus lost.[5] Accurate statistics of the number of MZ twin conceptions would probably reveal a much higher number of MZ twins being conceived than are born. Unfortunately for our purposes such statistics are not available. Only intact twin pairs are counted to create twinning statistics and the

---

a   MZ twins sharing a placenta

b.   DZ or MZ twins with separate placentas

incidence of twin conceptions is quite another matter. It was only when twin conceptions were counted that we discovered the secret story behind the twinning rate.[6] In the majority of cases, the lost twins are probably MZ twins for they are the most vulnerable. This means that the majority of womb twin survivors are MZ. If you are possibly a womb twin survivor but in search of more clues in order to be a little more certain, this may be important for you to consider.

A season for twin births

The season of your birth may be another clue to the secrets of your mother's pregnancy with you. The birth of twins does show a seasonal cycle with peaks in spring and autumn.[8] It is probably no coincidence that Gemini, the astrological sign dedicated to twins, is for people born from 22nd of May to 21st of June. If you were naturally conceived and you were born under the sign of Gemini, then this may be another clue.

> *I guess it was four years ago that I heard for the first time that I was a twin. But I did not realize what it meant for me. I told my friend that I was one of a twin. For me it was funny because also my constellation is Gemini, the twins, so I am a double twin. My father told me that my mother was having a miscarriage and when they recovered it, it was a child. My father asked the doctor what he should do with it. The doctor said flush the toilet and that is what he did. My mother went to the hospital and there they discovered that she was still pregnant - with me.*
> *Nancy, Holland*

Assisted reproduction produces twins and multiples

We have already seen how the various artificial methods of conception are strongly associated with the conception of twins or more. If your mother needed medical help to conceive you, then even in the absence of any other clues it is highly likely that you are a womb twin survivor.

> *I am seventeen and an only child. My mother had difficulty conceiving. I can remember my mother always telling me that I had a twin, and that it died because I overcrowded it and "ate" it. Ever since then, I have always had this strong will to be the best at everything. I feel that if I am not perfect, then I don't deserve to live, that my twin should have survived instead and that my parents regret me surviving instead of my twin.*
> *Beth, USA*

107

Fertility drugs

Taking fertility drugs greatly increases the chances of conceiving DZ twins. Where there is a multiple conception we also know there is an increased chance of MZ twinning. The most popular fertility drug used today is Clomiphene Citrate, sold under the brand names of Clomid, Milophene and Serophen. This drug was first used in the 1960s and is still used today. If your mother took a fertility drug, the chances are that she ovulated more than once. More than one embryo may have been conceived as a result.

> *My mother did take drugs to get pregnant. A few years ago I began to read about VTS and recognized so many characteristics that it shocked me very much. My whole life I am looking for a soul-mate and every time I get close to someone I find a way to sabotage the friendship. I am unbelievably scared that something will happen to him and I cannot bear the feeling to lose him again.*
> Jan, Holland

A problem pregnancy

If you were conceived in Europe or the USA between 1940-70 and your mother had a history of miscarriage or premature birth, then she may have been given Diethylstilbestrol (DES). It was the standard drug treatment for problem pregnancies during that time. As this drug is given after conception, it is not related to the conception of twins or multiples but the problems in pregnancy, for which DES was routinely prescribed, may be a sign that you were once a twin. If your mother's pregnancy was fraught with problems, this could be another tiny clue that you are a womb twin survivor.

The sub-optimal pregnancy

The concept of a sub-optimal pregnancy was created to provide a way to assess pregnancies as they progress. Twin or multiple pregnancies are usually classed as sub-optimal, in that they are more likely to be complicated by such problems as pre-eclampsia, diabetes, high blood pressure, the death of one or more twins, toxaemia, premature delivery or lower birth weight. Knowledge of the "vanishing" twin is expanding and more and more studies are being carried out, particularly among children of IVF. As a result it is becoming clear that when one twin dies in the early weeks of pregnancy there are likely to be problems for the mother during the remainder of her pregnancy.[9] So here is another clue: if your mother had complications of pregnancy, even if she did not have any bleeding or other symptoms typical of a "vanishing" twin pregnancy, she may have been carrying twins during the early stages of her pregnancy with you.

Nausea and vomiting

In a twin or multiple pregnancy, morning sickness and vomiting may be worse than in a normal pregnancy. This is particularly strong in a partial molar pregnancy and may affect as many as 25% of molar pregnancies because the pregnancy hormone levels are very high.[10] There is some evidence that extreme nausea and vomiting in pregnancy requiring hospitalization, known as *hyperemesis gravidarum*, is also more likely in twin pregnancies. This may be due to an excess of Human Chorionic Gonadotropin or HCG, the hormone responsible for maintaining a healthy placenta. This hormone is produced in unusually high quantities in twin pregnancies.[11] The effect of constant vomiting on the foetus is drastically to reduce the supply of nutrients via the placenta. The mother is effectively starving and so is her baby. The combined effect of constant vomiting and the nutritional drain on the mother's system can be devastating for the mother, who may lose as much as 5% of her body weight. Babies born to a mother with extreme vomiting are more likely to be under-weight at birth.[12] If there is a twin pregnancy and extreme nausea starts, it is unlikely that there will be enough food to keep more than one baby alive to term. Vomiting in early pregnancy, that resolves naturally by the end of the third month, may be a clue that a twin pregnancy did begin but could not be maintained, because there were not enough nutrients for two babies.

HCG hormone levels

In IVF and high-risk pregnancies, the levels of HCG hormone are carefully monitored. If the levels are seen to fall, the pregnancy is at risk. In the first few weeks of pregnancy, levels of this hormone can be unusually high and this has been associated with the loss of one or more embryos. A raised HGC level is also associated with chromosomal abnormalities such as Down's syndrome. Until this was known, it lead in many cases to a misdiagnosis of Down's syndrome and an early termination.[13]

Fatigue in early pregnancy

A twin pregnancy puts a strain on the mother's body. Some mothers carrying twins get very tired, become anaemic and need extra rest and iron. Twin pairs are born to taller, stronger women because these mothers have the necessary constitution to carry them both. If a small, slim woman conceives twins she will need a lot of help in carrying them both to birth and may lose one of them at some stage.

First trimester weight gain

During the first three months of pregnancy with twins, pregnant women gain more weight than would be expected if they were carrying just one baby. If your mother quickly grew very large around the waist in the first trimester, this may be another clue to the existence of your lost twin.

An unusually enlarged womb

Your mother's doctor may have suspected a twin pregnancy if her uterus was larger than it should have been for the stage of pregnancy reached. In the weeks before an ultrasound scan is made, an internal examination of the uterus may be carried out via the vagina to establish the state of the pregnancy. In this way, a doctor can determine the size, position and shape of the uterus and make an early guess at the duration of the pregnancy. He may be surprised by the large size of the uterus and guess that there are more than one embryos developing. When on the scan only one foetus is found, the doctor may assume that he was mistaken.

> *My mother was told she carried me ten months instead of nine. The reason for this is because she was so large early on that they thought she was further along than she actually was. I was a normal sized newborn, 7 lbs 8 oz and there were no signs of me having been a month overdue as they had thought I was. As far as I know there was nothing unusual about me, or the placenta, at birth. This was in 1968 so there weren't any ultrasounds done.*
> *Mike, UK*

Clues around the time of delivery

There are more clues to be found at the time of birth, even if the pregnancy has been symptom-free until then.

Birth trauma

Birth trauma of various kinds is commonly reported among womb twin survivors. If your birth was traumatic, this may be a factor to consider.

> *I was born almost dead. I was pulled out by forceps, had the cord around my throat and had drunk the amniotic liquid. I didn't cry, I had to be taken to cold water to cry. It was a very long delivery. My mother was in a lot of pain and I just wouldn't come out.*
>
> *Veronica, Portugal*

Birth trauma may include a long labour, foetal distress, an abnormal presentation, a "breech" birth, a forceps delivery or a Caesarean section. Birth trauma does not always leave any long-term physical effects on the baby, for new-born babies are remarkably resilient and soon recover. In the last thirty years, despite being very risky for both mother and child, a planned Caesarean delivery for a breech or transverse presentation has become more and more popular. It is considered less risky than a vaginal delivery for these babies. [14]

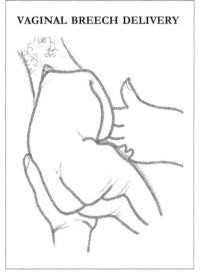

VAGINAL BREECH DELIVERY

> *I came out with my forehead first. I was about five hours in the expulsive phase of delivery, which was extremely difficult for my mother, rather than for me. I had no negative physical consequences, apart from a melon-shaped head in the first days.*
>
> *Jacki, UK*

Extreme birth trauma may leave some physical effects on both mother and child. This may include a very rapid, drug-assisted delivery, skeletal or head injury caused by the delivery method, birth triggered by sudden trauma or the umbilical cord around the baby's neck. There may be injury to the baby's head, shoulder or neck during delivery. A lasting effect of extreme birth trauma may be that both baby and mother are traumatized. This can adversely affect their relationship.

My mother told me that I was a "problem child" even before I was born. I lay transverse in the womb and was placenta previa. Hence I was born out of an emergency Caesarean. I was small for a full-term baby, barely four pounds. My mother said she did not believe I was her child when I was handed to her. She was never able to breast-feed me.
Eliz, Ireland

Small for dates

In a study carried out in the USA, womb twin survivors were found to be more likely to be of low weight, delivered prematurely and be a small size for their gestational age compared with twins born in a complete pair. [15] A Danish study carried out in 2004 with babies conceived by IVF found that 10% of them were womb twin survivors, of whom 66% had lost their twin in the first eight weeks. [16] These babies had significantly lower birth weights and gestational ages than naturally-conceived children, and it was clear that monochorionic MZ pregnancies were at greatest risk. If you were tiny at birth and much smaller than expected, or if you were born prematurely but there was no sign of your twin, these may be more tiny clues.

Abortion attempts

If your mother tried to end the pregnancy by abortion, that may have adversely affected the rest of her pregnancy. She may have made several attempts to end the pregnancy, assuming that the first attempt didn't work and not realising you were still there. A deliberately-induced miscarriage, especially if is it repeated, can disrupt the placenta of the surviving twin. This can trigger episodes of bleeding and slow down foetal growth, so that the baby may be smaller than expected at birth.

Bodily signs of a lost twin

If none of these clues have been helpful to you, then there may be more to learn: in the next chapter we will look for clues in your body and the way it is made.

10

Bodily evidence of a womb twin

I often do things left-handedly, even though I officially write with my right hand. Despite feeling often very feminine, I have some very masculine interests such as karate - I can't even explain my fascination with that! I don't know if all this means I was once a twin; I have no proof beyond a feeling, which could be explained by any number of issues....

Malcolm, UK

Perhaps it is not possible for you to find out any information about your mother's pregnancy. Perhaps there was no sign that she was at some stage carrying twins when she was pregnant with you. Yet this idea of womb twin survivors resonates strongly with you and you wish there was some clue, however vague and uncertain, that may substantiate your deep sense of truth about this idea. This chapter will set out for consideration some of the more compelling associations with twinning, which by extension could concern the sole survivors of twin or multiple conceptions. These clues are to be found in your body and in the way it is made.

Gender

There appears to be a huge advantage in being a female foetus. Most conjoined twins are females, which suggests that the conjoined males do not manage to survive.[1] Of the people with evidence of their twin who completed the Womb Twin Research Project questionnaire, 80% were female.

The fragile male

We may assume that there is as much chance of a male being conceived as a female. So, as we find an excess of females among womb twin survivors, it is probably the fact that male foetuses do not manage to survive that makes the difference. Male babies are also more likely to be born prematurely, with all the concomitant risks, some of which are fatal.[2] According to one report, even at conception the male embryo is more vulnerable than the female. From this point on, the prognosis

113

is not good. With gentle humour, one doctor has hinted that maleness itself could be considered a genetic disorder.[3] The fragility of the male continues throughout life. Men live less long than women and are more likely to die of a stroke.[4] The loss of male foetuses has been hard to understand. Various studies and reports have been published to attempt to explain why the number of males being born varies so much over time and across continents. The study of womb twin survivors suggests that when it comes to sharing limited resources, the battle of the sexes can occur in the womb as much as in born life.

Women need less food

It is known that females manage on less food than males. If you are a woman who has ever tried a slimming diet, then you will know that men are allowed more calories even if they weigh the same as you. Even in times of famine and shortage of food, the women are able to carry babies to term and breast-feed them while maintaining their health and strength on a minimal diet. Men do not seem to be made in quite the same way as women and it has been so from the very beginning of life. Male foetuses develop faster than female foetuses.[5] This can be a major disadvantage in a marginal twin pregnancy. If you are a female DZ womb twin survivor who once had a male twin, then it could be that you both shared a plentiful supply of nutrients at the start but your twin brother grew faster than you. In those first critical weeks he took the lion's share so you had to adapt to getting less food. It would not be long before your faster-growing, nutrient-needy twin would find the available food supplies insufficient for his survival. Where the nutrient supply is marginal, it is the twin who can manage on less food who will survive.

Characteristics of the opposite sex

As twin embryos develop into foetuses, the boy in a boy/girl pair of DZ twins seems to benefit from the presence of a girl in the pair. The male in a boy/girl DZ pair is less likely to die in the womb or around birth than one of a pair of male DZ twins.[6] Research has found that girl/boy DZ twins are very different in their make-up from same-sex DZ twins. Among twins, girl/boy DZ twins have been described as a distinct and separate group.[7] The reason is that there can be a mutual transfer of sex hormones when girl/boy DZ twin's placentas become fused.

As a result, womb twin survivors who once had an opposite sex DZ twin may have some of the characteristics of the opposite sex. Studies among opposite-sex DZ twin calves, show that a transfer of hormones affects the development of the female more than the male. The female twin calf has poorly-developed or missing ovaries and is infertile, whereas the male twin calf is normal and fertile. This is known as the "freemartin" effect and is thought also to take place in humans when several embryos implant close together. [8]

I am a woman and feminine and masculine at the same time. I actually enjoy it. I dress like a woman, with a few masculine details.
Roni, Portugal

Hormone transfer between human twins is possible. The sex hormones, oestrogen (female) and testosterone (male) can pass from one placenta to the other, as well as from the foetus into the amniotic fluid. [9]

Female DZ womb twin survivors with extra male hormones
Some female DZ womb twin survivors do seem to carry extra male hormones and this affects both their bodies and their behaviour. Among DZ twins, the females tend to develop polycystic ovary syndrome (PCOS) which can render them infertile. Their high levels of testosterone make them bold and adventurous with a strong sex drive, like a man. They also prefer more masculine pursuits and like to wear masculine clothing.

I prefer male company to female. I'm very masculine and married a man who appears effeminate sometimes. I have a high sex drive. I was diagnosed with polycystic ovaries and high testosterone levels.
Drew, UK

If you are a woman with polycystic ovaries, if you have had a problem conceiving or if you "wear the trousers" in relationships with men, this may be another set of clues to your identity as a womb twin survivor. You may be this way because you are a DZ womb twin survivor and once shared a placenta with your opposite-sex twin.

I have high testosterone levels and a metabolic hormonal disorder. I am barren and cannot have children. I am broad-shouldered and masculine in build. I have a preference for masculine habits, hobbies and interests.
Shelley, USA

115

In an intact opposite-sex DZ twin pair, it can often be observed that the girl is the more dominant of the two, as if her extra dose of testosterone provides her with a portion of male power.[10]

A test for testosterone

Did you receive a dose of opposite-sex hormone before birth? If you are female, there may be a way to find out. Examining the length of your fingers is one way.[11] It has been known for more than 100 years that the length of the index finger compared with the ring finger is different, according to whether one is male or female. However, this ratio varies among individuals and in 1998 it was found that this ratio is a reflection of how much testosterone a person has been exposed to.[12] The shorter the index finger (the second) relative to the ring finger (the fourth), the more testosterone you have been exposed to. This is known as the "2D-4D ratio."[13] The same ratio has been found to exist in female foetuses as young as nine weeks, probably due to early exposure to testosterone in the womb.[14] If you are female, take a look at your fingers: the pictures below may reveal how much testosterone you received in the womb. It may be worth trying, even though some doubt has been cast upon it recently.[15]

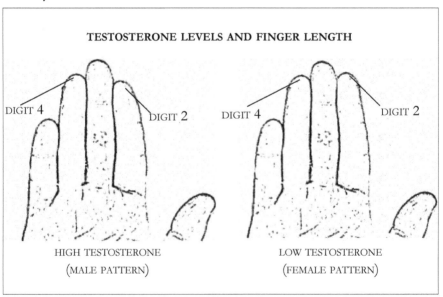

TESTOSTERONE LEVELS AND FINGER LENGTH

DIGIT 4   DIGIT 2   DIGIT 4   DIGIT 2

HIGH TESTOSTERONE
(MALE PATTERN)

LOW TESTOSTERONE
(FEMALE PATTERN)

Studies have related the 2D-4D finger-length ratio to various aspects of human physique and behaviour. For instance, a high testosterone finger length is linked to an athletic body and sporting prowess in women. Otherwise, correlations have been found between the 2D-4D ratio and sperm counts, family size, musical genius, autism, depression, homosexuality, heart attacks and breast cancer.[16] A connection is known to exist between a high testosterone ratio and polycystic ovary syndrome, which happens to women who have too much male hormone.[17] If your 2D-4D ratio is not as it should be according to your gender, the reason may be that you were exposed to opposite-sex hormones while in the womb. If you have no DZ twin now, this hormonal effect may have come from an opposite-sex DZ womb twin whose placenta once overlapped with yours, a very long time ago.

Gender confusion

Some male womb twin survivors, although fully male and with no infertility problems, may experience some inner confusion. They may be confused about which gender they prefer for intimate relationships or what gender they truly are. This can apply to women too. Your gender confusion (if any) may cause you to wonder if you are homosexual, trans-gender or even inter-sex. Adolescence, when sexuality begins to develop rapidly, can be a very difficult time indeed for those DZ womb twin survivors who received a pre-birth dose of opposite-sex hormone.

> *I have had some experience, not with gender confusion but with gender ambiguity. I am a straight male, but as a child and teenager I had an extremely close relationship with my mother and went shopping, got manicures, and other stuff like that. I'm six feet tall and weigh 190 pounds, I constantly stay in shape - in my first semester I ran six miles a day.*
> *Greg, USA*

With such a strong affinity to the opposite sex, some DZ womb twin survivors may begin to wonder if they are truly male or female. For some individuals it is not enough to find a long-term partner with whom one can share one's particular balance of gender energy: they feel like two people in one and they are not sure which one is real. If you are a DZ womb twin survivor you may have experimented with living as a person of the opposite sex in order to discover your true self. Clarifying their own gender can be a lifelong struggle for some womb twin survivors.

I am torn in completely different directions in life in every respect. My sexual identity is so confusing, that to make it easier I've gone celibate, and I'm so torn between science and art I'm terrified of what I'll do for college. I know whichever I pick, I will feel like I have made the wrong decision the rest of my life and I will always regret it. I am often mistaken for a eunuch, and my friends frequently tell me I am very masculine at times, or very androgynous.
Lesley, USA

If this has been your story and your fight, it may be a clue to your identity as a womb twin survivor. The small number of inter-sexed individuals who have participated in the Womb Twin research project have found this explanation helpful in making sense of their dual identity.

I feel much more feminine than masculine, even though outwardly I appear very male. I have a strong female sense of self and since I started living as a female, I have been able to achieve many things that my former self was unable to. As a guy I never was consistent as a person. It was almost as though I was a made-up person. I didn't know how to be a guy. I was trying to be something I wasn't. Now that I am living as a female, I do feel some sense of loss at not expressing my male self. It's hard to explain, I have no desire to be or act male, but at the same time I know that I am male as well as female, because I'm inter-sexed. I almost feel like two different people. The female wears the pants in this body, but I do have male energy in me.
Ky, USA

Same-sex attraction

If your sense of your own gender is a bit shaky you may have wondered which gender you would prefer to choose for an intimate, sexual partner. If you have ever been physically attracted to the same sex, then this may be another expression of the opposite-sex hormones that exist in your body and yet another tiny clue to the possible existence of your womb twin.

Males attracted to males
If this is your story, other males are of more interest to you than females but you have all the equipment and ordinary physical desires of a male.

118

My female side is stronger than my masculine side although I'm a very masculine guy, not effeminate. It's so difficult for me to have love relationships. It's because I have some sort of wish of giving everything to the other guy, like he is a god, or something to be adored. When I fall in love I want to be with that person all the time. I felt always that I have to look for someone I lost in a past life or something, and that I have to find him because something tells me he is out there somewhere. I feel some pain in my left side all the time when I think about that lost one. The doctor didn't find a cause for that pain, he says it's psychological.
Miguel, Mexico

You are not a woman but somehow you react to some other males as if you were a female. You want to nurture and gently caress the partner of your choice. You find that the best way for you to express your feminine side is to be the passive partner in aggressive sexual acts, which may become abusive. Alternatively, you may create a long-term partnership with another man and keep house for him as if you were female, enjoying such things as cooking and interior decoration. In that case women probably find you easy to be with, but in a completely non-sexual way.

Females attracted to females
If you are a female attracted to other females, you are a woman with a strong male side. You find a truly feminine partner ideal, for this sets you free from the woman's role in society to express your dominant male energy in archetypal male ways. Many top female executives have a great deal of testosterone in their bodies and love to go out to work, leaving the domestic tasks such as food preparation and housework to their female partner, who remains at home.

Physical weakness

Some womb twin survivors feel as if they are dying by inches, as if they are slowly sinking into a permanently weakened state from which there is no prospect of recovery. This may be diagnosed as fibromyalgia or chronic fatigue. Fibromyalgia in particular seems to be a common complaint among womb twin survivors. This strange disease, which many doctors do not believe is a physical condition at all, is suffered by millions of people worldwide, mostly women. Most womb twin survivors are female and it would seem that there is some other connection between this condition

119

and the pre-birth loss of a twin. The symptoms known to be associated with fibromyalgia do seem to have a strong genetic background.[17] Also a connection has been found between stress hormones and the pain of fibromyalgia, in particular the hormones produced by the body when under long-term psychological stress.[1] It is known that after an extended period of extreme stress there is often a sudden health breakdown. There are normally three stages: - shock, adaptation and exhaustion.[19] Fibromyalgia may be an example of this kind of physical and emotional exhaustion. People with fibromyalgia do experience anxiety and depression but this could be the result rather than the cause of fibromyalgia. The two go together, to drag you down until you are no longer able to function normally.

I am left-handed, and my doctor believes I have many fibromyalgia symptoms but I am too young to diagnose. I get very emotional when I see siblings, and I feel deep connections with boys, as if I am trying to seek out a brother to replace the one that left me in the womb. This has been torturing me my whole life.
Lesley, USA

If you feel permanently exhausted, sleep very badly, have indefinable symptoms such as sharp pains and sensitivity in various parts of your body that change and shift over time and feel as if you are slowly dying by inches, then these may be more clues. Perhaps you have always carried a deeply-felt psychological stress that dates back to the very beginning of your life. It has been suggested that certain personalities are more prone to develop fibromyalgia. They are intense, meticulous, perfectionist personalities, with very high standards, no ability to delegate and very harsh critics of their own performance.[20] They take on too much, physically and emotionally, and carry the psychological burdens of others. Many womb twin survivors feel and behave this way.

There's definitely a psychological component to fibromyalgia. I know that if I get stressed, I get more pain. And when I have more pain, I get depressed, which causes even more pain. It can be a nasty downward spiral. My osteopath describes my whole body as being inflamed, and he says that it's a result of stress, rather than stress being caused by ill-health. Makes sense to me.
Bernie, Australia

Perhaps fibromyalgia is a psycho-spiritual malaise, expressed in physical symptoms. The diseases of the body can naturally produce psychological distress and the effects of psychological distress can cause the symptoms of disease.

Handedness

It has been found that there are more left-handed people among same-sex twins than in the general population. [21] The majority of these same-sex twins are monozygotic (MZ) twins. As a result there is a long-standing, assumed connection between left-handedness and twinning.

Mirror-image twins

We learned in Chapter Two that the creation of MZ twins varies in outcome according to when the single zygote splits. If the split occurs after 12 days or so, the twins share an amniotic sac, chorion and placenta. At that time there is an increased chance that the twins will be mirror-images of each other. [22] It frequently happens that one will be right-handed and the other left-handed. [23] For many years, left-handedness has been linked to having had a "vanishing" twin. It has been known for a long time that

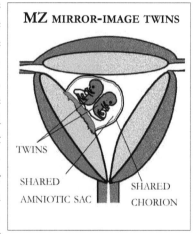

MZ twins are prone to various conditions that are related to unequal brain symmetry development (this decides which side of your brain will be dominant.) [24] The concept of mirror-image twins has developed into the notion that left-handed people are the sole survivors of an MZ mirror-image twin pair. Some MZ twins do look and act as if they were mirror-images of each other.

> *I only recently heard about mirror twins and "vanishing" twins, but as soon as I did a bit of research I was really freaked out by it. I'm a left-hander and have always had feelings that something has been missing in my life and that I'm not like other people.*
> Lucille, UK

121

In conjoined twins it is frequently seen that one twin is a mirror image of the other. This is sometimes obvious in looking at their faces, but it is clearest when we consider their internal organs. Many of our organs come in pairs so it is hard to tell if they are mirrored or not, but some organs are single and found on one particular side of the body. For instance, the heart normally lies on the left and the spleen on the right. Some people have their heart on the right side of their body instead of on their left side. This is known as *situs inversus*. [a] Even in the absence of any other clues, it can be safely assumed that any individual with their heart on the left either has a living mirror twin, or is the sole survivor of a mirror-image twin pair. The layout of your organs may not be clear to you unless you have had an X-ray or scan of your body. For example, Janet Frame, the famous New Zealand poet, knew all her life that she had been a twin, but it was finally made clear when a kidney specialist examined her and told her she had "mirrored organs." [25]

The advantages of being left-handed

When intact twin pairs are studied, there does seem to be some small advantage to being the left handed-twin of an MZ pair. One study found that in tests for cognitive performance the left-handed twin in a living MZ pair did better than the right-handed twin. [26] This could be a sign of a better-developed brain. In the highly-competitive situation of twin embryos sharing a placenta, a better brain may also indicate being better-developed in other ways, so the left-handed twin survives. When the right-handed twin of a mirror-image twin pair is left alone following the death of their left-handed twin in the womb, they would of course not be included in any study of left-handed people or of mirror-image twins. Consequently, we have no idea how many right-handed people in the population may also be MZ mirror-image twin survivors.

Mixed-handedness

Mixed-handed people are neither right-handed nor left-handed. They may cut their meat with a knife held in their right hand but kick a football with their left foot. They may look through a telescope with their left eye and write with their right hand. Sometimes they may use their left and

---

a. The heart and other organs of the body are on the opposite (left or right) side.

right hands interchangeably for the same task.

I am left-handed for writing or using scissors. I cannot use left-handed scissors, though. I also throw a ball or use a hammer with my left hand, but bat, hold a racquet, and use a golf club right-handed (left-handed feels weird). Someone at work told me about the "vanishing" twin syndrome and that's the first I've heard of it.
James, USA

Handedness seems to occur in a continuum ranging from strong right-handedness at one extreme, mixed-handedness at the centre, and strong left-handedness at the other extreme. [27] In the Womb Twin research project, just 14% of the participants described themselves as left-handed but 20% described themselves as "ambidextrous," which is a term commonly used for mixed-handedness. [b] It is possible therefore that mixed-handedness may be a better indicator of being a womb twin survivor than left-handedness.

Mixed-handedness and dyslexia

Dyslexia is most noticeable when reading or writing but there are many people with dyslexia who can read well, if perhaps a little slowly. People with dyslexia are often highly intelligent and creative and find ways around their problems in order to succeed. Samuel T. Orton, a neurologist in the USA who became interested in the problems of learning to read in the 1920s, was one of the first scientific investigators of dyslexia. Orton noted that many dyslexics are left-handed or mixed-handed and that they often have trouble telling left from right. [28] This finding has often been replicated and the association between dyslexia and mixed-handedness is now well-established, so this could be another clue worth noticing.

Mirror writing

If you can use both hands equally well it follows that you could, if you wished, write in either direction. If you find it easy to write backwards - that is, from right to left - this is called mirror writing. It may be related to being an MZ mirror-image twin survivor.

My mother has reversed lower organs, her appendix is on the wrong side and her colon goes the wrong way. She and my father are left-handed. I was born with

---

b. The Womb Twin research project is described in Part Four

a "caul" or blood clot over my eyes. I ended up being right-handed. As a teen I figured out I could do most things with my left hand also. I use both hands interchangeably as an adult. I was also diagnosed with numerical dyslexia after almost failing Accounting. When I'm stressed, I often mirror-write my first name and numbers without thinking about it. If I try to write like that on purpose, I can't.
Jen, USA

Grief and loss

Even if no signs of a "vanished" twin are to be found in your mother's pregnancy or your body, this does not have to be the end of your search for clues to your identity as a womb twin survivor. In the chapters to come, you may yet find the affirmation that you seek. It is now time to look at the psychological effects on the survivor when a co-twin dies during pregnancy or close to birth. Somewhere deep inside your psyche, there may be a deep sense of grief and loss that seems to have no explanation, so that is where we will begin.

PART THREE

The grief of a lone twin

A Lonely Heart

I shed a tear for you, my half, my twin.
A tear for toys we never got to share.
A tear for fights we'll never get to win.
A tear because we can't play Truth or Dare?

A salty tear for you, my twin, my half.
A tear for hugs we'll never give or get.
A tear, for we will never share that laugh.
A tear because I'll never once forget.

Another tear for you, my half, my twin.
A tear, for matching clothes were never worn.
A tear for empty feelings are within.
A tear because that day you were not born.

Those tears, they soak my pillow every night.
I think, "We never had a pillow fight."

Evelyn Burdette

11
The grief of a lone twin

My twin was such an integral part of me that when she died, I was lost: I had
to reconsider my whole sense of myself.
Kath, UK

This chapter will explore various aspects of the grief of the lone twin.
If your twin died, it will hopefully also reassure you that it is natural in
the circumstances to have feelings of grief about your twin. The grief
of twin-loss is completely different from the grief engendered by other
family bereavement experiences such as the death of a parent, sister or
brother. Few people understand this difference. If you are the only
womb twin survivor in the family you may end up totally isolated in your
grief. The death of your co-twin at any age is a catastrophe. Your entire
inner world, constructed since conception around your personal role as a
twin, is completely shattered.

My sister, my fraternal twin, had a heart condition where the blood would not go
completely through the heart valves. There was a blockage of some sort. She died
thirteen days after we were born. When I was really young I asked my parents
if I ever had a sibling or if I could have a sibling (at least that is my memory of
it.) And they told me of her. When I was nine, for three years I went through
this horrible mourning period for her. And ever since then I have been in this
depressed state in my life or something like that.
Minnie, USA

The twin bond

The grief that twins experience when their twin dies is without equal
anywhere in the field of human relations, for nowhere else in human
life is the love so deep. We grieve as much as we love and the bond
between twins is the closest bond in Nature, so it is extremely painful for
a surviving twin when the twin bond is broken by death. The twin bond
differs from all other possible attachment bonds formed in the lifetime
of a human being.[1] Twins live entwined lives at every level imaginable.
For a twin, the twin bond is the primary and deepest attachment bond to

which all other attachment bonds are subservient. It begins at conception and lasts a lifetime. It truly is life-long and transcends even death.[2] The intrauterine twin bond is not created in the same way as other attachment bonds formed in born life. It is formed out of the experience of a consistent Presence since the very beginning of life and includes the belief that the bond will last a lifetime. It has been pointed out that this deep childhood attachment is particularly strong between MZ[a] twins.[3] Like all other strong human attachments, the twin bond is necessary for the development of both twins throughout their lives.[4]

A preoccupation with the co-twin

For twins, the whole idea of twinning itself is a major preoccupation, with particular emphasis on their own pair. DZ[b] twins differ markedly from MZ twins in the way they relate to others, such as in the way they make and share their friends. MZ twins may share as many as half of their friends, but then they share so much already and have always done so since their earliest days. DZ twins share fewer - about 25% for same sex and only 5% for opposite sex.[5] Opposite-sex twins may end up at different schools and spend much of their lives living separately. The bond between opposite sex DZ twins is much less intimate than same-sex DZ twins and MZ twins. MZ twins sometimes end up marrying another set of MZ twins and living very close to each other. Clearly, only another MZ twin would understand and empathize with the need to speak to one's co-twin several times a day.

Alpha and Beta twins

There can be developmental differences between twins of either zygosity for much depends of how much nourishment each twin can obtain from the placenta. This has a psychological effect, because in every twin pair there is always the dominant, Alpha twin who tends to initiate activities.[c] In a pair of opposite-sex DZ twins when there has been an exchange of hormones, the Alpha/Beta relationship may not be quite what one may expect. The female twin with extra male hormones may be the first-born, take the dominant role and become the Alpha twin of the pair.

---

a. Monozygotic twins, formed from one zygote

b. Dizygotic twins, formed from two separate zygotes

c. For more about Alpha and Beta twins see page 31

128

Meanwhile, the male Beta twin with his dose of female hormones may be quiet and compliant by comparison. This difference may go against the social mores in a patriarchal society where to be male and compliant may be seen as shaming, but the twin relationship is primary. The male Beta twin remains quietly compliant nonetheless, at least when in relationship to his Alpha sister.

A survival struggle

The twin survival struggle seems to be strongest between MZ twins. They tend to identify with each other and copy each other more than DZ twins. Even so, each MZ twin is extremely careful to maintain some sense of their own individuality within the twin pair. This creates a kind of paradoxical intimacy or survival struggle.[6] In Marjorie Wallace's book *The Silent Twins,* June and Jennifer Gibbons, two MZ twin sisters, were so taken up with their twin survival struggle that even when young they lived separate from their family in an upstairs room at home.[7] They had their own language and spoke to hardly anyone else. They tried to maintain some kind of equality between them but Jennifer was born ten minutes after June, which created a lifelong problem. As the first-born, Alpha twin, June assumed dominance within the pair. Jennifer the Beta twin struggled desperately to create equality but without success. The twins kept obsessive diaries in tiny print that revealed their claustrophobic love-hate relationship. Something had to give and eventually Jennifer died from a mysterious heart condition at the age of twenty-nine.[8] This example shows how creating equality while maintaining individuality can be a difficult balance to maintain between twins. It requires moment-by-moment concentration on the state of the twin bond, often at the expense of other relationships.

The twin identity

The nature of each twin bond is expressed by each individual twin as their personal twin identity. Every twin is an individual but has also acquired their twin identity. This expresses where each twin stands within the twin pair. Six different twin identities have been described and are listed below.[9] We will see how the way the bond is formed decides how each twin copes with separation from their co-twin, either through particular circumstances or by the death of one twin.

Twins as a unit
Each twin gladly adopts a "half-of-a-whole" personality. This sounds like monoaminiotic MZ twins, formed from a single zygote which split after eight days. The twins shared the same zygote, the same sac and the same food supply from the very beginning of their existence. Naturally, they would want to continue that in born life and would find separation devastating.

Twins as interdependent
These twins share a healthy, symbiotic relationship. This sounds like MZ twins who equitably share a placenta but each has their own amniotic sac. Separation is very difficult but if they both remain in close proximity and communicate regularly, then all is well.

An unequal pair of twins
Where twins perceive inequalities within the pair, the twins define themselves polar opposites, such as "good/bad" or "strong/weak." This can set up antagonism, or even hatred, between them. This sounds like MZ or DZ twins who get an unequal share of the available resources in the womb. Separation may be seen as beneficial as each resents and blames the other for the fact that the desired twin bond doesn't work.

Twins in parallel
For this group, the identity of either twin develops in parallel with that of the other but each retains an appreciation of the differences between them. This sounds like dichorionic MZ or DZ twins whose placentas were fused, but in such as way as to let them develop equally. Separation is not too difficult but there has to be a constant check to make sure that both sides remain equal in every respect.

Twins with personal space
To this group, being twins is the most important aspect of their lives but they find separation from each other a little difficult. This sounds like dichorionic MZ twins who were not in direct competition with each other for space or resources because each had their own personal space and placenta.

Twinning as a sibling attachment
These twins develop very separate identities and have a relationship

similar to that of very close siblings. This sounds like dichorionic DZ twins who had their own living space (amniotic sac) and separate placenta. Separation is no problem. These twins can tolerate living at opposite ends of the world so the death of one twin is not such a catastrophe.

Whenever I lie quietly and just try to feel anything I can about this, I get a sense of my twin being older than me by just a bit, and that if she'd lived she'd have been born perhaps six or seven minutes before me. She was my protector, my shield from the world. I'm so tired of being alone.
Stephanie, USA

MZ lone twins seeking individuality

Developing a sense of individual identity is hard for MZ twins. This difficulty can be seen even in young children. One three-year-old MZ twin asked about her living twin sister: "But why two? Is she me or am I her?"[10] It has been said that after the death of their twin the sole survivors feel a terrible draining away of themselves.[11] When your twin died it may have felt as if some part of you also died.

I feel spiritually dead inside. My dreams and ambitions have somehow left me. I don't do anything because I feel that the very act of wanting itself is bad.
Kit, USA

The identity of a twin is forged right from the very first days and weeks of life. For MZ twins the bond is created at conception but each twin has slightly different genes and womb environment. They are distinct individuals but because of their strong bond there is no clear sense of individuality. It is only in the struggle for survival and the interaction between them that a pair of MZ twins can each find themselves. After an MZ twin dies there is no way to carve out that sense of individuality.

Boundaries and bereavement

A research study has shown that twins have to manage the boundaries within their relationship in life and after the death of one twin.[12] When one twin dies, the survivor tends to perpetuate the original twin boundary regardless of how other people now see them. Even when a twin dies before birth, these same effects can be seen, in the way the womb twin survivor has a sense of once having been in a twin relationship.

Separate individuals

These twins are seen by others as a pair but each twin wishes to be separate and feels allowed to exist as a separate individual. After the death of one twin the sole survivor is self-contained. In this case the missing person remains in some sense close by in the mind of the survivor.

A pair

The twins are seen by others as a single entity." No sense of individuality is promoted by parents. After the death of one twin, the survivor is distraught and has a sense of being only half-alive. The real sense of existence has always relied on being half of a pair.

A womb twin survivor

When a twin dies at birth or before, the sole survivor is seen by others as "an individual" but there is always the shadow of the dead twin somewhere near. The sole survivor tries to occupy all of the original shared space and tries to be "two people in one." The personal boundary is often willingly breached in order to invite others in to share the most intimate space, which was once shared with the twin.

BOUNDARIES
IN A TWIN PAIR

TWINS AS
SEPARATE INDIVIDUALS

TWINS AS A PAIR

WOMB TWIN SURVIVOR

Support for grieving lone twins

When it comes to grieving the loss of a twin it seems that zygosity does matter. An on-going study of twin loss, conducted by Nancy Segal for California State University, revealed that MZ twins take longer than DZ twins to get over their grief after their twin has died. This is perhaps not so surprising, for the MZ twin bond is so strong.[13] That is not to say that the loss of a DZ twin is any less devastating, but the pain of loss has a different quality for MZ twins: there is a definite correlation between genetic relatedness and the intensity of grief.[14] For a DZ twin there will always be a gap where that companion, who was always there from the beginning, remains only as a sense of Something Missing. For an MZ twin, the one person who made you feel whole is no longer there - that is the difference. The grief of twin loss has for far too long been underestimated and misunderstood by the 90% of the population who are not lone twins or womb twin survivors. After many generations of neglect, in the 1980s, in the UK and the USA two sole surviving twins on either side of the Atlantic decided to do something about it.

The Lone Twin Network

Joan Woodward, a psychoanalyst whose MZ twin died when they were three years old, carried out a study of 200 bereaved twins in the 1980s. The severity of the grief reaction was found to be greater among MZ or same-sex twins. [15] One participant described, "An intense loneliness that nothing quenches…" [16]

> *My twin, also male, was stillborn. He was buried in unsanctified ground because at that time the church refused to baptize stillborn children. I have always known I had a twin brother. He couldn't have a religious burial so my father had to take the coffin in the car and bury the body himself. I liked it when people spoke about my twin. It was very rare, but it made me feel as if he really existed.*
>
> *Mike, France*

Joan Woodward's study led to the creation of the Lone Twin Network in 1989. [17] The Lone Twin group still meets regularly and is a vital form of help for lone twins in the UK. It helps to spend time with others who have known for themselves the tragic breaking of this unique bond. In this way, the Lone Twin Network does a great deal of good.

Twinless Twins International

The Twinless Twins Support Group International was started in the USA by Raymond Brandt in 1986. He was an MZ twin whose twin was killed aged 20 in 1949. For many years afterwards he struggled with his own identity. Was he still a twin? With the help of other twins he was able finally to discover that, "once a twin, always a twin." Overjoyed at this discovery he founded Twinless Twins International in 1986 as a support group and directed it until his death in 2001.[18]

My mother and I talked about my twin briefly about twelve years ago. It was then that I connected the fact that I have always had this huge gaping hole in me and have always felt like something was missing in my life. It wasn't until earlier this year that I was told hat I was a "twin-less" twin. This brought forth some very deep emotions for me. I cry anytime I think about having lost my other half.
Christopher, USA

Simply to know that there is a name for a person whose twin died at birth, or before, can be validating and a great relief for sole surviving twins. To be silenced and pathologized for one's natural feelings of grief serves only to increase the sense of isolation and pain that comes with the death of one's co-twin before or around birth.[19]

My Mother told me that my twin brother was stillborn and that he died at four months in the womb and I was actually born a week early and very small. I've spent my whole life looking for a soul-mate but yet every relationship I got into, after two weeks it just seemed empty and I left. Now I finally know why.
Chrissie, USA

Mourning for a lost twin

It seem that lone twins live their lives accompanied by a perpetual sense of loss. John Bowlby (1907-1990) who was a psychoanalyst, was the first to write about affectional bonds.[20] He recognized the pain that arises out of the breaking of an intimate bond. It does seem that the attachment and affection in the twin-twin relationship is unrivalled among all other possible human relationships. It follows then, that when a twin dies this must create a sense of loss in the survivor that is catastrophic in its intensity.

Unbearable pain

The painful feelings of the surviving twin may be so strong that he or she needs lifelong support in order to bear them.[21] The pain lies in the loss of that very special and particular form of emotional support that only a twin can provide, particularly an MZ twin. Recourse to a dear friend, a loving relative, a highly empathetic therapist or a bereavement counsellor can enable the lone twin to survive psychologically.

A need for empathy

In a support group, comfort is made available through fellow lone twins who know exactly how it feels. That is very important, for any relationship lacking in empathy just emphasizes the pain of being abandoned by your twin and left to manage your pain for yourself. The unspoken empathetic understanding that your twin once provided was always there for you but is now beyond reach. Just finding a way to share the pain with another empathetic individual, human or animal, can provide a comforting echo of the lost twin bond.

Forever misunderstood

The unique nature of the twin bond can lead people who were not conceived as twins to unwittingly act insensitively in relation to twin-less twins and womb twin survivors.[d] People of a single conception cannot possibly understand the depth of the twin bond.

> *When I was about thirty I tried to find my twin - I phoned hospitals in the area where I was born. I had been told that my twin, although stillborn, was perfect as a specimen for the age of the foetus and so my mother had allowed him to be put in a jar and preserved for medical purposes. I wish I had proper acknowledgement of his death. They did name him but then they gave him to science. I had no luck finding him. I could not do the burial that I wanted.*
> Clare, UK

A lack of understanding on the part of others can badly hurt a twin-less twin or womb twin survivor. Having to explain how they feel is very difficult because twins and womb twin survivors are "hard-wired" to expect the empathetic understanding they once received from their twin. That wordless relationship cannot be duplicated anywhere in born life.

---

d. The term "twin-less twin" used here refers to the survivor when a co-twin is lost after birth. A "womb twin survivor" is the survivor when a co-twin is lost before or around birth. There is an overlap in the use of these terms when the co-twin is stillborn or dies within four weeks of birth.

Private pain

A major problem for the survivor when a co-twin dies is the extremely private nature of the twin-twin relationship. The relationship was carved out in a private, enclosed space where outsiders were strictly not admitted. This is particularly so among MZ twins. When a twin-less twin grieves, he or she believes that no one else can possibly know how it feels to be them, not even another twin-less twin. The pain lies in the sad fact that there once was someone who did truly understand without anyone having to say anything.

> *I learned at an early age that I had a twin that died at birth. However, I have never been given details about how she died. I have an old clipping from a newsletter about it, but that's all I know. Anytime the subject came up in my family, the subject was always changed. I constantly feel like something is missing from my life, though I can never figure out what it is. I'm always wondering what it would have been like to have a sister my age...*
> Chris, USA

Re-inventing the self

If two members of a twin pair have never developed a separate identity then after the death of one twin, the survivor has no such source of strength in order to build a new identity as a twin-less twin. Joan Woodward remarks in her book *The Lone Twin* that all her life she has felt the need to make up for being "only half" by being "much more than half."[22] Elvis Presley, whose twin was still-born, was always larger than life. He died young after many years of frenetic performances, from what may have been sheer exhaustion.[23] Twin-less twins have to discover who they are as independent human beings for the first time, and a first step might be to stop trying so hard to be two people at once.

Early memories of twin loss also bring grief

It is time now to explore the possibility that a twin lost during pregnancy can be remembered. We need to explore what form those memories might take, so that we can learn to recognize them.

12

A womb twin remembered

I have always been fascinated with twins, and have always felt somehow out
of place. I remember when I was little I would search my mother's drawers,
hoping to find a birth certificate/ death certificate or adoption papers.
Wendy, USA

This book depends absolutely on a single assumption, that at a very early
stage in your development you were capable of some kind of awareness
of being in the womb. This chapter will describe some of the research in
this area and the astonishing conclusions that have been reached. Despite
widespread ignorance on this topic it is generally believed that we do
not remember life in the womb. Of course, this is not a memory in
the usual sense of the word but a vague and confused impression, more
like a dream. Many decades of research has revealed that the unborn
child is capable of awareness and learning. Exactly how early in life that
awareness begins has been the subject of debate for a long time, but
research studies are revealing more and more about the extraordinary
abilities of the developing human, even in the first few weeks of life in
the womb.

My most vivid, cherished and beautiful memory is being in the womb with my
sister. We are together, playing, in contact, a slow rolling motion between us.
If I have only that memory to hold onto forever - it is enough.
Jean, USA

The perceptions of the unborn child

It would be a mistake to imagine the womb as a kind of flotation tank
in absolute darkness and silence. You lived in a small bubble of fluid
where the everyday noises of the world were audible. In sunlight it was
not altogether dark, and in the night or the daytime it was never silent.
Thomas Verney, in his book *The Secret Life of the Unborn Child* wrote, "The
foetus can see, hear, experience, taste and, on a primitive level, even learn
in utero." [1]

Touch

You had been alive in the womb for only about 29 days when your first skin was formed, served by neurones that could detect temperature and texture. Anything that came into contact with your skin would have stimulated you. It is known that, if anything enters the womb and touches the skin of an unborn child enough to wound, it causes pain. It was established in 1980 that an unborn child can feel the prick of a needle and would require anaesthesia for intra-uterine surgery: researchers have found that unborn babies pricked with a needle show changes in heart rate and an increase in bodily movement.[3] Until then it had been assumed that unborn children did not feel pain.

Taste and Smell

Your sense of taste and smell was developed at about four weeks from conception. Just because you lived in a bubble of amniotic fluid does not mean to say there was nothing to taste or smell. Various organic compounds crossed the placenta into amniotic sac and it is reasonable to suppose that you were aware of them. It is well known that smells evoke emotional memories and it is also known that emotional memories are the most enduring. It follows then that the smells we each find most agreeable may in some way be related to the tastes and smells of those long-ago days in the womb.

Hearing

The womb was never silent. The beating of your mother's heart and the sound of her food and drink churning through her digestive system went on continuously. Only a few membranes and muscle tissue lay between you and the outside world. Sounds, voices and music could be heard without much distortion. As you grew and your hearing developed you became aware of your mother's voice. It reverberated through her body. If there was a sudden loud sound, you literally leaped in the womb. You were particularly sensitive to vibrations of various kinds.[4]

Vision

Your eyelids did not open until you had been in the womb for about seven months, but your skin was so thin and transparent that light could easily get through. Unborn babies have been observed to cover their eyes or shrink way from bright lights. At about 14 weeks or so, a foetus is aware of an amniocentesis needle entering the amniotic sac and can be observed on ultrasound to shrink away or attack it with a fist.[5]

A dawning awareness

By the end of the third week of your life your central nervous system was laid down. A few weeks later you had muscles and could react physically. Where there is a reasonably well-organized nervous system there can be a reaction, and where there is reaction there must be awareness of the most primitive kind. We can measure the changes of foetal heart rate, measure stress hormones and observe muscle twitches on ultrasound, so we know that a foetus is capable of reacting to stimuli. We can therefore assume that there was a gradually dawning awareness of yourself and your environment. Naturally, it would have been very vague and confused

Activity

Activity gave you the ability to make things happen in your tiny little world. Once you had learned to move you could begin to actively exercise your most fundamental human gift - curiosity. You could spend your time jumping and bouncing off the wall of the womb, swimming about, somersaulting in the amniotic fluid and touching everything you encountered - including the umbilical cord, which you could grab and hold onto.

Autonomy

Every moment, you were learning new things about how to handle your body. This is the very start of autonomy which means being a separate person with a will of your own. If you were observed on ultrasound, your own characteristic behaviour towards your twin would have been distinctly recognizable. If you were the Alpha twin for example, the dominant behaviour that is now part of your character would have been noticeable to observers.[6]

Discovery

In the womb, new activities were discovered quite by chance to be an advantage. For instance, if the womb is compressed in any way, the foetus experiences compression. As a foetus, the first time you felt compressed you had a choice: just lie there and take it, or move. By chance, you tried moving and at once felt more comfortable. Until this happened for the first time, your awareness had not included the concept of "Being Compressed." From then on, thanks to this discovery, getting more comfortable in this way quickly became part of The Way Things Are.

Learning to adapt

Over a hundred years ago, Sigmund Freud and his contemporary psychologists regarded intrauterine life as a time of bliss, untroubled by need. For this reason the Freudians have assumed that we all yearn to return to the womb to experience that blissful state once more. Today we think otherwise. With the help of ultrasound, modern science and technology, we have learned a great deal about life in the womb. We now know it was far from blissful. The womb was not a padded, unchanging cocoon and you were not held there in a state of total sensory deprivation.[7] Variations of temperature, oxygen levels, glucose levels, toxin levels etc. were being registered and reacted to by your new, rapidly-developing neurones. Simply by surviving a series of slight changes in the environment of the womb and adapting to them, your brain was eventually "wired" to maintain a healthy balance throughout your whole body. The adjustment was done through the autonomic nervous system, which is a primitive system of connected neurones linked to a series of biofeedback mechanisms. Almost from the very start, your personal biofeedback system has orchestrated a complex series of hormonal reactions in every moment of your life: it is, for example, the system whereby your heart keeps beating. Your mother's womb was a flexible, ever-changing environment and you had to adapt to those changes in order to survive. When your mother went swimming, cycling or running so did you. When she was cold, hot, anxious or in pain, you shared the effect of her hormones via the placenta. You adapted to danger even then, by moving in alarm or freezing in fear.[8] Learning to adapt and cope with environmental changes during your time in the womb was an important part of learning how to survive in born life.

Your foetal memory matrix

No one knows how memory really works. It is generally believed that memory is somehow held in particular neuronal circuits. Conscious awareness is believed to be a function of the central nervous system but those ideas are still held in doubt. The true nature of memory and how it is created remains a mystery.[9] Nevertheless, we can begin to imagine how the foetal memory matrix develops. As soon as your brain and nervous system began to develop, information began to enter your brain through your nerves, both from inside your body and from outside. That information still remains somewhere in your body in what is often called "body" memory. In the first few weeks of your life there was no way of processing the various data entering your neural circuits, so it was all in a confused muddle. Smell, taste, sight and hearing were all mixed together. A little later, once you started to move, things became more interesting. Now there was output, because the electricity in your brain enabled you to do things. Memories of those things you did also made up part of your foetal memory matrix. At first you moved because your muscles twitched all by themselves. You were not in charge at that stage of your early life: you just moved about at random. You were passive and had no autonomy. Things just happened to you over which you had no control.

Neurones

Your central nervous system is made up of millions of neurons, each one a single branching cell. The number of branches varies with the kind of neuron it is. For example, the motor neurones that control muscle activity have many hundreds of branches. Neurons are linked together in chains which enable electrical impulses to pass back and forth between them. Neurones enabled you to react to stimuli from various parts of your body. They are specially designed to do that for they have hundreds of tiny branches

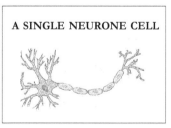

A SINGLE NEURONE CELL

at either end with which to make countless different connections with other neurons. This process creates a neural network, which is a circuit based on electrical and chemical changes between the cells. As the number of neurones increases the network of inter-connected neurones begins to grow, with countless connections. Neurones tend to develop more branches and increase in number more rapidly in the presence of outside sources of stimulation. A complex, interacting feedback mechanism was formed, based on a system of networks of interconnected neurons which formed your foetal brain. Stimulation created more connections between neurones and connections are essential, so the more neurones you developed, the better. As a result of the stimulation you received in the womb, you now have a unique and individual impression of your earliest days "hard-wired" into your neural networks. Furthermore,

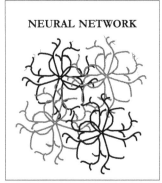

NEURAL NETWORK

by the 57th day of your life, your brain had developed the capacity to shape itself according to experience. This has given you the essential characteristics of versatility and adaptability which have enabled you to adapt to your environment and survive until this moment.

A foetus is capable of learning

Peter Hepper, Psychology Professor at Queens University Belfast, has for many years made a careful study of the foetus in order to discover more about the early development of human behaviour. Hepper has come to the conclusion that the foetus can learn. According to his research, unborn babies can learn by discovery, habituation and classical conditioning. Pepper has received an award for his work, but even so he finds the psychology profession rather sceptical of his conclusions. The idea of foetal learning implies foetal memory and for some professionals agreement with that idea would be like "opening Pandora's box".[10]

Stimulation and response

As a twin embryo, your new neurones were growing at such a rate that you were much more sensitive to your environment than you are now. You were hyper-sensitive and hyper-aware. Information was pouring in about what was going on around you, including the tiny twitches made by your twin. The slightest change or movement in the womb stimulated a response in you. In the womb you continuously explored your environment, discovering things all the time. By moving about in a fairly random fashion, at some point you found the boundary of your space. Your sac boundary and placenta were more often encountered than any other objects in the sac, because the cord twirled around with you: this was the stimulation you needed to enable you to learn.

Discovery learning

By a random process of trial and error, new things can be discovered. For example, ultrasound scans show the unborn child interacting with the umbilical cord. This is not consistent, for the cord is flexible and moves when touched. The placenta is more solid and reliable, because it is fixed to the womb wall. The amniotic membrane yields just a bit when kicked but stays approximately in place. By means of ultrasound, we can observe how actively the foetus bounces and kicks at the boundaries of his little womb world, learning all about it by random chance encounters: this is discovery learning.

Habituation

When you began to explore you discovered a quality of responsiveness in the objects around you. Where objects reacted consistently, a new assumption began to form: "When I do THIS with my body, THAT always happens." A specific action produced a specific response. When that had happened a sufficient number of times, it became a habit: that is the process of habituation. It is the way you "got used to" the various recurring events that occurred in the womb. For instance, the very first time in your life you heard a specific loud noise, you would have reacted with alarm and some bodily movement. After hearing that same noise several times, you would be habituated and would no longer be alarmed. You would remember the event having happened before, so it would no longer be a shock. Many pregnant women notice habituation in their babies, who can be felt to react but gradually adapt to new noises.

My mother had a difficult pregnancy with me (and my twin). She bled for the entire pregnancy. By the third week of July, my mother started to haemorrhage and she had to stay in the hospital for a week. She said it must have been my twin but she didn't know it then. I asked my mother if anything happened to her in late July when she was pregnant with me. I dreaded late July because every year something bad happened. A relationship would end, a job would end, a big upset/upheaval would happen, some significant loss, some major ending. I was absolutely stunned to hear about my mother's experience.
Jan, USA

Training the unborn

Unborn children of thirty weeks or more can be repeatedly told a specific story by their mother or played a specific piece of music. When they are born they can be observed reacting strongly to that specific story or piece of music more than any other. They seem to remember it. [11]

The fact that unborn babies can be trained in this way was once used to great effect in Venezuela. In the 1970s the population of that country was 85% illiterate. In an effort to improve matters the President created a Minister for the Development of Human Intelligence in the person of Luis Alberto Machado. In 1979 he was given an office, a secretary, a very small budget and the mission to somehow raise the level of intelligence of the entire population. Efforts were made to improve education in schools and colleges but it was with the unborn children that the project was most successful. Machado created the "Family" Project lead by Beatriz Manrique, who had previously worked on a project in the USA that was successfully raising the intelligence of children by means of prenatal stimulation. Beatriz Manrique wanted new parents to learn how to foster the fullest possible development of their children. Most importantly, prospective parents were taught how to stimulate their unborn babies. After birth, these children were different. From the very moment of birth, babies of the experimental group were more alert and turned their head when they heard their parents' voices. They recognized the music they heard when they were in the womb. A report said, "These are dynamic and relaxed children, they have initiative and are very curious." [12] This positive effect was long-lasting. Six years later, the IQ of the stimulated children was several points higher than the rest of the population. They showed more common sense and were better at everyday problem solving, observation and analysis. Clearly, intrauterine stimulation helps to develop the foetal brain. This research has spawned a variety of projects to help parents create a "prenatal classroom." [13]

Trained by Mother

Your mother was your first trainer, even before you were born, as research has shown. Speech is learned from the interaction of the unborn child with the womb environment and Mother's voice is an important part of that. [14] Your mother's hormones circulated in your body, so if your mother was agitated then so were you. Attunement between you and your mother was the start of your training.

Trained by your twin

Twins train each other to be responsive and aware of other people. Unborn twins have been observed on ultrasound responding in reaction to stimulation from each other. This interaction has been seen to begin at 65 days from conception.[15] Twins do not require an outside source of stimulation to strengthen their neural networks, for each receives plenty of stimulation from the other.

Making friends

Humans are created as social beings and they want to make friends. We cannot survive for long in isolation for the need for society is written into our human genetic make-up. In the womb you were genetically predisposed to build relationships but not yet capable of choosing between one object and another. As soon as you were able you reached out in pure curiosity to make friends with everything in your immediate environment. Your acute hypersensitivity helped you to discern what happened when you reached out. Perhaps when you moved your arms and legs you felt the amniotic fluid move around you. When your twin moved, so did you. When you moved, your twin moved in response. Your early attempts at building relationships in the womb remain in your memory as a template for how you relate to others, even today.

Developing a personality

The unborn child, once regarded by scientists as a witless tadpole, a clean slate, or even a placid, dependent, fragile vegetable, is in fact a distinct personality.[16] Any mother of several children will testify that every one of her pregnancies was different. Every unborn child has its own personality and way of being in the womb. Allesandra Piontelli, author of *Twins: from Fetus to Child* wrote that babies come into this world with a wealth of sophisticated competencies which enable them to adapt to the complexities of post-natal life.[17] At birth, after all those months in the womb learning how to be a person, you were precipitated into a brand new world. What you have made of your new-born world has depended very much on your experience of what came before birth.

Healthy scepticism

If these ideas are new to you, then make sure you keep a mind of your own on how it was for you in your mother's womb. Healthy scepticism is a logical and intelligent tactic for you to apply at this stage, especially if you are exploring these ideas with a view to making up your own mind about whether or not you are a womb twin survivor.

The womb twin survivor theory comes in handy: it would give me something to explain a lot of the things I experience and have experienced in life. But that shouldn't be the reason to accept it as the truth, should it? The questionnaire suggests from the personality aspects that it could be true. Maybe I'm not ready to either accept or reject the idea.
Helen, Canada

If you are easily lead into false ideas you would do well to follow the sceptical belief system and demand scientific evidence of your twin. Some womb twin survivors are afraid of being caught up in a web of delusions, but that is unlikely if you are well- informed. As long as you think for yourself and make up your own mind, then your personal truth will emerge in time.

I have thought a lot about the womb twin survivor idea. Being pretty pragmatic, it seems too me that in the absence of definite proof - and I haven't got any, one way or the other - then this theory is persuasive. At the very least, it paints a coherent picture that allows me to account for my way of being. I find it easy to imagine a situation in the womb that would account for my particular psychological sensitivities. It is quite imaginable to me that there was a fundamental pre-birth "driver" which would have shaped my very earliest way of being and world view.
Tony, UK

After several years of occasionally revisiting these ideas, it may be that tiny shreds of evidence will begin to gather. Eventually, a personal conviction will begin to grow and the requirement for specific medical evidence will diminish. Many womb twin survivors with no evidence whatever of their twin have been able to make beneficial changes in their lives, simply by accepting the possibility that they did once have a twin, when they were in their mother's womb, but their twin died.

146

Discovering that I am a surviving twin has not been - and still is not- an easy trip. I still don't have any "proof" but I do have so many symptoms that I don't have to have the proof. I am in therapy now with a prenatal therapist and I am moving in strides toward healing.

Lena, Canada

Children just know

If you have no proof but deep down you have a sense that there may be some truth in this for you, then continue to keep an open mind. If you are the parent of a womb twin survivor you may have already encountered the way children "just know." In the next chapter we will explore how parents cope with having a young womb twin survivor in the family.

13

My child is a womb twin survivor

*I am very sure she was a twin. She is six months old now and is
very needy. She has to be in constant skin contact with someone
all the time. She will not sleep unless you are holding her or lying
down with her. She is beautiful, healthy and happy.*
Helga, USA

This chapter will explore how it feels to be the parent of a young womb
twin survivor. Some parents find it hard to cope with their own loss, some
are not sure of the best way to tell their child about their twin and some
experience difficulties in parenting their child. A research study carried
out in 2003 in the USA with a group of over 50 surviving twins reached
the conclusion that the lost twin should be openly talked about, right
from the beginning.[1] The study report made several useful suggestions
about the best way for parents to deal with having a womb twin survivor
in the family:

- Give information truthfully
- Allow feelings to be expressed
- Encourage openness of communication
- Educate the medical profession
- Educate the public that the lost twin is a real problem

The loss of one twin at birth is devastating for the parents. Twin
pregnancies are increasingly the result of lengthy, laborious and costly
fertility treatments and are all the more precious because of that.[2] Earlier
on in the pregnancy there is still a sense of loss when one twin dies. Many
parents discover early on that they are expecting twins or more and get to
know each baby very well. After birth, because of the realities of caring
for one or more survivors, parents are typically unable to grieve properly.
In the case of MZ twins, the memory of the lost twin is kept alive in
the person of the survivor. The loss of a twin is a tragedy for everyone
involved but young children have a particular problem because they do
not understand what has happened.

Support for grieving parents of twins

Parents badly need support in their grief but it is only in the last forty years or so that such support has been provided. If you are a womb twin survivor born forty years ago or more, then your parents were probably left alone and unsupported after the loss of your twin.

The Center for Loss in Multiple Birth (CLIMB) [3]
Jean Kollantai lost one of her twins at birth. She resolved that thereafter no parent would ever have to survive such a tragedy unsupported. She once said that her introduction to parenthood was holding two full-term babies where one was alive and one was dead. [4] She created CLIMB in 1998 as a local support network with excellent information. There are now branches all over the world. [5]

Stillbirth and Neonatal Death Support (SANDS) [6]
In the UK in 1975 two parents with stillborn children decided to do something about the fact that most parents were not allowed to see or hold their babies and they were not told where their babies were buried. If you are the parent of a stillborn twin born in the UK before 1984 it was probably normal practice at that time to whisk the baby away sight unseen. Today in the UK there is SANDS, founded in 1984 as a charity supporting parents bereaved by the loss of one or more babies at any time from the second trimester until around birth. They produce leaflets suggesting best practice for professionals involved with stillbirth.

Good information for bereaved parents
There is an increasing amount of information now generally available for parents of stillborn babies, including parents of womb twin survivors. The Twins and Multiple Births Association (TAMBA) was created in the UK in 1978. [7] They have a bereavement support group for parents who had a twin or multiple pregnancy but one or more babies died. In the USA there is the material written by Elizabeth Pector, a medical doctor and the parent of a sole surviving twin. She has created a web site with resources for parents. [8,9]

Baby memorials
Today after the stillbirth or neonatal death of one twin, parents are offered the chance to hold their dead child, take a photograph and carefully

keep some mementoes of the baby. This can be helpful to the parents and the surviving twin.[10] There are now some printed resources to help chaplains and others to create Christian services of prayer and memorial for babies who have died during pregnancy or around birth.[11] It is also considered suitable for the siblings of the baby to attend the funeral or memorial service: it is their loss too.[12]

Death in the womb - a real loss
If it has been hard to obtain public recognition for a stillborn baby, it is even harder for the public to recognize the death of a baby in the womb as a real loss for the parents. The very idea of grieving for a miscarried baby has been considered unreasonable by some professionals, who have been concerned that parents and others may magnify miscarriage into a "tragedy."[13] Nonetheless, it is now clear how important it is for professionals to keep parents informed when their baby dies in the womb and take account of their feelings of loss.[14] The same imperative applies to giving full information to the surviving twins. They must and should be told in the kindest way possible. The knowledge that one was once a twin is a very important piece of personal information. Every womb twin survivor has a right to know their origins as one of a twin pair or multiple group but it is very hard to talk about.

Telling your child about their twin

Parents are often at a loss about how to talk to the survivors about their deceased siblings, which is understandable, but there are ways to tell the story that can help to diminish the distress on both sides.

When silence seems the best policy
Some adults subjected to the horrors of war have lived their lives since then in a mild state of post-traumatic tress, an important element of which is to avoid any associated places or events. This is an important element in surviving horrific situations but the result can be a perpetual denial of the event. In the same way, even before ultrasound was available, doctors and midwives may have felt the presence of a multiple pregnancy in the womb but avoided saying anything about it until the next examination, when things were a bit more developed and certain. This policy probably arose out of the fact that twin or multiple pregnancies are highly likely to

fail in the first few weeks. In fact, for many years the emotional aspects of miscarriage and stillbirth have been largely ignored by the professionals involved in childbirth, even though miscarriage can affect both parents very deeply.[15] One can always make up the excuse that not speaking about the loss of a baby "avoids upsetting the parents." If you are the parent of a womb twin survivor there may be good personal reasons for you to remain permanently silent on the subject: there is a strong shock and grief reaction after stillbirth and miscarriage, particularly in the first few weeks after the event.[16] This could be enough to make you unwilling ever to speak about it again.

> *My parents had me very late in life. My mother was, as far as I've been told,*
> *huge during her pregnancy. As I grew up I never, ever felt like I belonged.*
> *I was a strange kid, drawn to stuff others avoid/ignore. My mother never*
> *seemed to have a lot of patience with me, almost as if she "blamed" me for*
> *something but she would never say anything.*
> Barbara, Canada

After an abortion, it has been found that there is a long-lasting avoidance reaction on the part of the parents.[17] That would be enough to prevent any open and frank discussion with anyone, let alone the survivor of a twin pregnancy where only one twin was taken.

> *My Mom had no idea she was having twins until we were born. My sister*
> *and I had one heartbeat through the whole pregnancy. When she came first she*
> *was full size but stillborn. Then three minutes later I came out. They told her,*
> *"Hey! You have another baby coming!" When I was two my Mom told me*
> *about my twin, that I had one and she was not here with us. She never wanted*
> *to talk about her. To this day we do not talk to each other about my twin.*
> Liz, USA

If you did not have access to ultrasound or any other method of diagnosing twins, the arrival of two babies may have come as a complete surprise. If you had made no plans for two babies then the loss of one of them at birth would have been very confusing. In that case, your lost twin baby, never expected and hardly known, would seem to be easy to forget. However, you may still be carrying unresolved feelings about your own loss, so that talking about the event to the surviving twin might reawaken them. In that case you would probably prefer not to revisit that experience by openly speaking about it. In turn, your child may be aware of your difficulty and hence keep silent on the subject.

> *I remember the time Mom first told me the truth. I was really young and didn't understand at the time and I remember asking dumb questions like, "Did we talk alike? Or walk alike?" It wasn't till I was older that I really began to understand. That's when I began to ask the real questions like, "How did she die and why?" My Mom answered all the questions of course, but then she began to cry. I felt so guilty afterwards and though she tells me I can talk to her about anything, I don't have the heart to bring the subject up again.*
> Laurie, USA

As a parent, you may have mistakenly assumed that your child's feelings would be very similar to your own. In fact, your child may be glad to hear the story and may want to know more details as they grow up.

Will it help my child to be told?
Telling your child will help both of you. If carrying and delivering your twins was traumatic you may still be suffering some of the symptoms of post-traumatic stress without realising it. The symptoms include avoidance of any connection to the original event and can last for many years.

> *I am 40 years old and two weeks ago Mom told me that I had a twin who died in the womb. I have known that she had a complicated pregnancy and been told the story that they thought I was dead - that Mom had miscarried. It was a couple of months after this "miscarriage" that she felt movement – that was me. I want to move away from where my family is even though we are on good terms. I suffer from PTSD and depression.*
> Mel, USA

We know that recalling the details of the original event helps to heal trauma and that includes a traumatic delivery. Sharing the story can be a relief, at least for the parent concerned. Also some womb twin survivors suffer trauma at birth, so trauma may be experienced by both parties.

Will my child be upset?
It is normal for a bereaved twin to have feelings of loneliness, emptiness and sorrow and that goes for womb twin survivors too. So rather than

leave your child with unexplained, difficult feelings, tell him or her about the lost twin. Make it real, because that really helps. When the time comes to speak, it is important for both parents to be in agreement about what to say and whether to say anything at all.

> *My Mum told me casually one day that when she was expecting me, the doctor told her after the ultrasound that she was expecting twins. But when I was born, I came out alone. She did not say any more than this. I have never tried to ask my mother more details about my birth. I've always felt she was responsible for telling me such (potentially) important things, not me asking her.*
> Stuart, Singapore

Lynne Schulz, who is the founder and coordinator of the Murraylands Lutheran Stillborn Infant Support Service in South Australia, is mother to Rhys, a womb twin survivor. In her book about him, called simply *The Survivor*, she writes, "It is more common for a surviving twins to show curiosity about their unique situation rather then be emotional distraught by it. If parents are aware if this then they can feel encouraged to share their story with their children rather then trying to shield them from events in life that they feel may cause too much upset." [18]

My child is only a baby, so when should I tell the story?
Being a womb twin survivor will always be part of your child's nature. Research has shown that it is helpful to tell your child the truth of what happened to their twin as soon as possible, in the calmest and most natural way. Surviving twins do experience an inevitable sense of loss but the greatest pain is to have their loss ignored or underestimated. [19]

> *I was raised with the twin issue being a massive secret kept from me. It certainly has been the taboo subject in my family. I have deep down always known, that secret way twins know, about my brother.*
> Leslie, Canada

Tell your child early in life, but make sure you are well informed about the details of your pregnancy. You may find that, as they grow up, your child will want to know more and more about what happened. Right from the start make your little lost twin part of your family so your child feels natural talking about him or her. A Portuguese mother and her seven-year-old daughter were together one day when the girl, who had always

153

known about her womb twin, began to tell her story, "She got smaller and smaller until she was a little dot." Together they created a little illustrated booklet for young womb twin survivors. [20]

If you decide to remain silent on the subject this may magnify your grief out of all proportion, creating a place of private pain for you to carry. Your baby may sense it in you and become anxious that something terrible is wrong. Even very young womb twin survivors are very empathetic and sense hidden feelings in others.

If you delay telling your child until adulthood it can become more and more difficult to talk about. Once you have spoken, your son or daughter may be very hurt that this important personal information has been withheld for so long. Be sure to apologise for the delay. The saddest situation for a womb twin survivor is never to know of their twin because both parents have died. If you have decided to remain silent for life about it that is of course your right, but it would be helpful to put a note with your will, so that your child will discover the truth eventually.

Bringing up a young womb twin survivor

Here follows some of the typical characteristics of young womb twin survivors, as revealed by the Womb Twin research project. [a]

My child is hypersensitive
If you have a hypersensitive child then that sensitivity may have become a problem. You may be struggling with their eating problems, shyness, nightmares, constant worrying and emotional outbursts. [21]

> *My daughter had a very severe retardation in her whole development: she sat late, she crawled late, she walked when she was 22 months old, she only started talking when she was three and a half years old. I feel there is a very deep sadness in her. She has had eating problems since she was a little child, always eating too much. Nowadays she steals food and when she is caught she cries a lot and says, "This feeling is stronger than herself." She is extremely sensitive to what others tell her.*
> *Diane, Belgium*

My child does not like to sleep alone in the dark
Being alone in the dark seems to be a major problem for young womb

---

a.   The Womb Twin research project is described in Part Four.

twin survivors and this can continue into adulthood. If your child is very young, this persistent need for company may be misinterpreted as manipulation to get more attention - particularly at bed time.

I am an only child. When I was little, I always asked for a brother for my birthday. My mum always told me that it wasn't possible and I felt very sad and angry because of it. Playing with other children was very nice, but I'd also need to spend time on my own. I liked to read books, or I'd play with stuffed animals and 'talk' to imaginary friends, but never in my own room, as I felt very afraid of being all alone in an empty room, or in the dark at night. Many times my mother had to comfort me because I was so scared to be alone in my bed.
Julia, Holland

My child is unusually aware of how people are feeling
If your chid is a womb twin survivor they may act as a "family barometer." Some womb twin survivors can easily sense an atmosphere in a room and are acutely aware of the nuances of body language. If people are unhappy or distressed in any way your child, even as a baby, will probably cry in empathy with that feeling.

People have always told me that I was too sensitive. As a child, as a teenager and still as an adult, they say I am "too sensitive." I care too much. I want to make things right, etc. Recently I have found out that I am indeed sensitive and often I know exactly how other people feel. This can be physical or emotional.
Joanne, Australia

My child has a rich, creative imagination
Womb twin survivors, even when young, are able to create imaginary stories and can have a hard time separating fiction from real life. When they are able to speak and write clearly they are often gifted in their use of words. They are not usually bored, for they have creative minds.

I remember when I was six years old I told a friend at school that "I had a twin brother who got lost." I would also constantly talk to Mum about this and she was often puzzled by why I was mentioning such a thing at a young age. When I would play with my cousins and friends, we would pretend to be our favourite superheroes or TV characters, I would always make up a twin for the main character.
Aleena, UK

155

My child talks a lot about death and dying

A rather worrying aspect of living with a young womb twin survivor is their preoccupation with death. They ask blunt, uncomfortable questions about dead people and if someone dies, they worry that they too will die. If they encounter death in a close relative at a young age, this can have a profound and unsettling effect on them.

> *My mother passed away when I was thirteen. I am the eldest of three children. After my mother's death I felt responsible for my siblings. I regularly wished that it had been me that died of cancer instead of my mother. I felt an overwhelming sense of sadness frequently. I would cry almost daily for years - often for no apparent reason.*
> Mel, USA

My child is extremely upset when a family member or pet dies

Young womb twin survivors can become unreasonably grief-stricken when a beloved person or pet dies. They may grieve for a very long time and even need professional help.

> *My brother and my father died in the same year two years ago. My daughter still cries for each of them every day. She is just so dear, she mothers everyone. Before she'll eat the last cookie she has to ask everyone in the entire family if they want it. It was strange seeing your list of symptoms. She has them all.*
> Katrina, USA

My child loves animals and yearns for a pet

With their extraordinary awareness of non-verbal signals, young womb twin survivors can relate well to animals. They know intuitively how to handle them and communicate with them. They may yearn to have a pet of their own, particularly one who loves to be handled and cuddled and is prepared to sleep in the same bed. On the other hand, they may be so acutely aware of animal suffering that they rescue any neglected animal they happen to come across.

> *I have a horrible problem with my empathy, and I am constantly trying to fix or heal anyone and everyone I can. It goes so far that I have the same problem with animals. I will go out of my way, to my detriment, to rescue animals.*
> Renie, USA

My child is different from other children

Womb twin survivors are rare and unusual people and the difference may vary from subtle to blatant. Research seems to suggest that this is because their unusual pre-birth experience has formed their character. The difference will be more evident if your child is a womb twin survivor but you were always a singleton.

> *I know from what my mother tells me that I was somewhat different as a child. My Mum has always lovingly joked that I was and am still very different emotionally. I've always unwittingly taken a path that is somehow different or out of the ordinary.*
> Julie, UK

My child has a double identity

Some parents of womb twin survivors say that their child is like two people in one. Your child may change from dark to light and back again over the years, or even within the space of one day. If your child is good and polite at home but terribly rude at school (or the other way about) then be assured that this is quite normal for a womb twin survivor.

My child seems too mature, like he or she has "been here before"

When you first looked at your own little womb twin survivor, did they look back at you like an "old soul" as if they already knew their way about in the world? That is a wonderful characteristic found in some womb twin survivors and is worth celebrating as a great gift.

> *My daughter has always been very mature for her age, she doesn't act silly like most kids or like her sisters. She's always been very nurturing with her two younger sisters. She gets very frightened when she hears loud noises. She tends to be quiet, reserved and somewhat clingy. Sometimes when she cries she says that no one loves her and no one understands her.*
> Sue, Ireland

My child has an imaginary friend

Creating an imaginary friend is quite normal for a womb twin survivor and can be an excellent way to find comfort when alone. It is common among lone twins, and more than half of the respondents to the Womb Twin research project questionnaire had an imaginary friend as a child.

My son is eight years old. He has an imaginary friend that he says is exactly his age, has known him since they were in my tummy and he states that his "imaginary friend" floated off into the air when they were cut out of my tummy. He doesn't know I had a Caesarian delivery. When I try talking to him about his imaginary friend he gets very emotional and doesn't want to talk about it.
Shena, USA

My child often seems lost and alone

Most womb twin survivors can feel alone even when other people are around. This begins early in life. A shy, withdrawn child will be ignored if the parents' attempts to make contact are repeatedly blocked, yet the same child can look disconsolate and hurt when left alone.

I've always felt different from others and very misunderstood. This has forced me to become withdrawn. Even until today, almost all of all the thoughts that I think about I do not speak to anyone.
Stuart, Singapore

My child is a womb twin survivor - should I be worried?

Research seems to indicate that if an individual knows for sure from the beginning that they once had a twin, they understand their feelings better if they do become upset at any time. They can be reassured that they are responding perfectly normally to the genuine loss of their "other half." Living in a loving family with lots of encouragement and displays of affection seems to help a great deal. Generally speaking, the loss of a twin is worth keeping in mind as a potential effect on your child's development as an individual. Most womb twin survivors are highly sensitive and empathetic. As a result of their extreme sensitivity they have a special need for steadiness and reassurance. They are often vulnerable and afraid but they are strong survivors nonetheless.

I was told that I was a twin in the womb when I was about eight. When I was young I would frequently have strong feelings, mostly when I was alone, that I couldn't explain, where I would just simply feel like I shouldn't be here, alive, on this planet.
Greg, USA

Once the truth of the lost twin has been absorbed and fully understood, the fact that your womb twin survivor child is "different" can be celebrated as a special gift rather than a source of concern. With your help to come to terms with their pre-birth loss, your child will hopefully develop to their full potential. Whatever happens, your love for them will never change. That is all a parent can ever do, and it is enough.

A primal experience

There are many parents who choose not to tell their young womb twin survivor the truth about their pre-birth origins. However, this primal experience is too powerful to remain hidden. In the next chapter we will explore some of the many ways in which womb twin survivors, who have lived all their lives unaware, have discovered their lost twin.

14

A womb twin discovered

I'd been searching, searching, searching for her all my life
But I had no idea of where to find her;
I'd been hurting, hurting, hurting all my life,
But felt sure that she would make it better.
Andy, Ireland

If it is true that for every pair of twins born there are at least ten womb twin survivors, then there are 600 million womb twin survivors in the world. About half of them are adults and one of them may be you. If you were never told when you were a child that you once had a twin, there are still many ways in which you might discover your own womb twin for yourself. In this chapter we will review some of the ways in which a womb twin may be discovered for the first time by the sole survivor.

When an infant is aware

We learned in the last chapter how some young womb twin survivors, almost as soon as they could talk, ask their mother for a twin. This can sometimes pre-empt the mother's intention to tell their child. For instance, Maxim who is now 12 years old has no recollection of the fact that at three years old he talked about his twin sister. "When I was in Mummy's tummy there was a little girl there. We used to talk, then one day she disappeared." Similarly Lisa, who was not told about her twin until she was 14, remembers sitting half-way up the stairs from the age of two or three, chatting to her twin. Young womb twin survivors seem to have some uncanny knowledge about their twin. For example, Evelyn was a teenager when she wondered about her twin's name and the name Meredith kept coming to her. She asked her mother what she was going to call her twin, and her mother said, "Meredith."

The mark of a lost twin

There may be a physical scar as a reminder of your lost twin. If you are a womb twin survivor and you had a dermoid cyst, a teratoma or a *foetus in foetu* (a twin-in-a-twin) there is probably a scar where your twin was taken away. If this happened when you were very young, the scar may be a disturbing mystery if it is not properly explained. Every time the scar is noticed it will be a perpetual reminder to all concerned.

The ultrasound at the beginning of the pregnancy showed us as two twins in our own sacs, side by side. Then at about the fifth month of my mother's pregnancy she felt something was wrong. She went to the doctor and they did another ultrasound and they discovered that, by a way as yet undetermined, my twin and her sac was growing inside of me. My Mom will not let me have ultrasound pictures, I guess she is still missing her. I had surgery at two days old to remove her from me. I guess that is what makes me think of her all the time, because I see this scar and it reminds me of when they took her away.
Lin, USA

A dawning awareness

Even after the parents have told their child, naturally and gently, leaving them to process the information in their own way, the fact of the lost twin can remain a mysterious secret for many years, giving the child's rich imagination full play. The fantasies that arise sometimes include a sense of somehow being responsible for the death of your twin. Such thoughts have been described as: "Confused delusions about a supposed murderous foetal life."[1] Where some reassurance is not provided, these thoughts can be disturbing for a young womb twin survivor. It is not enough to simply mention it, because as the child grows the true significance of this loss will gradually become clear and there will be more questions to be asked.

When I asked my mother about having a twin, she started crying and ran out of the room. Ten years later I asked her again on the phone. She got very angry and hung up on me. She has never talked to me about it.
Sue, UK

Even when a child has been told, the original memories can be lost for many years, surfacing in a disguised form in writing, art, dance or other creative activities. These vague impressions from the time before birth may not be recognized as being based in a real memory until a moment of realisation occurs some time later.

I found out about my twin when I was about six years old, but it took me ten more years to understand it, when I told my friend about my twin. The moment I mentioned it, some things fell into place for me. I knew there was an old ultrasound picture and I found it. It clearly shows that there were two embryos at seven weeks. I felt so sad looking at it. I can't really describe it.

Anja, Germany

Triggers to a lost memory

The moment of realisation can be triggered by a chance encounter with a friend who talks about twins, or less directly by a television programme, a radio broadcast, a magazine article or a book.

I read the book "Twins - Genes, Environment and The Mystery of Identity" by Lawrence Wright and in it I first came across "Vanishing Twin" syndrome and immediately thought, "I think that's what happened to me!"

Bridget, Australia

The pre-birth memory of a twin may be triggered by dreams of remarkable clarity. It is possible of course to dismiss these thoughts as a complete fantasy but the biological details are often surprisingly accurate.

Sometimes when I dream, I dream of Michael, my twin. He died in utero at the end of the first trimester. My birth mother doesn't believe me when I talk to her about him, but I know deep down he was real. In my dreams, Michael and I are floating in a pink womb. We are playing and kicking each other and we have long cords coming out of our tummies that are fun to pull on. The fluid that we drink is salty. One day, when I kick Michael he doesn't move. I remember feeling confused. Why isn't he moving? After a while as I get bigger, Michael gets smaller. One day he isn't there anymore.

Queenie, USA

A body memory revealed

We all have a body memory, which holds pre-birth impressions, particularly traumatic experiences, such as a difficult birth. The memories of the womb are entangled with deep, primitive feelings. Various physical therapies have evolved in the last forty years to help people rediscover body memories. When these treatments are applied they re-stimulate the original trauma. If a memory surfaces intact there can be a sudden and unmistakable whole body response - physical, hormonal, emotional and spiritual. This is experienced as an "Aha!" moment.

Chiropractic treatment

Chiropractic treatment is based on the diagnosis and manipulative treatment of misalignments of the joints, mostly in the spinal column, which cause other disorders by affecting the nerves, muscles and organs. The basic idea is that when the spine is misaligned the whole body is thrown out of balance. The injuries caused by a traumatic birth, such as a forceps delivery, can be corrected by a chiropractor. The treatment can be very profound, for within the spine lies the spinal cord. Emerging from the spinal cord are 31 pairs of spinal nerves that permeate the entire body. Manipulation of the spine can therefore affect and sometime correct aspects of the nervous system.

Kinesiology

Kinesiology is a branch of chiropractic that involves testing the body's responses when applying slight pressure to a large muscle. Sometimes emotional issues show up, such as the grief of losing a twin.

> *The kinesiologist was testing me last night and I showed up for grief in utero. I never heard of this before but I have always felt alone, like something was missing in me. I longed for a twin to share everything with, but I never had one. I suffer with depression and an eating disorder. I have a deep sadness that never shifts. I have nice home, family, friends and job, and yet inside I am so sad and lonely all the time.*
> *Deidrie, South Africa*

Neuro-emotional Technique (NET)

This is a technique developed by Dr. Scott Walker, a chiropractor in California, USA. NET uses the same techniques as kinesiology but applies these to emotional rather than physical conditions. Dr Brent Babcock experienced NET with Dr Walker for the first time in 1991. He later wrote about this experience: "When the origin of the feeling was pinpointed as 'in utero' my heart began to pound, my mind raced, and my feelings came to the surface. What was determined then, on that warm sunny afternoon, was that I was a survivor of a "vanished" twin." [2]

I have been suffering a lot of strange issues for many years. I am a chiropractor who recently started studying NET where we found this idea to be a part of the problem. When I asked my mother about this idea she almost fainted and confirmed the doctor's and her thoughts that she was having twins. When I realized that the "vanished twin" thing was a possibility, I knew it was true and broke down with grief.
Matt, USA

According to Dr Babcock, NET practitioners use muscle testing and body reflexes in such a way as to recall the specific emotions associated with "an original significant emotional event." This may be a physical trauma such as an accident or a fall, but equally this can be an emotional trauma such as the death of a co-twin. NET does seem to be particularly effective in revealing pre-birth trauma and NET practitioners encounter issues in their clients related to a "vanished" twin on a regular basis. [3]

I have consciously known that I am a womb twin survivor since my doctor used NET (Neuro-Emotional Technique) to diagnose emotional reasons for the physical health problems I was having. My mother subsequently confirmed she had bleeding during the first three months of pregnancy.
Amy, USA

Psychotherapy and counselling

You may have spent many years moving from one psychotherapist to another in search of answers. If you find a therapist who is a womb twin survivor they may help you to discover your twin. At some point, you may say or do something that hints that you too are a womb twin survivor and the possibility may be suggested. This may be enough suddenly to awaken the memory of your twin, or at least set you wondering.

I've had over thirty jobs, changed my name by deed poll; broke contact with all my family and friends in an effort to "sort myself out." Of course none of this worked and I spent over twenty years in therapy, seeing personal development gurus, doing personal development courses. I've just had a two-hour session with the therapist who told me about the womb twin web site - the first time I've worked with my womb twin.
Andy, Ireland

Some psychotherapists have voiced concerns that the idea of a twin lost before birth may be taken on by any individual in therapy as an easy and useful explanation for how they happen to feel. Alternatively, therapists who are new to this idea may imagine they have detected "signs of a lost twin" in almost all their clients. After all, when one is given a bright new hammer to play with everything can start looking like a nail!

Pre- and perinatal therapies

Some forms of therapy have evolved in the last fifty years that focus attention on birth and the prenatal period.

Primal therapy

Primal therapy was pioneered by Arthur Janov in 1971, who happened to believe that memories of trauma from birth or before persist into adulthood.[4] If you go to a primal therapist you will be encouraged to experience "primals" and literally relive your birth trauma and any traumatic pre-birth experiences. Unfortunately, Janov does not mention the lost of a twin in the womb so this style of therapy may not be helpful for womb twin survivors.

Primal integration

Primal integration embraces a range of therapies to help the client to come to terms with pre-birth trauma and integrate it into their lives.[5] There are also several other psychotherapeutic techniques now specialising in healing the trauma associated with events in the womb. If you were to undergo therapy with a pre- and perinatal psychotherapist it would soon be clear whether or not you had a twin before you were born.[a]

Transpersonal psychology

This form of therapy embraces not only human experience but also wider insights into human development, suffering, healing and the spiritual search. It includes elements such as ritual, forgiveness and acceptance that would normally not be practiced in other forms of psychotherapy. For example, workers at the Crucible Valley Centre in Australia practice transpersonal therapy with clients and in a great many cases they find that a twin has been lost before birth. They have found that the pre-birth loss of a twin has a profound impact on the living twin for their whole life.[6]

---

a. There is more detail about pre- and perinatal psychotherapy in Chapter 15

Hypnotherapy

This form of therapy involves being taken into a hypnotic trance by a hypnotherapist. Some people can be regressed under hypnosis back to a childhood state or even back into the womb. By this means they are able to access prenatal memories, that are remarkably accurate. David Chamberlain worked for many years as a hypnotherapist specialising in uncovering prenatal memories. One of his clients suffered from insomnia and came to him for hypnotherapy. [7] In a hypnotic trance, she was able to recall a near-death experience in the womb. She felt as if she had needed a "high-powered adrenalized action to stay alive" during that experience. Slipping into sleep felt like slipping into death so she forced herself to stay awake. She also said she saw "body parts" in her nightmares. She said she didn't want to be alone for it didn't seem right to be alone. In the process of this therapy she recognized that an attempted abortion had killed her twin sister. The body parts she saw in her dreams belonged to her twin sister who had slowly disintegrated after her death. This had not been a nightmare at all but a traumatic memory of a real event. Chamberlain says that pre-birth memory is never lost. Far from being lost in the depths of the unconscious, memories of past trauma are "knocking at the door." [8]

Family constellation therapy

Family constellation therapy is a therapeutic tool devised by Bert Hellinger, who is a psychotherapist living in Germany. It is one of the most effective means to reveal the previous existence of the lost and un-mourned members of a family, including a stillbirth, abortion or a lost twin. The method requires a group of people to represent members of a particular family and intuitively act out their relationships with each other. Alfred Austermann, a family constellation expert working in Germany, wrote: "A constellation is another means of finding out whether a client has or has not been alone inside the womb. With some experience and based on the reactions it is possible to clearly see whether or not a twin has existed." [9] It often happens that a lost twin can "appear" quite unexpectedly in a family constellation created for another, separate purpose. For the womb twin survivor concerned this can be their moment of discovery.

Although there are no indications according to my mother that she was carrying twins, I am certain now that I had a twin brother. It came out a few years ago during a family constellation but I could not believe it right away. The question I asked the constellation was, "It is so difficult for me to have a healthy, strong and fulfilling relationship." And there he was, my twin brother.
Anna, Holland

Healing workshops

Some womb twin survivors use various forms of healing therapies to uncover and heal their emotional symptoms.

I have only recently found out through someone within a healing workshop that this actually had the name. It has been a relief for me as it answered so much of what I have felt for most of my life, the searching and longing I have felt and how painful it has been along the way. I would like to heal this part of myself and not have to search outside of me for something I am never going to find.
Denise, Australia

Ancestral healing is a form of healing that works with the way that family pain is handed down from generation to generation. Jim Cogley, a priest and psychotherapist working in Ireland, focuses mainly on ancestral healing. He came across the "missing twin" in his clients in the 1980s. Today, he helps womb twin survivors and others to heal by using a series of hand-made wooden sculptures.[10]

Using intuition

To know one had a twin in the womb is almost always a huge relief but that knowledge alone is normally insufficient to facilitate deep healing. Some newly-aware womb twin survivors, fearful of being considered weird or crazy by their families, eschew all forms of therapy and try to go it alone. For these people - and this may include you - their own intuition is the only available tool to understanding their feelings. Womb twin survivors are highly intuitive. An intuitive person seems to have the ability to access a body of knowledge about the world and other people that lies somewhere below the threshold of conscious awareness. Some people clearly know "more than they know".[11] It would seem that twins have the intuitive ability to "tune in" to each other at a deep level. It is common for twins to know intuitively that their twin is hurt, afraid or has died. Twins are involved with each other from conception, negotiating for space in full awareness of one another every day of their lives. Therefore, they are in a position to gather many millions of clues about each other and use them to practice formulating guesses about how the other is thinking or feeling. This is how practice makes perfect. Twins learn to make accurate intuitive guesses about each other. The use of intuition seems to explain how "twin-talk" works as a language without a real vocabulary, for where words fail, intuition can work just as well. Where twins have a speech difficulty, they prefer "twin-talk." [12] It follows therefore that womb twin survivors will have been exposed to that same level of intimate interaction in the womb during the time when their twin was alive. They too will have had a pre-birth opportunity to develop their intuition. Many womb twin survivors become therapists themselves and make good use of this gift. Intuition can also inform them of their own twin, even without therapy.

> *I recently went to an intuitive healer. He told me I did have a sister who died and my immediate reaction was "I knew it!" He said she could have been a twin, but he wasn't sure. This information has really resonated with me since then. My intuition is telling me that she was my twin, but whether she died in the womb, or we were separated at birth and then she died, I do not know for sure because I was adopted, so I can't find out. Truly, I feel I know the answer in my heart...I had a twin sister and I lost her somehow.*
> Hilary, USA

The lost memory in a dream

As the possibility of being a womb twin survivor is ever more widely discussed, the womb twin survivors of the future will not have to spend so many years in therapy searching for evidence of their twin. Rather, news of their twin will be brought to them while they are still young. When they do hear the news they will probably not be surprised, for the memory of their twin already lies in their Dream of the Womb. Everyone who was ever born has a Dream of the Womb but womb twin survivors have a particularly interesting story to tell. That story will be the subject of our next chapter.

15

The lost twin in the Dream of the Womb

One of the questions in therapy was, "If you imagined the perfect
place for you, where would you be perfectly happy?"
The only thing I could think of was the womb.
Robert, Belgium

Many decades of research and exploration have revealed that an imprint of your time in the womb still remains, deeply rooted in the most primitive part of your brain. This vague and ineffable impression is known as "The Dream of the Womb" for it cannot be described as a "memory" exactly. In this chapter we will explore how a hundred years of studying the Dream of the Womb did not reveal the lost womb twins until we developed the technology to see into the womb. Only then did we fully recognize that some people have always had a lost twin – or more – in their Dream of the Womb. Like everyone else on this planet you have a Dream of the Womb, which is constantly being re-enacted in your life. Nothing in the world is more important than that. Your Dream drives your choices, fuels your desires and controls your fears. It is a strange place but everyone has a Dream like this. It seems to be at the very back of your mind, as deep and primitive as can be. Yet at the same time, it is just behind your eyes and creates a kind of prism through which you see the world and everything in it. It is a memory of long ago but it seems to be happening right now.

Hard-wired

Your Dream was built as your brain was built. The whole pre-birth experience is "hard-wired" into the neurones of your brain. It is integral to your personality, written into your mind and seemingly inescapable. Your whole life so far has consisted of keeping your Dream alive. If you are a womb twin survivor then the life and the untimely death of your womb twin is in your Dream of the Womb and constantly re-enacted. This imprint of "Someone Else" lies somewhere just below the lowest threshold of memory. However, it has not passed out of sight and out of

169

mind for all time. There is evidence from womb twin survivors themselves that the imprint is expressed in the body, mind and spirit of the survivor as a kind of lifelong, coded message. We now have the key to that code, thanks to ultrasound technology.

The Dream of Hell

For womb twin survivors, the Dream of the Womb is a restless, unquiet place. In the Dream is not only the time spent together with your twin, but also the time when your twin died and you were left alone. Your foetal assumptions about "The Way Things Are" were completely overturned.

> *My mother suddenly miscarried my twin. I have memories of being in the womb and feeling joy, everything is mustard-coloured and there are two of us in a warm, gushy place and I feel whole and content. There is another memory of a black screen (so to speak, it's difficult to put feelings into words) an emptiness after a sort of gushy sensation. This for me is when loneliness begins.*
> Tania, UK

For most womb twin survivors the Dream is not a pleasant memory of floating with your twin in intrauterine bliss: rather it is a nightmare of loss, loneliness and utter helplessness. You may be living a happy life but deep down you may have a nagging feeling of Something Terribly Wrong. The Toltecs of 15th century Mexico were familiar with a Dream of Hell, which was a place of great suffering. The following description is adapted from the Toltec writings about the Dream of Hell.[1] It makes a compelling description of a womb twin survivor's Dream of the Womb.

Just behind my eyes, my Dream of the Womb is like a matrix through which I see the world. Like a dark, mysterious cloud whirling through the primal places of my unconscious mind, this Dream is my way of being. It is with me always. I cannot remember a time without this Dream. In the dark hours of solitude when there is no one there and all is emptiness and stillness, out of the corner of my eye, I catch the faintest glimmer of gold. It is elusive but it is always there, and it gives me hope. It is like a light to show me what came before the Dream. But I am convinced nothing existed before the Dream. It is all I have.

170

The way to end any nightmare is simply to wake up. To end the Dream of Hell that you may be experiencing as a womb twin survivor, you need to awaken to the reality that lies behind it. Your Dream began in the womb, so now we will explore the psychological impressions that remain in all our minds, from that long-forgotten period of our lives. The Dream of the Womb has been in the background since psychology was invented but to mention all the individuals who have played a significant part in bringing this idea into the light would require another volume entirely. Instead, here is a brief description of how the existence of these elusive, pre-birth memories has gradually been brought into the public consciousness.

Early days

Before prebirth memories and prenatal awareness were recognised as such, a variety of explanations were put forward by people who were struggling to understand the workings of the human psyche. Unfortunately, they did not have the window on the womb that we have today, or they might have come to some very different conclusions.

Sigmund Freud (1856 –1939) The Unconscious Mind

Sigmund Freud got very close to recognising the Dream of the Womb, but he had no access to ultrasound scanning as we do today. He had to make do with what his small group of patients told him of their memories and feelings and make what he could of them. However he once wrote "There is much more continuity between intrauterine life and earliest infancy than the impressive caesura of the act of birth would have us believe." [2] Unfortunately, he did not develop this idea any further. Freud was always aware of how easily the human imagination could create fantasies and illusions, especially in the matter of incest. He decided that only if a patient remembered events in early life after the age of about three, would this be a real memory. Despite overwhelming evidence to the contrary, this arbitrary decision, made in relative ignorance of developmental neurology, is still regarded as a fact. Freud imagined that any professed "memories" of infancy must lie in the unconscious mind. According to Freud, this part of your mind consists of repressed memories of shameful or traumatic events, which are too terrible to acknowledge

171

and are therefore kept denied and buried. They surface later in disguised form, in what he called "neurosis." For those following Freudian theory today, the unconscious processes at work in the lives of neurotic patients have to be interpreted by someone trained to understand the workings of the unconscious. Because these memories are inaccessible to you, it is supposed that only a properly-trained expert can understand them.

> *How do you get to the bottom of guilt that you know you have but do not really feel? I try to be positive, I really do, I try to look at things with perspective but always I am paranoid and fearful. What is the point of having this thing when you can't tell anyone about it, conventional psychotherapy does not even acknowledge it, and so everyone just thinks you're a nutcase and there is nothing you can say?*
> *Jack, Australia*

Carl Jung (1875-1961) The Collective Unconscious

A contemporary of Freud but with some very different ideas, Carl Jung dreamed up the notion of The Collective Unconscious, which is a system of images and archetypes that all humans seem to have in the very back of their minds. These archetypes are, according to Jung, an important driver of human attitudes and behaviour. It seems that Jung was very close to describing the Dream of the Womb. He was always in search of a "final cause" for neurosis. He insisted that psychological phenomena had some purpose and meaning that lay far beyond the ideas that were current at the time. Modern-day Jungians have created some concepts similar to the Dream of the Womb, such as a "magical level of consciousness" which is a persistent but naïve way of apprehending the world. One example is, *I do not exist because no one is acknowledging my presence.* In an infant, "magical" thinking could be considered normal, but not in an adult. Jungians view "magical" thinking as "a persistent complex from the past" with no seeming cause. Is this the Dream of the Womb?

Otto Rank (1884-1939) The Trauma of Birth

In the 1920s, Otto Rank, a Freudian–trained psychoanalyst, had the sudden insight that in psychoanalytic work the relationship with the analyst reproduces the process of birth. The patient "enters the womb" with the analyst and is only able to leave psychoanalysis when he or she is ready to be "born." Leaving is very traumatic. Rank developed this idea and in 1929 named a traumatic birth as a major cause of neurosis.[3]

Nandor Fodor (1895-1964) Prenatal Conditioning
Nando Fodor was a Hungarian journalist who trained as a psychoanalyst and who wrote extensively about spiritualism. He began to explore the psychological basis of spiritualism. This lead him to consider the influence of pre-birth events on human psychology. His book *The Search for the Beloved: A Clinical Investigation of the Trauma of Birth and Prenatal Conditioning* was published in 1949.[4] In this context, the "beloved" is said to be the mother. According to Fodor, we are constantly trying to get back to our mother's womb where all our needs were once met. Of course, for womb twin survivors the "beloved" is their lost twin.

A prenatal mental life
Thanks to the work of all these brilliant pioneers, by the 1950s some people were at last beginning to believe that some kind of prenatal mental life might actually exist.[5]

Ronald David Laing (1927-1989) An Inner World Based in Reality
In the 1960s, R.D.Laing, a maverick psychiatrist whose personal life was chaotic but who had an intuitive understanding of madness, suggested that people with so-called "mental illness" are in fact living in an inner world of their own construction. Laing believed that within these fantasies there must be some kind of reality. Unfortunately, he blamed the family for the mental health problems of their children.[6] However, by the end of his life he was attempting to explore the psychological effects on the adult of the time in the womb, as far back as conception. He wrote: "It seems to me credible, at least, that all our experience in our life cycle, from cell one, is absorbed and stored from the beginning, perhaps especially in the beginning. How that may happen, I do not know."[7] Were he alive today, Laing would have seen ultrasound scans of twins interacting. He would have witnessed womb twin survivors describing their lost twins. It seems that he already had an intuitive understanding of the lost twin in the Dream of the Womb, but was born too soon and with too little knowledge to comprehend it fully.

Frank Lake (1914-1982) The Maternal-Foetal Distress Syndrome
Frank Lake, a psychiatrist who in the 1970s began working with clergy
in pastoral counselling, came to his conclusions when working with
patients who seemed to be re-experiencing pre-birth memories. He
hypothesized that the mother's distress went straight through the
umbilical cord to the developing foetus. The foetus experienced the
distress and was also capable of an individual response to it. He called
this the Maternal-Foetal-Distress Syndrome. He wrote: "Affliction in
its worst forms strikes in the first three months after conception."[8]
Unfortunately, Lake never fully grasped the prevalence and psychological
impact of a twin lost before birth.

Arthur Janov (1924-) The Primal Scream
Arthur Janov developed a form of therapy where people physically re-
experience the earlier parts of their lives that were presumably lost to
memory. In 1973 he wrote *The Primal Scream*.[9] His patients were forced
to face and not turn from their "lifelong core of pain" by means of
"primals." These were an absolutely open expression of stored feelings,
memories and pain from an original trauma. The patient then followed
these feelings to their origins. As years passed, Janov realized that his own
clients were telling him that their birth was in fact their earliest trauma.

In 2000 Janov admitted that he had been incorrectly informed
that it was impossible to relive birth experiences, because such memories
were "impossible to store."[10] He was then ready to be open-minded to
new approaches.[11] Meanwhile, the idea of the trauma of birth being a
major cause of neurosis has lead to the new "gentle birthing" practices,
which have been adopted in an attempt to reduce birth trauma.[11]

> *I believe that my brother died quite late in the pregnancy. My mother said she
> knew something was wrong with one of the babies. My mother said that if he had
> survived he would have been very disabled. A lot of fluid collected around Alex,
> and so I was squashed. I do feel that my birth was very traumatic. It sounds
> funny - I get very freaked out by seeing anything to do with pot-holing. The fear
> of being stuck, of not being able to breathe is very strong. Those images trigger
> those feelings. I've also had dreams like that. When I was born I had jaundice
> and was curved round from being squashed. My dad said I looked like a banana!*
> *Ivan, UK*

Stanislav Grof (1931-) Basic Perinatal Matrices
In his work and writing, Stanislav Grof focuses on pre-born life and describes Basic Perinatal Matrices. He describes a kind of "oceanic bliss" experienced by the foetus. Occasionally this is disturbed by maternal stress or by noxious substances, such as nicotine, crossing the placental barrier. Later in pregnancy, there is a feeling of being very cramped and short of space, followed by the difficult experience of being forced down the birth canal. Then there is the triumphant emergence from the womb during the birth process. According to Grof the trauma doesn't stop there: loud noises in the labour room and any rough handling can leave a deep and lifelong impression in the mind of the newborn child.[13] Grof's work does not directly address the experience of losing a twin before birth.

Graham Farrant (1933-1993) Prenatal Imprinting
Graham Farrant was an abortion survivor himself but as far as we know, never connected it to being a womb twin survivor.[14] He learned about birth trauma from Janov in the 1970s. He took things further back into the pregnancy and gave much consideration to the idea that pre-birth memory begins very early indeed. In the 1980s, he was working in "primal" therapy in Australia. He practiced regression, helping his clients to rediscover "lost memories" of childhood traumas, birth trauma and the prenatal imprinting of the mother's psyche, even the mother's feelings at the time of conception. He placed great emphasis on the importance of parents consciously preparing for the act of conception.[15]

The birth of Pre- and Perinatal psychology
By the 1980s it was time for these ideas to come of age: Thomas Verney was at that time a psychiatrist practising in the USA. He had developed a great interest in the unborn child and founded the Association for Pre- and Perinatal Psychology and Health (APPPAH) in 1983.[16] The papers given at the first congress in 1983 were published as an introductory book in the same year.[17] According to APPPAH, the unborn child is an aware, communicative and vulnerable human being. Furthermore, parenthood begins in the intent to conceive.[18] By the 1990s it was clear that the unborn child's experiences in the womb had more influence on personality development than anyone had previously imagined. Today, in this emerging science, the hidden connections between the quality of

conception, pregnancy and birth and the psychology of the born child, are becoming clearer every year. Pre- and perinatal psychologists often encounter the lost twin in their work with clients. Many of them are womb twin survivors themselves, drawn to this work by their own pre-birth experience.

Scepticism and incredulity

Thanks to these open-minded pioneers, it is now widely accepted that our experiences in the womb exist as real memories, not imagined memories. Today, terms such as "false memory syndrome" or "recovered memory" are used to describe imagined memories. It is true that some impressionable people can be made to believe almost anything if it is explained persuasively enough or there is a great incentive in believing it. Unfortunately the idea of "false memory" has persisted and is still occasionally invoked to cast doubt on all aspects of pre-birth psychology. This is a natural response for the 90% of the population who are not womb twin survivors and it is certainly very difficult indeed to separate fantasy from reality when dealing with the vague and inchoate material that lies in the Dream of the Womb. It has been a difficult task for pre- and perinatal psychologists to counter widespread public scepticism and incredulity. However, if you are a womb twin survivor you probably need no scientific theory to convince you that you have vague memory of your twin in your Dream of the Womb.

> *To tell you the truth, I felt so relieved when I put this together. But I do not think anyone really believes me. They think all of it is just circumstantial evidence and I am trying to put it together the way I want! Even people who do (sort of) believe me do not realize what it means. They don't know what its like to feel alone when you are surrounded by people.*
> Dee, USA

Unfortunately, the possibility of a pre-birth memory is still looked upon with suspicion by people working in some forms of psychotherapy. This means that if you are still trying to work out what psychological impact the loss of your twin has had on you, there will be only a few therapists prepared to take you seriously.

The lost twin in the Dream of the Womb

Anyone seeing twins interact on an ultrasound scan will recognize the bond between them.[19] Yet the idea still prevails that the loss of a twin at birth cannot possibly leave a real impression on the sole survivor. For example, Joan Woodward, whose identical twin died when they were three years old, was taken when very young to see two different child psychoanalysts because she had feelings that did not seem to be shared with her singleton friends. Neither of these professionals considered the death of her twin as having any great significance in her life.[20] Later she was surprised to discover how traumatic the early loss of a twin can be.[21] Nonetheless, she had her own explanations for this, arising out of her training as a psychotherapist specialising in Attachment Theory, which was developed by John Bowlby in the 1930s.[22]

A reluctant acknowledgement

Elizabeth Pector, medical doctor and mother to a womb twin survivor, has always trodden carefully in what she writes about the feelings expressed by sole surviving twins. On her web site she refers to Elizabeth Noble's book *Primal Connections*[23] which was published in 1993: "Controversial techniques discussed in Noble's book, including primal therapy and hypnotic regression, produce troubling accounts from patients who relived, under therapy, prenatal emotional trauma purportedly caused by the death of their co-twin."[24] Pector insists that most adult surviving multiples are psychologically well-adjusted, although some have "a very real sense of loneliness or something missing." Indeed, it cannot be said often enough that womb twin survivors are psychologically well-adjusted.

What is in your Dream of the Womb?

Your Dream has in it certain vague characteristics that reflect the original vagueness of your prenatal awareness. It is very difficult to interpret as a Dream, because it has always been your view of normality. However once the idea of a lost twin is discovered, a wide range of previously inexplicable behaviours begin to make some kind of sense. They are a constant re-enactment of the Dream of the Womb.

Whenever I'm at my low points, I tend to want to cling to a male friend. I have several repetitive dreams. They always occur in the same location: at my old primary/elementary school and I'm a little girl again. Oddly enough, there is always a dominant male character in the dreams. Most times he takes the form of a close male friend or my "substitute twin."
Anim, USA

A physical sensation in your body

Your missing twin can feel so close that it is like a physical sensation. If there is a physical sign like a scar on your body, then that may be an ever-present reminder. Lyn, whose twin was a *foetus in foetu*, said: "I am the reason that my twin is gone because she was growing inside of me. I like being with her in my dreams but I don't want to wake up because I know she won't be here." Womb twin survivors are often sensitive to touch and the sensation may in itself be a memory that goes back to the time in the womb when they were so close to their twin that their twins' death was perceptible. As a foetus they could not have any real concept of death but there would have been physical changes in the body of their twin, such as stillness and coldness, which would remain in their memory.

My twin brother died in the womb, I was born first and he was still-born. My parents never spoke to me about his death, but I remember when he died, as he went very cold, and I remember that coldness.
Jane, USA

An imprint in your neural network

A vague imprint of events in the womb, hard-wired into your brain, may circle endlessly until it is understood as a real memory. These vague memories tend to surface in the time between sleep and waking. If the impressions surface sufficiently clearly they can be interpreted as a story.

I remember her somehow, clear yet vague at the same time, and yet, she left me. I feel that she once existed, but she was never present in my actual lifetime. I don't "remember" her, but I know she was once with me. At the suggestion by my mother that I could have had a twin that died in the womb everything seemed to click.
Anna, Canada

An impulse to express

Many womb twin survivors are artists or writers. Once they understand about their Dream, they are able to look back and see the coded theme of the lost twin behind almost all of their work. The desire to express the inexpressible is a driving creative force for many womb twin survivors. They seem to be in search of some answers, or want to tell a mysterious story.

> *I am a professional artist, I paint childish images. I paint quickly as there is always another painting bursting out of me. Sometimes I paint in a kind of dream and don't know what I am painting until I step back from it and look. It is almost as if someone else has painted it through me.*
> Nicola, UK

A timeless story

Some womb twin survivors, usually those who have talked with a therapist about it, are well aware of how they constantly recycle the timeless, never-ending story of their lost twin in various areas of their life.

> *I get into relationships where I recreate myself as being "the dying twin" - subconsciously of course - then I try to push myself out of the "womb space" I've created with this person or other, and leave the relationship - and then when the other person does fine without me and is successful in "living" - I have a weird thing of getting suicidally depressed. It's as if one of us has to metaphorically die. It is a strong feeling and one that I am going through right now. I want to live and not feel guilty about it - it is hard to even see it as guilt about surviving - I just have these deep subconscious unwritten laws that are like, if I live, someone close has to die.*
> Frances, USA

The Womb Twin research project

We have come to the end of our exploration of the grief of a lone twin. It is time now to move onto the next stage of our journey, which is to review the results of the Womb Twin research project. It began in 2003 and has been providing information, help and support to womb twin survivors ever since.

179

PART FOUR

Being a womb twin survivor

You Were A Spinning Seed

You were a spinning seed
Torn from my hand.
Now I have taken root
In this thin land,
Fixed here forever by your absence from me.

I keep the faith, seeing what you should see,
Breathing familiar air, each breath
For you as well as me.

I am the treasure chest
Left in the lane,
Under the leaves,
Waiting here just the same,
Knowing, as you do not, what I contain.

Linda Clark

16

The Womb Twin research project

I've reacted to most of what I've read on the subject so far with "Aha!" type amazement. So much of what I've felt, of what I am, makes sense now.

Victoria, UK

The whole idea of the Womb Twin research project has been to find womb twin survivors and ask them how it feels to be a womb twin survivor. This chapter will review some of the main developments since the project began in 2003.

Womb twin survivors revealed

In 1995, Charles Boklage concluded from his research that for every twin pair born intact there are at least ten sole survivors.[1] It took another ten years for the impact of this statistic to be fully realized, but gradually, the idea entered into the public consciousness. Two years later, in 1997, a web site about "The vanishing twin phenomenon" was created by Caryl Dennis in the USA. She writes that she began her work: "...after finding out not only that I am a surviving twin, but also that my fraternal twin siblings probably began as triplets, and that my youngest brother was a surviving 'mirror' identical twin."[3] Four years later in 2001 the idea caught the attention of the popular scientific press. By 2005, pre- and perinatal psychology was well-established as a science in California, USA. One expert described the lost twin issue as "..a little known but very commonplace phenomenon."[5]

I didn't know that there was so much information about "vanishing" twins or that it is so common. It's making me take a different look at my own life.
Christina, USA

Finding womb twin survivors

Until the 1980s there was no way of identifying womb twin survivors, simply because few people had any idea they existed. By 2003 modern technology had made it possible to find a sufficient number of womb twin survivors to carry out this research at minimal cost. It was possible to recruit a large number of womb twin survivors via the Internet. To that end, the first womb twin web site was created in 2003. Until then, it had not been possible to go out and find womb twin survivors but now they came to the site. One by one, they began to tell their stories.

This web site speaks for itself. It is undoubtedly an inspiring beacon in the lives of many twin survivors out there.
Kris, Belgium

The Womb Twin hypothesis

Within a few months of launching the web site it was clear that womb twin survivors do have a specific psychological make-up, which appears to be related to the loss of their twin. On that basis, the Womb Twin hypothesis was formulated:

> **Womb twin survivors spend their lives re-enacting the life and death of their womb twin. Nothing is more important than that - even life itself. Once the real pre-birth scene, which is constantly being re-enacted, is made clear, then the re-enactment tends to diminish or cease altogether, greatly to the benefit of the individual.**

It has not been necessary to amend the hypothesis in any way since it was formulated in 2003. In fact, repeated analyses of various versions of the Womb Twin research questionnaire have consistently supported it. At first, it seemed an extraordinary idea that the loss of a twin at birth or before could be the cause of a variety of psychological problems. As time passed however, more and more womb twin survivors came forward, each with a similar story of misery and loss, which was clearly explained by the womb twin hypothesis. It now seems that the psychological effects on the sole survivor when a twin is lost around birth or before, have been hidden in plain sight for generations. At last, we have learned how to recognise these effects and describe them.

It means so much to me to know that it's not a figment of my imagination or wishful thinking, and that there are other people out there who have gone through similar experiences.
Valerie, Canada

Scepticism

Most people are not womb twin survivors. The idea that the loss of a twin before birth can have any kind of psychological effect on the survivor is greeted by many of them with scepticism and scorn. For instance, the term "Wombtwin survivor" was entered on the Wikipedia web site in 2006. The first discussion comment was, "That wombtwin survival stuff is totally bogus, on the same level as star-sign astrology and alien mind control. It doesn't really deserve mentioning in an article about a medical phenomenon."

Evidently, the Womb Twin research project was going to be a very small voice in the world of scientific research. Therefore, an early policy decision was to work exclusively with the 10% of the population who are womb twin survivors. They were delighted to have the truth of their inner experience recognised at last.

Many times growing up I felt that I did not fit in, had no friends, and felt the empty hole in my life, and now I know why that hole was there.
Krista, USA

Creating a questionnaire

The original purpose of the Womb Twin research questionnaire, first created in 2003, was to clarify the subjective experience of womb twin survivors. At the time, there was no way of knowing whether womb twin survivors felt any differently from the rest of the human race. The only feelings that had been mentioned in other research with the sole survivors of twin or multiple conceptions were "loneliness" and "a sense of something missing." As we have seen from the stories in previous chapters, the feelings associated with the pre- or perinatal loss of a twin or multiple are not often openly discussed. Where they are heard, they are frequently misunderstood. In any case, they are often too vague to articulate clearly.

I don't know if any of this means I'm a womb twin survivor, but it feels good to know that the person reading it will at least empathise and possibly even understand.
Anonymous, Australia

185

Part of the work of the Womb Twin research project has been to try and put the Dream of the Womb into words. To do that has required a great deal of negotiation with hundreds of womb twin survivors over several years.

> *All the things mentioned in the questionnaire are just ME! I didn't realize some things could be to do with this. I have been looking for a web site like this for some time.*
> *Molly, Australia*

The many e-mails that arrived via the web site were a written testimony of how people truly feel about being a womb twin survivor and this was rare and precious material. If anything useful was to be learned from these e-mails, there were just two options: the first was to create a list of the most commonly-used statements in the e-mails and form them into a questionnaire, in order to find the statements most often agreed to and therefore most characteristic of womb twin survivors generally. The other option was to collect all the e-mails and analyse each one to discover the most commonly-stated ideas, according to the tenets of Critical Interpretive research.[1] This is particularly useful in areas of study where the use of questionnaires with fixed responses may be limiting. The Womb Twin study aims to characterize how people experience the world, so it is necessarily open-ended.

No possible control group

In 2003 when the Womb Twin research project began, it was immediately clear that however much good data was collected the traditional scientific method of testing an hypothesis was not going to work in this case. The scientific method would have required a significant number of people to come forward voluntarily to act as a control group. They would have to know they were definitely not womb twin survivors and they would have to complete the same questionnaire under the same conditions. The main difficulty was that in an unknown number of cases the loss of a twin before birth is symptom-free, so any control group would doubtless include an unknown number of womb twin survivors. It was decided that the only reliable way to discover the psychological effect of losing a twin before birth was to rate a list of statements commonly made by womb twin survivors about their feelings, behaviours and attitudes.

186

The list of statements would be available as an online form. Womb twin survivors visiting the web site would then rate each statement according to the strength of their agreement with it. As more was learned from the stories received, the list of statements was amended and extended over the next four years.

It was almost like an awakening. A huge burden has been lifted from my shoulders and a light is truly at the end of my tunnel.
Sarah, USA

It remained to draw up a list of evidence, signs and indications of a lost twin and include them in the questionnaire, so that a group of people could be found who were able to provide evidence of their lost twin. (See Appendix A). From February 2007 to July 2009, 500 completed questionnaires in the final version were collected. Of these, about half were completed by womb twin survivors who were able to provide evidence of their lost twin. The first 500 of the completed questionnaires were sent for analysis to the University of Hertfordshire in Hatfield, England. A preliminary professional analysis of the results was carried out in 2009 by the Statistics Department. (See Appendix B). The analysis was based solely on the respondents able to provide evidence of their twin. Of these, only the strongest responses to the statements were counted.

Exploring the results

It is now time to explore the results of this research and discuss each statement in detail. On the way, we will meet some of the many hundreds of womb twin survivors who were honest and open enough to reveal their innermost feelings about their lost twin. Without them, this research would not have been possible. Without this research project, the womb twin hypothesis would still be only an intuitive guess and this book would have no substance.

17

An unusual person

I feel like not only does nobody around me really "get" me, but that nobody in the entirety of the universe does. It's exacerbated by the feeling that there's supposed to be someone who is so incredibly in tune with me that I don't really even need to say anything for them to know what's going on with me.

Stephanie, UK

This chapter will focus on the questionnaire statements that suggest an unusual person. The table below shows what proportion of the selected respondents[a] agreed strongly with each of these statements.[b]

AN UNUSUAL PERSON - QUESTIONNAIRE RESPONSES	
Out of the ordinary	**%**
I feel different from other people	67.4
I am paranoid	22.5
I am dyslexic	7.4
Specially gifted	
I have a great desire to heal the world, and everyone in it	49.6
I am so intuitive and empathetic that it is a problem for me	48.1
I think I am psychic	35.5
I feel very privileged, simply to be alive	27.2
Gender issues	
I am a female with a strong male side	31.9
I am male but I have a strong female side	8.1

a. The respondents able to provide evidence of their twin.

b. The levels of agreement were 1-5. The term "agreed strongly" refers only to the respondents who checked "1" as the strongest possible agreement with the statement. This explanation applies to all statistics provided for the statements described in this chapter, except where indicated.

OUT OF THE ORDINARY

Womb twin survivors comprise only about 10% of the population, so it stands to reason that they will appear to be out of the ordinary.

I feel different from other people

It is not easy feeling different. As a newly-aware womb twin survivor, you may have returned home from a workshop or therapy session, full of relief that at last your psychological problems have been explained, only to have this amazing new idea dismissed by your family as "nonsense."

> *This has always been bizarre to me. I usually don't share it because no one has ever understood what I am saying, including me. I also have a lot of nagging in my soul. It keeps me searching. I never really feel I fit in anywhere.*
> Beth, Canada

Prenatal psychology is not yet widely accepted as a science. Some therapists and mental health professionals may assume that the idea of "being a womb twin survivor" is at best another ingredient in an eccentricity of character. At worst, they may call it a delusion.

> *I thought I was weird, thinking like I do and becoming so aware of my twin. Yes I do always feel weird - like an outsider, that I'm not as good as others.*
> Elizabeth, USA

PAULA: ALWAYS CONSIDERED WEIRD

All through her childhood, Paula was called "weird." The other children at school avoided her. Her parents just looked baffled and didn't seem to understand her at all. She had few friends as a result. She felt guilty for being so different but wondered why she had to change for the sake of others.

You may have close friends but perhaps it is necessary to put on a false face and keep private your strange, secret feelings. You may have learned how to conform to every nuance of human behaviour in your peer group, always fitting in like a chameleon.

> *I feel that I have two distinct personalities and have for the majority of my life played certain social roles.*
> Terry, USA

189

Your strange, secret feelings may seem to defy explanation and grow out of all proportion into what seems to be a "Shadow." It may be possible to drown your feelings in constant activity. However, as soon as there is some quiet space, the feelings immediately surface and the sense of "being different" is at its greatest.

> *I already know that I had a twin who died in the womb. I've known that for as long as I've known anything. I've always wondered if the reason why it's so easy for me to get lonely is because I don't have my twin. To everyone else, I'm happy. It's when I actually sit still and don't keep my mind occupied on something that I just feel horrible inside. The worst part is that no one understands it. I don't know who I am or what I feel sometimes. That's a hard enough thing to explain, let alone understand.*
> Sabrina, Canada

Some womb twin survivors make a point of being different. They defiantly proclaim their individuality through dress, manner and beliefs. They cultivate eccentricity. If you are deliberately eccentric as a way of proclaiming to the world who you are, then this could be a reflection of your pre-birth story. If your twin was opposite to you in every way, then that mismatch may be reflected in every part of your life. [c] Perhaps your twin developed in some strange way quite differently from yourself, and that difference was incompatible with life. In that case, difference itself would be a major emotional issue and it would be very important to be different but still be found acceptable.

> *I know I'm not normal in the way I relate to people and I have no idea why. I am not a nut, it's just me, I can't help it. It's not a matter of trying or anything like that, it's to do with what feels authentically ME. It's so very important that I can express myself fully, just the way I am and for that to be found acceptable by other people.*
> Henny, USA

I am paranoid

Paranoia is another side to hypersensitivity. It is an acute sensitivity to rebuff. It is a tendency to misconstrue the motives of others as hostile, easily feel suspicious and frequently assume that one is under threat.

---

c. For more on the differences between MZ twins, see page 26

Due to a condition known as "continuous low mood" I've been put on medication, as well as to ease constant anxiety and paranoia. However I often find means to be paranoid and anxious through reasoning and justification.
Natalie, UK

Paranoia is paradoxical. It seems to be associated with a feeling of vulnerability and helplessness, but paranoid behaviour is essentially defensive - a powerful feeling arising out of a sense of powerlessness.

> TONY: ENRAGED BY INCONVENIENCE
> Tony feels inwardly so vulnerable that he is acutely concerned with his personal welfare. He becomes enraged if he experiences the mildest form of inconvenience. A delayed train is seen as a personal slight.

Paranoia is essentially self-centred. If you are paranoid it probably feels to you like a perfectly justifiable form of self-protective anxiety. Even so, deep down, you are probably aware that it is self-inflicted.

I am dyslexic [d]

For generations, dyslexia has been misunderstood as a condition. It is much more than a problem with writing or spelling and certainly does not imply "laziness" or "stupidity."

I am possibly a chimera, my blood is type A2B. I was never diagnosed with dyslexia, but I had trouble learning to read, although later graduated college with honors.
Hannah, USA

The main problem for someone with dyslexia is that their inner world is at odds with the outer world they inhabit. They live in a dream world where the passage of time and the demands of outer reality seem to be of no consequence. The immediate moment is where everything happens, in a perpetual sense of "Now." The energy for life is focussed on the present moment, in an imagined temporal "bubble" in which time does not exist. Of course, in the Dream of the Womb there was no sense of time.

---

d. For more about the associations between dyslexia and twinning see page 123.

JANE: DYSLEXIC AND CHAOTIC

Jane exists in a dream world. At 23 she still lives with her parents, but far removed from reality. That means promises broken, missed appointments, forgotten tasks and general chaos reflected in the mess in the house. The wonder is that she manages to survive at all, but she is very good at recruiting help with her dyslexia. She is constantly rescued by others but oblivious to the amount of energy that others put in to sorting out her problems. She has no instinct for self-preservation, which would consist of taking time to create safety nets, make memoranda or carry out reality checks. In fact, Jane has a very high tolerance to chaos and has all kinds of clever strategies for coping with the chaotic environment that she creates for herself.

This may be Jane's Dream of the Womb: a twin pair of embryos floats in the same bubble of amniotic fluid, where there is no awareness of time and there are of course no words. One of the twins dies and begins to degenerate into a chaotic mass of cells. The survivor is left with the deep certainty of being the strong survivor but there is also an inner sense of helpless chaos. This may be why Jane deliberately re-creates that chaos in her home environment and seems helpless to organise it.

SPECIALLY GIFTED

All womb twin survivors share in a rare and extraordinary pre-birth experience: to be a womb twin survivor is a great gift.

I have a great desire to heal the world, and everyone in it

A desire to "heal the world" is strongly idealistic and obviously unrealistic, but it is a persistent idea among womb twin survivors. It arises out of a sense of "mission" and a deep desire to make a difference in other people's lives. The need to heal others runs so deep in some womb twin survivors that to them it doesn't feel altruistic. However, the necessary self-sacrifice can lead to becoming totally exhausted.

---

e.   For a diagram of this situation see page 64.

When someone was suffering I felt a lot of confusing emotions with them.
I tried to help them, listening to them and doing things that were too tiring for me.
I try to take care of me before taking care of others. I'm not always successful.
Ana, Portugal

Of course, the "world" that womb twin survivors wish to "heal" is not the outer world of people and things. It is their own inner world, their Dream of the Womb, and for you it may be yours. If your little lost womb mates in your Dream could be restored to health and strength, then the original conception scenario where everyone was alive together could be restored. The idea of "healing the world" feels like a strong, noble and self-sacrificing mission but perhaps it is only a dream. There are countless healers and therapists in the world, but healing is a choice made by the suffering individual concerned: it cannot be provided by any healer.

I think that it may be possible that I can help or heal other people; perhaps I do
have something special to offer.
Tina, USA

I am so intuitive and empathetic that it is a problem for me

Empathy is an innate capacity of every human person. It is by means of empathy that we form intimate relationships. It is a way of using your imagination to guess how another person is feeling. The drive behind the wish to be empathetic is a kind of mental "reaching out." It began in the womb and you are still doing it.

I am constantly trying to be a peacemaker for all relationships. I sometimes
wonder why other people do not have the empathy that I do. They constantly are
thinking of number one, while if something happens to someone, I automatically
put myself in their shoes, and feel the pain with them.
Greta, Netherlands

It seems that the experience of being with a womb twin in the earliest weeks of life heightens empathy in the survivor. Using empathy with others is very similar to reaching out in curiosity to another embryo in the womb, who can't be seen, heard or touched but seems to be out there. The shared womb experience that awakens the capacity for empathy also sharpens intuition. This is a combination of two distinct capacities; an

193

acute sensitivity to a million tiny clues in the environment and the ability to process all these tiny clues and formulate a guess.[f] As we have seen, a twin foetus develops extra neurons because of the additional stimulation received from a twin in the early days of development.[g] The end result is a heightened sensitivity to everything in the womb environment. A twin foetus who has learnt how to discern the tiniest movement of their twin through ripples in the amniotic fluid would naturally end up as an untuitive and intuitive person.

> *I always was considered odd, strange, quiet, shy. I abuse drugs to help me feel*
> *normal. I talk to myself all the time, always have. In a strange way I feel more*
> *sensitive to life than others.*
> Mark, USA

Prenatal lessons are not easily forgotten and this may be difficult for you as a womb twin survivor. You may pick up feelings from others just because of your heightened awareness and empathy. Empathy taken to extremes is a curse, known as "hypersensitivity." For hypersensitive people, their awareness of other people is so strong as to be almost overwhelming: they need time alone after any social contact.[1] If hypersensitivity is your problem and you tend to withdraw, you may seem to others to be lacking in emotion. You will know however, that time spent away from relationship with other people is the only way for you to survive in society.

> *I am still struggling with trusting people and letting my guard down, and other*
> *times I can be too open and sensitive to other people's emotions that I feel*
> *drained and an emotional wreck.*
> Tara, Ireland

I think I am psychic

We have already seen that womb twin survivors are very intuitive and aware of other people. They pick up on millions of tiny signals that are not noticed by others. This very strong intuition is helpful in dealing with people and can make some womb twin survivors feel "psychic." Some womb twin survivors do seem to be extraordinarily gifted, particularly in relationship to other people.

---

f. For more about intuition see page 167
g. For more on the development of the neural networks, see page 141

I am set apart, I have gifts that other people don't have. I recognize that in many ways I am superior to other people in the way that I can do things or the way I think so clearly or quickly.
Freya, USA

Another "psychic" effect may be created by a strong sense of the real presence of the lost twin, which can begin in childhood with imaginary friends and continue into adulthood with a sense of being watched over.

I have accepted that I did lose a dear person. He is still with me though. I believe he's been with me all my life. Perhaps I felt his presence when I was little, perhaps I talked to him, not knowing it was him. Maybe he was my imaginary friend. I don't know. But yes, I do believe he's with me, and I am not scared anymore.
Joy, Holland

You may have a strong, pre-birth memory of life with your twin and a desire for reconnection after death. If you process these using your creative imagination, you may experience all kinds of visions, voices, manifestations and strange kinds of knowing. Such extraordinary and baffling experiences may seem to require a supernatural explanation.

I feel very privileged, simply to be alive

The very act of living could be a joy for womb twin survivors, who so very nearly did not make it into this life at all. A sense of privilege at being alive suggests that a tinge of survivor guilt is moderating the joy. As we will see in a later chapter, survivor guilt is a major issue for womb twin survivors. If you are a womb twin survivor and you have come to see your life as "a burden gladly borne" then you are already well on the way to feeling joy in living but there is no need for life itself to be a burden: you can lift that burden by overcoming survivor guilt.

GENDER ISSUES

Unusual gender issues among womb twin survivors were highlighted by the Womb Twin research project. To begin the discussion of the next set of statements we will explore what is considered to be the biological norm in terms of the expression of gender energy. In the last hundred thousand years of evolution, humans have lived as hunter-gatherers. The last five thousand years or so saw the first civilizations, but that is only a moment in geological time. Consequently, men and women are still expressing their in-built gender energy in ways that have prevailed for millennia and have enabled the human species to thrive.

Human in-built gender energy in action
This is how it works: the woman bears and raises the children. The man protects the woman and their children from danger, fights battles on their behalf and is prepared to risk his life for his family. The woman is always busy in and near to the home with preparing food, teaching the children about society and keeping the home together. The man goes out from the home, often covering huge distances. He obtains food and goods to nourish and protect the family.

Archetypal male energy
As a result of our genetic programming, male energy is active, often physical. It tends to be aggressive, powerful and strong. It is robust and uncompromising. In anger it is hot and destructive. It can be focussed on fighting and dying for the sake of others. Male energy deconstructs in order to rebuild, it endures extreme physical pain and injury, it confronts and challenges, it builds large structures and carries into action ambitious, broadly-based ideas.

Archetypal female energy
Female energy tends to be passive and yielding, gentle and pliable. It is more delicate and fragile. It creates, nurtures, unites and conciliates. Female energy is sacrificial of personal happiness. It endures emotional pain, is focussed on maintaining good relationships and concerned with immediate, detailed, small-scale projects, at which women are particularly skilled.

When the trouble starts
The two very different kinds of energy at work in the lives of men and women are usually complementary, and this makes for excellent team-work between them. If each partner uses their own genetically in-built energy to the full, then things will work well. The trouble starts if men start behaving like women and women start behaving like men. That can happen among opposite-sex DZ womb twin survivors who choose to live

together. Each carries some of the opposite-sex hormones from their lost twin.

I am a female with a strong male side

The respondents who agreed strongly with this statement are probably the female opposite-sex DZ womb twin survivors who received a prenatal dose of male hormones. We have seen in a previous chapter how fraternal (DZ) twins can share their gender hormones in the womb. [h]

JULIET: EXTRA MALE HORMONES IN A FEMALE

In her police career, Juliet has always been in a male environment. Despite the fact that she likes being female, male energy has always over-shadowed her, especially when she needs physical power, strength or aggression for her job. It shows in defiance and stubbornness if she is pushed too far. Juliet is goal-oriented and speaks about her views in a pushy way, despite trying hard not to. She has worked hard as a woman to prove she can be as good, if not better, than men.

You may be a female DZ womb twin survivor carrying male energy but you cannot ever be a man. Even so, as a result of your extra male hormones, you may behave or think like a man.

My mum said I may have had a twin, she says it's a girl. I think it might explain my deep resentment of women and girls, my distrust in them. I have always liked boys and men more than women. I think maybe my twin was a boy, it explains my occasional lesbian stages, every six months or so, and my being drawn to male things.

Emma, Australia

The presence of extra male hormones could thwart your genetically-in-built feminine desire to conciliate with others as a solution to conflict. As a masculine woman you may prefer aggressive manipulation over conciliation. On the one hand you may have an active and ambitious desire to drive a large project forward to completion, which requires male energy. On the other, there is your natural female desire to let things be and allow situations to grow organically. Your extra male energy may also

---

h. For the biological background to this see pages 114-5

be visible in your choice of clothing and favourite activities.

I'm a female and am not sexually attracted to females. Actually I'm not attracted to either sex. I don't care for frilly, pastel coloured clothing or high-heeled shoes. I'm not interested in feminine things such as jewellery and makeup. I am very practical. I also like "guy things" like cars and lawn mowers.
Barbara, USA

I am male but I have a strong female side[i]

Men with a strong female side are the opposite-sex DZ womb twin survivors who received a dose of female hormones while in the womb. A feminised man is not like other men: he doesn't really know what he wants in life and is not ambitious.

MIKE: EXTRA FEMALE HORMONES IN A MALE

As a male with a soft heart and having lost his twin sister before birth, Mike struggles with the additional female energy within him. He tends to help and conciliate when a direct and open challenge would be better. He does not express his anger or aggressively defend himself. His good-natured gentleness is often taken advantage of by any unscrupulous people he encounters. He routinely gives away his male power and finds himself greatly disadvantaged in the cut-throat world of work. He is always sacrificing his own ambitions to further the interests of female friends. He has taken his male, active energy and diverted it into an excessive number of nurturing, creative, helping projects that have drained him and left him less able to fulfil his male ambitions.

A man with extra female hormones may be overly concerned with his clothes and loves food. He may like to cook or work with food, for he loves to feed people. He may nurture people in other ways too, by being a carer or a therapist. He may seem to be an unusual man because he looks for pity from others when life gets tough. He may feel uncomfortable taking the lead in social situations. There are compensations, however: the feminised man has a touch of feminine intuition, which makes him a "people person." He is a good diplomat, with excellent negotiating

---

i.   For more about this see page 117.

skills, able to manage confrontation without the need for any aggression. On the other hand, every woman becomes a "sister" to him which can make sexual relationships difficult.

Although a man, I'm very emotional and tend to not understand other guys very well; in fact, I get along much more easily with women. I keep pursuing something, although I don't know what it is, and find myself always drawn to wanting to rid the world of suffering which is why I've entered a helping profession: first social work (typically a woman's field) then nursing (also typically a woman's field.)
Mark, Belgium

The suffering survivor

Being a womb twin survivor is much more than just being different: it can be very tough. Some womb twin survivors spend their lives in a secret state of deep suffering, that seems to have no rational explanation. Perhaps you have every reason to be happy with your life but deep down there is always a distressing sense of Something Wrong. If so, you will find the next chapter of particular interest.

199

18
Signs of psychological distress

I am famous for having been very distressed as a baby and
I cried an awful lot.
Kate, Ireland

This chapter will focus on the questionnaire statements that indicate psychological distress. The table below shows what proportion of the selected respondents [a] agreed strongly with each of these statements. [b]

PSYCHOLOGICAL DISTRESS - QUESTIONNAIRE RESPONSES	
Persistent emotional pain	%
All my life I have carried deeply felt emotional pain that persists, despite all my efforts to heal myself	54.8
I feel the pain of others as if it were my own	51.7
Death and dying	
I have wanted to commit suicide more than once in my life	40.0
I think a lot about death and dying	38.5
I have suffered for a long time from feeling vaguely unwell, as if I am slowly dying	30.1
A general feeling of distress	
I suffer from low self-esteem	51.8
I suffer from depression	48.7
I often find it difficult to fall asleep, even when very tired	45.3
I am a perfectionist	31.6
I get upset by silly little things	29.8

a.   The respondents who were able to provide evidence of their twin.

b.   The levels of agreement were 1-5. The term "agreed strongly" refers only to the respondents who checked "1" as the strongest possible agreement with the statement. This explanation applies to all statistics provided for the statements described in this chapter, except where indicated.

These statements, were drawn from what womb twin survivors were saying about themselves and 98% of the selected respondents to the questionnaire agreed strongly with at least one of the statements listed in the table on the previous page. Clearly, psychological distress is very common among womb twin survivors. It seems that womb twin survivors all share a particular sense of vague, mysterious suffering that lasts a lifetime. This "primal wound" is not accessible to healing unless it has been fully understood, so we will now explore it.

PERSISTENT EMOTIONAL PAIN

It is hard to define emotional pain. There is social pain such as rejection, and physical pain such as that caused by a physical injury. Emotional pain lies somewhere between the two.

All my life I have carried deeply-felt emotional pain that persists, despite all my efforts to heal myself

People who know that they lost a twin before birth carry an unending pain of grief and loneliness. Unaware womb twin survivors may carry a lifelong pain that has no name - that is, until they realize what it is. Grief can be healed, given sufficient understanding and perhaps an appropriate kind of therapy, but there is little specialist help available for sole surviving twins of any age, let alone womb twin survivors. Womb twin survivors may search in vain for years, moving from therapist to therapist, looking for someone who understands the nature of their emotional pain.

> *I have souvenirs of my birth and my identical twin's - the usual birth certificate and hair from first haircut etc. but I also have one that I don't want. That is my vision loss. It came as a result of our premature birth. Deep down, it is a daily reminder of that traumatic time of her death and the heavy burden I must carry. It is staring me in the face at all times. I cannot escape it. It's a heavy weight I have to deal with while my sister got off easy by just dying.*
> *Brenda, USA*

To let go of your pain would be to let go of your lost twin so it is not surprising that, however distressing the pain may be, there is a kind of comfort in it. As a result the pain, and the therapy to try and heal the pain, may go on for many years.

I feel the pain of others as if it were my own

Feeling the pain of others seems to be one of the many difficulties that come with being extremely empathetic and aware of other people. Coupled with the characteristic desire to heal the world that we discussed in the previous chapter, the result can be quite overwhelming if the pain you see in others does not diminish, however hard you try to help.

> *I would do anything for another not to be in pain. At one point I realized that I was so familiar with pain that if it helped someone for me to take it on, then I would. Then I accepted the suggestion that pain helps someone know they are alive. Even with this information I continued to become anxious when I saw suffering around me. The distress intensifies when I feel helpless to do anything.*
> Jean, USA

If you are a womb twin survivor you may have spent many years taking on the pain of others, believing that it will help. In fact, taking on another person's pain does not diminish their pain in any way. In the end there are two people suffering. You probably know this but still continue to adopt the pain of others as if it were your own. The reason for this may be the emotional pain inside you that you don't yet understand. Feeling pain on behalf of others may be as close as you have ever come to being able to express your own pain.

DEATH AND DYING

Womb twin survivors spend their lives re-enacting the life and death of their womb twin. For some people, that means death feels as if it is very near. They may have panic attacks, imagining they are *about to die any moment*. Others may have times when they *feel neither alive nor dead*. In fact, you are not dying and neither are you are about to die: this is a foetal assumption [c] based on a prenatal memory of death.

> *In my late teens I invented a perfect family where I felt loved and beautiful and I gave myself a twin brother in my stories. My whole life has been tormented with feelings that I can only describe as "death in the air." I was depressed and terribly anxious as a child and growing up and always felt that I somehow had witnessed death and that I was "bad" and going to be punished.*
> Bridie, USA

---

c. For more about foetal assumptions, see page 143.

Your particular concept of death may reflect a real memory of an actual event, long lost in your Dream of the Womb. You could not possibly have been able to understand death in the womb or near to birth but you would have probably noticed a change in your twin's behaviour. For example, your twin may have been lost in a complete miscarriage. In that case, your foetal assumption would probably be *death causes disappearance*. The idea that *death takes people away* may still be a major concern. On the other hand, the death of your twin may have been slow but inevitable, so that you may be more concerned about the process of dying than about being dead. If your twin existed only briefly, only to die and be totally resorbed, then your idea of death may be total annihilation of your self, as if you had never existed at all.

I have suffered for a long time from feeling vaguely unwell, as if I am slowly dying

If you are a womb twin survivor whose twin died slowly you may have identified a bit too closely with your dying womb twin and your foetal assumption may be *I am slowly dying*. You may develop all kinds of strange symptoms and have a sense of *dying by inches*.

> *I have always been totally fascinated by twins in general - conjoined twins, the mixed-race girls that ended up one very light and one very dark, all of them. The similarities and differences fascinate me. Details of some of my medical issues: I have fibromyalgia, chronic fatigue, insomnia, allergies, celiac sprue, dysautonomia. None of it will kill me directly but I feel like I am slowly dying a dribble at a time.*
>
> Cherry, USA

A persistent feeling of being unwell, sometimes with alarming symptoms that come and go, may take you repeatedly to the doctor's surgery. As there is no physical disease, the symptoms may be described as "psychosomatic" with the inference that you are "malingering" or "neurotic." In fact, you are expressing your Dream of the Womb in terms of bodily symptoms.

I think a lot about death and dying

In this case there are no physical symptoms, as in the previous section, but rather a preoccupation with death. If this is how you feel, then death "walks beside you." You think constantly about your own death. This preoccupation can also be about the death of other people and be expressed as a great interest in dead bodies, graveyards, funerals, gravestones or pathology.

> *When I was a teenager I drove throughout our rural county looking for grave yards and examining the tombstones when I found them. I never told anyone about those explorations because I thought I was crazy.*
> Kathy, USA

Alternatively, you may experience a form of "living death" like a kind of spiritual inertia. This is expressed as a resistance to change, growth or forward movement: it can totally block your healing. Your problem is spiritual inertia if you would rather settle for what is "good enough" than challenge your own abilities. You would decide to be content with your lot, rather than reach for the stars. You would choose to live on the surface rather than explore your inner self. If you have been in a state of inertia for some time, then the lifeless place in which you have chosen to live could be in your Dream. It may be a re-enactment of the tiny spark of life that you were able to perceive in the womb using your exquisite embryonic sensitivity. If your womb twin never had a chance of life how could it be fair if you have life to the fullest? Rather than come to the feast of life you just settle for a few crumbs every now and then - just enough to maintain your existence and no more.

I have wanted to commit suicide more than once in my life

The incidence of suicidal ideation[d] varies greatly across the world. One study of 40,000 subjects, drawn from the United States, Canada, Puerto Rico, France, West Germany, Lebanon, Taiwan, Korea and New Zealand found that the number of people who had thought of suicide at some stage in their life varied from 0.7% in Beirut to 18.51% in Christchurch, New Zealand.[1] The Womb Twin research project found that 40% of the selected respondents agreed strongly with this statement, which is more than double the New Zealand rate. It seems from this result that womb twin survivors think about suicide much more often than most people.

---

d.   The contemplation of committing suicide, with or without an actual attempt

I've had suicidal thoughts most of my life. Have attempted suicide once, and did a pretty bang up job, but they saved me, thank God.
Valerie, USA

Researchers are beginning to connect some mental health problems to events in the mother's pregnancy. In one study, suicidal behaviour (along with schizophrenia and violent crime) was linked to perinatal complications.[2] As we have seen, perinatal complications are strongly associated with twin or multiple conceptions.[e] Evidently, this is an area that may reward further exploration and research.

Birth trauma

Various studies are beginning to suggest that some mental health problems are connected to events in the mother's pregnancy, including birth trauma.[3] The advocates of primal therapy hold that the first trauma of our lives takes place during labour when we begin the journey from the womb into the world. They suggest that birth is essentially traumatic. Furthermore, they believe that all pain that occurs in born life relates to unresolved birth trauma and is thus magnified and perpetuated.[4] If you are a womb twin survivor and you had a traumatic birth, the memory of that time of suffering may be foremost in your mind. If your own birth trauma remains unresolved it could block access to the older, more subtle memories of your twin, which lie in deep in your Dream of the Womb. The Womb Twin research project found that one third of the selected respondents claimed to have had a "traumatic birth." Of course "traumatic" is a general term, open to many interpretations. Respondents were simply given the chance to say Yes or No to the statement, *"I had a traumatic birth."* A few gave additional medical details. A birth is regarded as traumatic to the baby if they sustained physical injury or psychological shock in the process of being born. The questionnaire produced conflicting results. To some respondents birth trauma meant medical intervention during labour, such as a forceps-assisted delivery, while for others a traumatic birth meant they were delivered prematurely and almost died. Premature babies are subjected to a series of painful and frightening medical interventions as soon as they are delivered. Such interventions are probably both physically and psychologically traumatic

---

e. For more on perinatal complications, see page 108

for the newborn baby. Research has found that survivors of a "vanishing" twin pregnancy are more likely to be born prematurely, so there may be other prenatal causes for a traumatic birth, such as being a womb twin survivor.[5]

Birth trauma and wanting to commit suicide

To establish what connection there may be between birth trauma and wanting to commit suicide, the selected respondents with evidence of their twin were then divided into two groups: one group of respondents who claimed to have experienced birth trauma and a second group who did not. Among those who had experienced a traumatic birth, only 35% strongly agreed[f] with the statement: "*I have wanted to commit suicide more than once in my life.*" It seems, therefore, at least among these womb twin survivors, that the experience of a traumatic birth is not

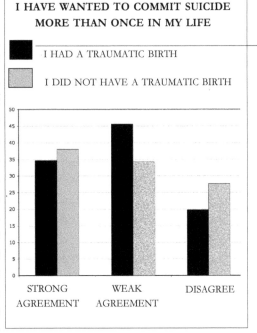

connected to suicidal ideation. In fact, in this study womb twin survivors who suffered no birth trauma at all were slightly more likely to agree with the statement than those who had experienced trauma at birth. Those who agreed less strongly with the statement were more likely to have experienced birth trauma. From this analysis it seems that there is far more to suicidal thoughts than a traumatic birth.

Other factors that have been linked to suicidal ideation include the pre- or perinatal loss of a co-twin. Intact twin pairs have a reduced risk of suicide, because of the support they can give each other.[6] On the

---

f. The levels of agreement were 1-5. For the purposes of this analysis, 1 & 2 indicated a strong agreement, 3 & 4 indicated a weak agreement, 5 indicated disagreement.

other hand, lone twins seem to be at a higher risk of suicide, as are all other bereaved people, especially those who are lonely and depressed.[7]

> *My mother's placenta weighed 25 pounds and she became very ill and then had my "brother" some time later in the form of a clump of hair, teeth and bones. I was and am still to a degree, pathologically shy and suicidal. In my past are three suicide attempts with the last being near fatal in my early twenties. I quit these efforts when I realized the pain I was causing others. I still feel strongly though that if there were no relatives that cared about me I would easily be able to kill myself given the "right" circumstances.*
> Roxanne, USA

Suicide attempts are not as random as they may seem. For example, a 1979 study of young people with a history of more than five suicide attempts each, showed that their suicide attempts always took place at the same time of year. In every case, the time of year coincided with the anniversary of their mothers' attempted abortion of the pregnancy.[8] Once these individuals had discovered that their suicide attempts were seasonal intrusions of a prenatal memory, they never attempted suicide again. It was generally assumed at the time that the trauma of the physical experience of an abortion was the trigger to suicidal thoughts but, perhaps, rather than die and leave this life, these abortion survivors simply wanted to go to the place where their twins had gone: to do this, they had to die.[9]

A GENERAL FEELING OF DISTRESS

We will now explore some common problems that you may not have previously associated with being a womb twin survivor but they have been mentioned again and again in the stories. Some womb twin survivors start life as problem children and may grow into troubled adults, with a persistent, distressing feeling of Something Wrong.

I often find it difficult to fall asleep, even when I am very tired

For many womb twin survivors, life is troubled and so is their sleep: almost half of the respondents with proof of their twin agreed strongly with this statement. They live in a state of hyper-vigilance, where Something Bad may happen at any moment and one has to be prepared. Going to sleep requires a quiet mind and a peaceful place. There are three main sleep disorders:- an inability to go to sleep; an inability to maintain sleep and an inability to return to sleeping after being awake for a short while. The first, the ability to go to sleep is of particular concern for womb twin survivors. Falling asleep requires a kind of trusting surrender that is totally at odds with hyper-vigilance. Sleep is like death and for some, falling asleep is like dying. The fear of one's own death - or a fear that someone dear will die soon - is an anxiety that comes straight out of the Dream of the Womb. Persistent insomnia has been closely connected to suicidal thoughts, sleeplessness and death. [10]

> *I have always been acutely aware of death and had insomnia as a child, fearing my parents would die in the night. I have had a lot of therapy all to no avail. I feel isolated and completely alone. I tried to fill the hole with lovers but they were not what was missing. I know now I cannot ever find what is missing - my beloved twin.*
> Pauline, USA

I get upset by silly little things

If you are acutely aware of every nuance of every situation and at the same time always watchful for danger or difficulty, then you are probably easily upset. If you are a womb twin survivor, that feeling of danger is an echo from your Dream of the Womb. Your tiny twin was too weak and fragile to survive and you are closely identified with that fragility. Out of a strange sense of utter vulnerability, it takes very little for you to feel wounded to the core. You may even become enraged.

> *My entire adult life I have battled depression and insomnia. Sometimes I get insanely angry over a small, sometimes imagined, slight and there is no reasoning with me until I calm down.*
> Becky, USA

Some womb twin survivors are rarely calm. Perhaps for you, normal life is being always agitated, worried or concerned, either for your own personal welfare or for the welfare of others. You may feel as if you "run the world" out of an exaggerated sense of responsibility for others. Such an agitated style of living seems to be a paradoxical response to coping with life, for it feels like you are "only just managing to survive", yet you possess enough strong, emotional energy to manage an agitated and aggressive response.

> NATALIE: CRYING UNCONTROLLABLY
>
> Natalie would cry uncontrollably if she had no ingredients available to make her friend's favourite cookies when she was ill. Then she would get absolutely furious and give herself an inner tirade of abuse because she could not remember where she put the car keys.

I am a perfectionist

Perfectionism is no virtue or ambition, it is a self-imposed life sentence. Some womb twin survivors have a deep need for orderliness and control. If you are like that, you are preoccupied with details and cannot tolerate even the slightest degree of messiness in others. This reveals an uneasiness with disorder, disintegration and mess, particularly within the home or workplace. There is a deeper agenda at work here, as is so often the case with womb twin survivors. Perfectionists don't have much fun, for this is serious work. In your Dream of the Womb, your Beta womb twin had some tiny flaw, which eventually and inevitably led to disintegration and death. You, the survivor, are left with a deep fear of anything imperfect, for imperfection leads to death.

> CRAIG: SUFFERING
>
> Craig says that he "suffers from perfectionism." As a brilliant artist, he feels as if nothing he does is good enough, yet everyone he meets is amazed by his accomplishments. No matter how great his success, he is quick to notice flaws in his own work. He knows he has very high expectations of himself or goals that are unrealistic, so he is doomed to fail. He makes a virtue of hard work and always strives to do his best, but pays no heed to his natural limitations.

I suffer from low self-esteem

To "suffer from low self-esteem" is a strangely illogical idea and in many ways paradoxical. It is self-imposed and if you have low self-esteem you will already know that there is no rational reason to feel that way.

When I started school I had very low self-esteem, despite being pretty and intelligent. I thought I was ugly, fat, unworthy, more stupid than my peers. I was exceptionally shy, fearing what my peers thought of me. Perhaps I tried too hard, or expected something deeper from friendships. From a very young age I would cry insatiably that I did not have a "best friend."
Susan, UK

You will probably find that being told you are wonderful may work for a while, but soon self-doubt sets in once more. You may find it very uncomfortable to be with people who treat you badly, but still you may find yourself "asking for punishment." After all, punishment can be a very useful way to express that inexplicable, vague sense of psychological distress that haunts you every day of your life. Your self-esteem cannot be lowered by unkind people, however much they taunt you, for your low level of self-esteem has been decided upon by you. You cannot be persuaded to hate yourself, unless of course it serves your secret purposes as a womb twin survivor. Even now, you may not have fully realized that this decision to hate yourself comes directly out of your Dream of the Womb. It could be that, when your womb twin seemed to turn away from you and would not relate to you any more, your foetal assumption was *no one is interested in me.* That un-tested assumption probably still underlies your deep sense of unworthiness, and is maintained as a self-inflicted wound.

I suffer from depression

As we have seen, suicidal thinking, feeling, and behaviour are core symptoms of depression, but no one is at all clear why some people become depressed. You may try to attribute your depression to something that is going on in your life, but it remains even when the bad times have passed. It may suddenly take you over and render you unable to function. Even then, you may have the clarity of thought to wonder why you feel so bad when you have so much that is good.

I was very depressed for a long time and even though I feel like I have finally conquered the depression, I still feel restless, yet fearful of moving, passionless and lost, empty and searching.
Heather, USA

210

Depression comes in waves. It can change from day to day or even from hour to hour. In the depth of a depressive episode it is like inhabiting a place filled with death, desolation and despair. You are trapped in it, and cannot escape, however hard you try. You may conquer it but it always feels as if a new wave of depression is never very far away. It is the prenatal memory of the death of your twin. It seems that R.D. Laing was very close to the Dream when he described depression as, "A state of sleep, of death, of socially-accepted madness, a womb state to which one has to die, from which one has to be born." [11]

The distress in the Dream

As a womb twin survivor yourself, you might have looked for professional help with your distress but probably you just keep on going, struggling to live a happy life. Never forget that your distress, however real it may seem to you, is all in your Dream of the Womb. In the Dream, there are a variety of very strong feelings which seem to have no basis in reality. This will be the subject of our next chapter.

19

Difficult feelings

When I was young I would frequently have strong feelings,
mostly when I was alone, that I couldn't explain.
Greg, USA

This chapter will explore the statements that relate to feelings, taken from the Womb Twin research questionnaire. The table below shows what proportion of the selected respondents[a] agreed strongly with each of these statements.[b]

DIFFICULT FEELINGS - QUESTIONNAIRE RESPONSES	%
Free-floating feelings	
I have a problem with expressing anger - either there is too much or too little	59.3
I always feel in some way unsatisfied but I don't know why	56.0
I grieve deeply and for a very long time after someone close to me, or a beloved pet, has died	49.6
I find disappointment very painful	48.4
I find it hard to forgive the people who have hurt me	43.8
Weakness and fear	
I generally lack energy and motivation	36.8
I frequently feel unable to cope with life	36.8
I am afraid of being alone in the dark	33.6
Guilt and shame	
I feel guilty about everything	35.9
I feel guilty about being alive at all	18.5

a.   The respondents who were able to provide evidence of their twin.

b.   The levels of agreement were 1-5. The term "agreed strongly" refers only to the respondents who checked "1" as the strongest possible agreement with the statement. This explanation applies to all statistics provided for the statements described in this chapter, except where indicated.

FREE-FLOATING FEELINGS

If you are a womb twin survivor and have not yet been able fully to unravel your Dream of the Womb, then your feelings may not make much sense to you at the moment. To make sense of them you will probably have created some seemingly irrational beliefs in order to find a place for these free-floating feelings to come to rest. Free-floating feelings are very disturbing and unsettling to experience and can make you feel as if you are going crazy. In this chapter we will see how they are in fact perfectly rational when considered in the context of the Dream of the Womb.

I have a problem with expressing anger - either there is too much or too little

Anger is a strong and powerful emotion. The appropriate expression of strength and personal power by means of anger is a problem for many womb twin survivors. Finding it difficult to express your personal power is related to the two-fold character of the womb twin survivor. If you are a womb twin survivor, you probably spend most of your life re-enacting the life of your weaker, Beta twin while knowing that you are the strong Alpha survivor. This dual existence creates an inner conflict about who you are and how to express your personal power. There are many subtle ways to resolve this split. For example, some people adopt the public false face of their weaker Beta twin and conceal their true Alpha feelings.

> IRENE: I NEVER GET ANGRY
>
> Irene has claimed for years that she "never gets angry." She avoids confrontation wherever she can. She just smiles and continues to "comply" in a false, exaggerated way. She seems to be completely unaware that her behaviour is very provocative. When other people are driven to anger by her false compliance, Irene is privately critical of their lack of control over their own anger. She admits no anger or irritation, only to "feeling disappointed" that people do not behave as calmly as she would wish.

When you deny your normal, angry feelings in this way to keep your Beta twin alive in your life, your powerful Alpha feelings will need to

213

find an outlet. However, to preserve your adopted "Beta status" they must remain hidden. Denied an outlet, angry feelings develop into a bitter indignation at having been "treated unfairly." If you can't remember some unfair or cruel treatment you can always exaggerate a small slight into a major episode of "rejection." Alternatively, if there is no place for your floating anger to settle, you may simply look for reasons to be angry with yourself.

> *I fear confrontation and this has had a severe impact on my marriage relationship as well as with my wider family. I feel a lot of resentment inside and I find it difficult to deal with this. I end up turning it in on myself and then go into the darkness of depression.*
> Tom, Ireland

Unresolved resentment is an excellent place to allow a floating feeling of anger to come to rest, as long as there is something to resent that can continue indefinitely. An ongoing vehicle for resentment, for example, would be to spend your life being unwillingly self-sacrificing. You could imagine you have been "forced" to become a servant to the world.

> *One thing I wonder about is my being extremely self-sacrificing but not in a good way. It builds up resentment. My husband can sprawl out on the bed, and I'll take up as little room as possible. If I'm in the center seat on an airplane, I'll use neither armrest, giving them up to those on either side who already have an armrest.*
> Tess, USA

I always feel in some way unsatisfied but I don't know why

Finding out why you feel so unsatisfied will be an important element in your healing. You may be running a "womb script"[c] about unmet needs, unanswered questions and frustrated desires.

> *I don't have many friends and none of my friendships lasted very long. When they end it, it leaves me utterly devastated. But it's always a silent suffering. I used to talk to my twin when I was little but it got too difficult to handle, so I stopped. Recently I began writing her letters in my journal but that's only made my yearning for her more difficult to bear.*
> Minnie, USA

---

c. A series of foetal assumptions arising out of your Dream of the Womb, see p. 215

If you are a womb twin survivor just beginning your healing journey, you may have felt for a long time that floating feeling of yearning for Something but never knew what would satisfy you. A good start may be to understand that you are yearning to be reunited with your lost twin, who is there just out of reach, in your Dream of the Womb.

I grieve deeply and for a very long time after someone close to me, or a beloved pet, has died

The loss of a loved person or pet in born life is probably too close to the loss of your womb twin. The Womb Twin research project found that among individuals where the zygosity of their lost twin was known, the MZ survivors were more likely than the DZ survivors to agree strongly

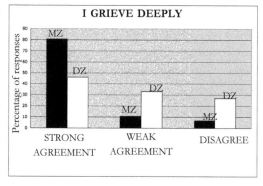

with this statement. A study of adult twins carried out in the USA in 2002 showed that higher levels of general bereavement-related behaviour were found among MZ twins than among DZ twins.[1]

> *I can only describe it as like having had a shrieking grief in my center behind my soul, not in the middle but behind it. Anguish like a part of me is dead and nothing solves it. On any day, there's a swath of grief in me that no one sees.*
> *Sean, USA*

If you are a womb twin survivor who grieves for a long time, you will know that yours is a complex form of grieving, which is heartfelt but inappropriately lengthy for the circumstances. Long-term, unresolved grief is a floating feeling from your Dream of the Womb.

> *I have trouble getting intimate with a man and when a relationship breaks I am on the edge of depression. My first love died of cancer when I was twenty years old. For me that pain was so deep that it prevented me from really living for the next twenty years. It was the trauma of my lost twin all over again.*
> *Tina, Canada*

215

A womb twin usually dies in the womb because he or she is the weaker one. The survivor is left in grief but inherits all the space and blood supply. In born life, many womb twin survivors feel deep resentment if someone close to them is weakened by sickness and dies. This is just a bit too close for comfort, because in their Dream of the Womb was a tiny twin who was too weak to stay alive.

I find disappointment very painful

A real disappointment, the origin of that painful feeling, is there to be found in your Dream of the Womb. The brief presence of a lively and stimulating womb companion who eventually stops moving and responding is a genuine disappointment for you, the sole survivor. Your initial foetal assumption would be *The Way Things Are is always having Something moving close by*. After the death of your twin, the assumption was completely overturned. The promise, that this situation would continue indefinitely, was broken. In time a new assumption was created: *The Something close by will stop moving and responding to me after a while and leave me alone.* This was your original prenatal disappointment. It has become a womb script, borrowed from your Dream of the Womb, generalized and applied widely thereafter in born life. A womb script is a section of your pre-birth story that is re-enacted again and again in born life. It perpetuates and solidifies that final foetal assumption you made about the Way Things Are. In this case the womb script that you live by is *I am always going to be disappointed.* Disappointment is the unfulfilled expectation of a positive feeling and there are plenty of subjects to be found in normal life that would make a great place for a floating feeling of disappointment to settle. A mechanism for preserving disappointment, used commonly by womb twin survivors, is to adopt very high expectations of others.

> *I know love isn't perfect, and sometimes I wonder if I'm expecting too much from my partner - having ridiculous expectations. I worry that I will feel this way my whole life and never really be happy inside, just always be pretending.*
> Julia, Australia

If you are a womb twin survivor and a perfectionist, your expectations of yourself, other people and the world in general, will be very high. You are guaranteed to live in a state of perpetual disappointment.

This may well suit your secret purposes, which are to keep alive the broken promises and disappointment that lie in your Dream of the Womb.

I find it hard to forgive the people who have hurt me

To find it hard to forgive is to hold on to hurt. The quickest way to hurt a womb twin survivor is to deny them love where love would normally be expected, such as from a member of the family or an intimate friend. If you are a womb twin survivor and there is someone in your life whose hurtful actions are very hard to forgive, then it may be worth considering exactly what it is you are holding on to.

> *No matter how much work I do on myself, I feel restless, irritable, tearful and depressed. I have a well of anger, bitterness and resentment that sits in my solar plexus, like a cesspit. Sometimes it rises up and spills out, but mostly it just sits there rotting. I'm acutely aware of it all the time. I want to be a kind, generous person and help others to heal, but the anger is preventing me.*
> Vicky, Australia

There are just two reasons why you are finding forgiveness difficult, and neither of them has to do with a "weakness of character." The first is that you probably have in your Dream of the Womb a sense of betrayal. Your twin was taken from you and it probably feels as if you are being punished for something you have not done. The sense of betrayal is probably another aspect of that disappointed foetal assumption, *my twin will stay with me forever.* Never to forgive a hurt would provide a seemingly reasonable place to settle a painful, floating feeling of betrayal and rage that still remains, in your Dream of the Womb.

WEAKNESS AND FEAR

Some womb twin survivors feel like two people. Their Alpha side is strong and powerful while their Beta side is weak and helpless. Their Dream of the Womb is a meld of these two feelings.

I generally lack energy and motivation

In this case, your energy may be physical or psychological. A lack of physical energy can be overcome with sufficient motivation: even the most exhausted individual will continue to strive and struggle if there is sufficient reason to do so. The critical element is psychological. To be aware of your lack of motivation is to know there is a lack of powerful, active psychological energy inside you. It is your Alpha energy, your inheritance as a womb twin survivor, that is lacking. Instead there is a lifeless, pointless feeling, based on your foetal assumption, *it's all too much for me to cope with, I am overwhelmed.* If you are a womb twin survivor who lacks motivation, it may feel as if some deterrent or encumbrance is preventing you from using your Alpha power and acting with efficacy. Perhaps you operate from a pessimistic belief about what is not possible. Yet deep inside you, there is a secret sense of your own power and mastery which may surface and become public from time to time.

> *There are times when I feel really energetic and motivated, but many times when I do have a general feeling of having no energy and motivation, although I have a great feeling of wanting to accomplish many things. Knowing that I can, and I very often do, accomplish many great things and am actually successful - and appear to be very successful to other people - is always looming in the background of the lack of energy and motivation.*
> May, USA

Womb twin survivors who adopt a truly "powerless" mode of being, have denied their Alpha energy. In order to emulate their Beta twin, they create an entire false Beta persona, which can be quite convincing. Some womb twin survivors truly are surviving Beta twins and this is their natural personality. How can you tell if your lack of energy and motivation is to do with denying your own Alpha energy or it is real Beta energy? The answer is in self-defeating behaviour and the strong resistance to changing it. That takes real motivation and plenty of energy! We will see later how strong your resistance to changing your behaviour can be, and this is where your Alpha energy will be revealed. [d]

I frequently feel unable to cope with life

True Beta twin characteristics such as weakness and a struggle to survive, would make it hard for you to cope with the ordinary stresses of everyday life. However, Beta womb twin survivors do not waste energy panicking or feeling fear. They are already equipped to surrender to forces far

---

d.   Self-defeating behaviour is described in Chapter 22

stronger than themselves. Meanwhile, false Beta womb twin survivors, who carry a floating feeling of weakness, depend on another person to use their Alpha energy to protect and preserve for them a quiet "half-life." They exaggerate small problems, such as losing a handkerchief, into a catastrophe, all because their foetal assumption is *I can't cope*. The outworking of assuming *I can't cope* has been called "learned helplessness" which is the effect of exposure to events which one cannot control.[2] Learned helplessness is a popular concept in psychology, but no one seems to be clear about where it originates. It could be attributed to any traumatic experience in which the individual is incapable of exerting control. In 1920 Sigmund Freud noticed in his patients, a compulsion to repeat a trauma.[3] Of course, endless repetition only serves to perpetuate the chronic feelings of helplessness that a trauma may bring. If you have a compulsion to repeat a trauma, this may be to settle a floating feeling of helplessness from your Dream of the Womb.

I am afraid of being alone in the dark

When alone in the dark, the connection with the Dream of the Womb can be very clear. As an embryo and a foetus, you spent every moment of your life accompanied by another responsive Something. Then one day you were left alone in the darkness of the womb.

> *I had a brother in the womb with me and he died early on. It is only in the last six or so years that I have begun to see and explore the true significance of this. As a child I remember terrible fear in the dark in my room, and that the walls and roof were being sucked away from me, and that I was shrinking smaller and smaller. I used to also have these visions that white cloth was billowing around and over me, that I was being suffocated and captured.*
> *Jerry, USA*

This feeling of being left alone can vary. It may feel like being the *terrified captive of Something Else that could be a Potential Threat*. It may be a memory of gradually outgrowing your weak little companion, who had ceased to respond. Or it could be a memory of being a forsaken and lonely little person, hanging off the side of the womb in an echoing darkness where once there was life.

219

GUILT AND SHAME

Guilt and shame are the most common of unpleasant experiences but also the least discussed, for we find them excruciatingly humiliating. These feelings are not the same. Guilt is an inner feeling related to something you have done or failed to do. Shame comes from contact with society, and is a feeling of disgrace and humiliation that is cast upon you by other people. Some womb twin survivors have within them a sense of toxic shame, which has created for them the identity of being a flawed and defective human being. If you are a womb twin survivor you may already have found several reasons to feel worthless. Toxic shame is self-imposed but it probably does not feel that way to you.

> *I was full of so much pain, was so terrified of life because of the rigid, perfectionistic, black and white perspective I had learned growing up. I was full of toxic shame, so sure that I was unworthy, unlovable, and truly a defective person.*
> John, UK

To preserve your self-respect you have to cover your toxic shame with pride. If you do that, every path you may wish to take in order to fulfil your life will be blocked by your own pride. The rigid structure that you will have created to protect yourself from shame will imprison you. You may choose to believe that this rigidity has been forced upon you, but in truth you willingly adopted it and this is where your Dream of the Womb is revealed. Your foetal assumption is *I am defective*, so you are living the life of your Beta twin. That means you are unable to live a full life, you have no real existence and you are captive by forces you don't understand. That is how you live and you are ashamed of yourself for living that way. This is how you have kept your Dream alive.

I feel guilty about everything

Womb twin survivors are very good at feeling guilty for no particular reason. Guilt floats about between womb twin survivors as they each seek out a receptacle for their floating guilt feelings. Some womb twin survivors feel a sense of responsibility to look after everyone. If anything should befall a loved one it must be their fault.

For a long time in my life I thought I have a right to live only if I care for others. I always had the feeling to be "too much" for others, to be unimportant or even disturbing or dangerous for others. When I fell in love with my husband, I was torn between extreme feelings of love and fear of losing him, between the wish to be close to him all the time and the panic to lose my own space. Often I thought I was not good for him, I often was close to ending the relationship (that has now lasted for ten years!) I always felt guilty for anything bad that happened to him, for any problems between us.
Petra, Germany

Irrational guilt feelings are taken straight from your Dream of the Womb. You were the only one able to survive, so out of a sense of survivor guilt you take responsibility for the welfare of the people you love and make great sacrifices on their behalf.

I feel guilty about being alive at all

Only 18.5% of the selected respondents agreed strongly with this statement, which is considerably less than the generalized sense of guilt described above. This was a surprising result, because a high incidence of survivor

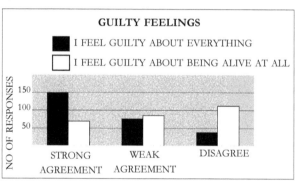

guilt was expected. However, when all of the stories were analysed, survivor guilt was found to be there as a strong undercurrent. For instance, some womb twin survivors feel that they "should not be here." They find it very hard to forgive themselves for being the one who lived.

To complicate things even further, my son is probably also a womb twin survivor. When I was pregnant with him, I had bleeding in the eighth week and the doctor who made an ultrasonic scan told me there were two embryos. My son developed a very similar attitude towards life as I have - "Why am I here? I shouldn't be here at all."
Anka, Germany

221

DAN: WASTING HIS LIFE

Dan is wasting his life, and he knows it. He is a caring, intelligent husband and father but he has a dead-end job, which does not bring in much money. He has to work long hours to earn what he does. When he finally does come home, he looks half dead. Meanwhile, his wife goes out to work to pay the bills and she and the children hardly see him to speak to. Dan is a womb twin survivor. He never realized it until recently but half of him is dead. He manages to be physically present at home with his family but he is usually asleep and generally uncommunicative. Only when he is outside the home does he come alive. When his wife sees him at work she is surprised how much energy he has and how respected he is.

If you are a womb twin survivor and you feel as if half of you is dead, your "dead half" is not you but your Beta womb twin. It is survivor guilt that holds you back, shrink-wrapped into a corner. You are living out only half a life, in a poignant re-enactment of the still body of your womb twin, who was squeezed into a corner of the womb as you grew. To atone for the sin of being the strong survivor, you have sacrificed half your life for your womb twin.

I have always been an extremely intelligent, artistic, and creative person. But along with everything that I excel in to the world is my deep dark depression that I have had since a very small child. After learning that I was a twin in my late twenties I have had an immense amount of guilt as to why I was the one that lived.
Wendy, USA

Womb twin survivors tend to wrap their floating feelings of guilt and shame in complex disguises. As they act out the brief life of their Beta twin they may feel worthless, invisible, pathetic, ridiculous or foolish. They then employ their Alpha energy to boost their self-esteem with addiction, denial, withdrawal, rage, perfectionism, exhibitionism and arrogance. As a result, in the eyes of others they appear to be immature, ridiculous or simply stupid. Subjected to scorn or contempt, they feel their self-esteem disappear. Nevertheless they remain unrepentant, for this process serves their secret purposes most excellently. By this means,

222

they can be Alpha and Beta at the same time. They carefully preserve a floating feeling of shame to make manifest the guilt feelings in their Dream of the Womb.

Re-enactment in relationships

In the next chapter we will examine how womb twin survivors re-enact their Dream of the Womb in their relationships, sometimes in ways that are remarkably complex but which accurately reflect a vague memory of pre-birth events.

20

A problem with relationships

I spend most of my time alone and have a difficult time connecting with others.
Heather, USA

This chapter will consider the statements from the Womb Twin research questionnaire concerned with relationships. The table below shows what proportion of the selected respondents[a] agreed strongly with each of these statements.[b]

A PROBLEM WITH RELATIONSHIPS - QUESTIONNAIRE RESPONSES	
Loneliness and isolation	%
I fear rejection	72.9
I fear abandonment	64.2
Deep down, I feel alone, even when I am among friends	62.2
Problems with intimacy	
I make a lot of effort to protect my privacy	46.9
I don't let other people get close to me	32.0
I spend a lot of time talking to myself in a mirror	28.4
Broken relationships	
I easily get into a love/hate relationship with individuals I want to get close to	40.1
I have been in an exploitative relationship with another person	34.0
Painful relationships	
I get very intense and involved at the start of a relationship but then I sabotage it somehow	47.8
It upsets me if I am unable to reduce the suffering of others	42.0

a.   The respondents able to provide evidence of their twin.

b.   The levels of agreement were 1-5. The term "agreed strongly" refers only to the respondents who checked "1" as the strongest possible agreement with the statement. This explanation applies to all statistics provided for the statements described in this chapter, except where indicated.

Truly to understand what being a womb twin survivor can do to your relationships, you have to take a look at the very first relationship you ever had. If you are a womb twin survivor, that first relationship was not with your parents, it was with your womb twin.[1] You came to birth with a template, already hard-wired into your brain, about what happens when you reach out to another living being. Depending on what that was like for you, your assumptions about every relationship since then have been based on your Dream of the Womb. All your life, you have re-enacted whatever style of relationship you had in the womb with your womb twin, in every close and intimate relationship.

LONELINESS AND ISOLATION

If you are a womb twin survivor, in your Dream of the Womb there is a feeling of aloneness that is vague and all-pervading. It finds expression in all your relationships in born life.

I fear rejection

This was the second most popular statement, according to the Womb Twin research analysis.[c] When compared with the fear of abandonment it was found that 168 respondents agreed strongly with both statements.

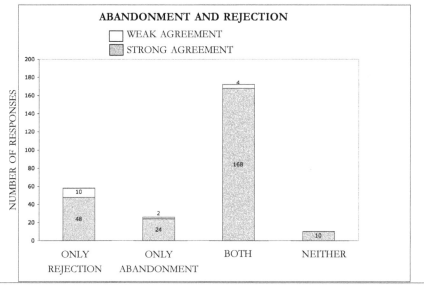

c.   For the full analysis see Appendix B

225

The term "rejection" has two meanings, both of which are suggestive of the Dream of the Womb. The medical term refers to an immune response to a tissue, so that the tissue fails to survive. The social term is to dismiss someone as a failure. Your womb twin was indeed unable to remain in the womb with you and failed to survive.

> *I often feel abandoned or shut out by everyone I meet, as if they're disgusted by me. I often long for a special kind of hug - not just a general one given by a mother but a more meaningful yet secretive one.*
> *Amy, USA*

In the mysterious muddle of pre-birth memories that make up your Dream of the Womb, there is no time or place and certainly no sense of who you are. It would be quite natural to assume that you are *dismissed as a failure,* for you carry a dim memory of your twin rejecting you - that is, ceasing to relate to you. Perhaps the assumption and the memory have become conflated in your mind. In born life, if a dear friend ceases to relate to you, that may trigger a memory of that original rejection. There are many ways to prevent yourself from being rejected: a common one is to work hard to create and carefully maintain close and intimate relationships with others. Another strategy is simply to remain alone, for then one cannot be rejected. The fear of rejection is so strong in some womb twin survivors that they feel unsafe in the company of other people. They are so fearful and withdrawn that their parents and friends may experience a sense of helpless frustration in trying to reach them and simply give up. From the womb twin survivor's point of view, that would be rejection. Being different can create a sense of *not being found acceptable,* which is another word for rejected. Some womb twin survivors find it very hard to be found acceptable to others and may try, a little bit too hard perhaps, to make people love them.

> *I'm a very depressive guy living always in a state of sadness, writing poetry or painting canvas. I fear rejection from my family and from my partners. I'm gay and I have always been looking for a guy to be more like my soul-brother than my partner. I always feel empty, unloved, rejected, and I want to give everything to others, even when I get nothing back.*
> *Miguel, Mexico*

A fear of commitment can arise out of the dread of close, intimate loving relationships coming to an end with subsequent feelings of rejection. A fear of commitment brings loneliness, so the Dream of the Womb is realized once again. Some womb twin survivors test close relationships because of their fear of rejection. They insist upon being un-cooperative, unhelpful and inconsiderate toward others. They badly need to discover just how much the other person is prepared to accept. This tendency to test intimate relationships to destruction keeps the Dream alive. Having exhausted everyone's patience, they will be left alone, rejected and friendless.

I fear abandonment

Some young babies are quite happy to be left alone and will lie quietly for a long time, looking around them. Others quickly become distressed if left alone. Probably, the second group are the womb twin survivors. [d]

> I know that there are other scenarios in life that warrant such emotional pain and depression, but it is this all-consuming and overwhelming struggle I have with attachment and abandonment that is still with me, despite all the healing that I've had. Deep inside of me I still feel different to other people. I struggle interminably with trusting people to want me around or like me. I always expect people to leave me.
>
> Jane, UK

Various explanations for a fear of abandonment have been put forward by experts. There is a general assumption among psychologists that the primary relationship for every baby is with the primary carers. It is thought that the breaking of the attachment bond with primary carers causes trauma, which triggers a fear of abandonment. [2] If you are a womb twin survivor, you will know that your primary bond was formed in the womb with your twin. [3] For you, experiences of physical abandonment in born life will of course be traumatic, and may include being torn away from your mother at birth and put into a nursery, given up for adoption or being left in foster care. These experiences are traumatic because they are reminiscent of being left forsaken and alone when your co-twin died.

---

d.   For more about young womb twin survivors, see Chapter 13

As a child I spent most of my time playing by myself, wandering in the woods. I didn't want company most of the time. When I did make friends, I tended to be fiercely possessive of them, and was jealous of any other friends they might have. I was afraid that I would lose them. As I got older, I continued to have those strong attachments, longings and fears of loss. I am still trying to learn to deal with them in ways other than shutting people out entirely.
Sara, USA

A whole new vocabulary has been created in the general literature to explain the fear of abandonment in adults. In 1997 a national study was made of a range of adult attachment styles.[4] Childhood maltreatment or neglect was found to be associated with a fearful way of relating to others, widely known as "anxious attachment," which is another way of describing a fear of abandonment. An intolerance of aloneness is also characteristic of people with borderline personality disorder (BPD).[5] To date, there has been no research study to test if people with BPD are womb twin survivors, but there is a considerable overlap in the characteristics of both groups.

Deep down, I feel alone, even when I am among friends

A feeling of being alone at a deep level inside yourself, regardless of how many wonderful friends you may have, is part of your Dream. After your twin died, there may have been many weeks and months when you were indeed alone in the womb.

I lost my soul mate thirteen years ago. I started to really work with this aspect of my life, intentionally healing. During all of this time, the only close relationships I have been able to sustain have been at a distance, and I have suffered horribly from losing my dear friend. Many times I have thought that loneliness was literally killing me, that the pain of being alone was completely unbearable.
Ella, USA

The loss of a co-twin at birth is no less isolating. Womb twin survivors display many of the same characteristics of twin-less twins, who were born together but one twin died at a much later stage in life. These include a feeling of painful loneliness.[e]

---

e. For more about the feelings of a twin-less twin see Chapter 11.

LAURA: A LONELY WOMB TWIN SURVIVOR

From an early age Laura wanted to be a twin. She had a great fascination with twins and twins run in her family. She has always been searching for something without knowing what. Throughout her teenage years she withdrew and was very depressed. She self-harmed by cutting and burning herself and developed severe anxiety. She often has difficult and very intense relationships with others. She much prefers to have close, intimate friendships with few people rather than many acquaintances, but she has always felt alone. As far as she knows, she is not autistic, but she does have some of the symptoms. She is highly intelligent, a dreamer, good at empathy, extremely perceptive and very lonely.

PROBLEMS WITH INTIMACY

All womb twin survivors know what it is to be alone. For some it is painful and may even be traumatic, so one way never to be left alone is to avoid intimate relationships of all kinds.

I make a lot of effort to protect my privacy.

If you had several weeks of interaction with your womb twin, you had a chance to be at least vaguely aware that there was *Someone Out There Somewhere*. In that case, your womb script will be this: you meet someone but, after the initial excitement of getting to know one another, the relationship *seems to die*. You somehow expect it, but you feel bound to remain with this person out of loyalty. Still, there is a feeling of being let down, for the good times were over so soon. In your Dream of the Womb is the foetal assumption that *love dies too soon*. The womb script demands that you avoid love altogether, to fulfil the assumption, *it won't last*. Womb twin survivors running a womb script of this kind will choose to remain private. They will create for themselves a safe, personal world where no one will come and hurt them or betray their trust with empty promises.

I have always felt outside looking in. I never let anyone get close to me and am often told that I always hold something back. I am very guarded about my life.
Mel, USA

229

In your private, inner world, the familiar sense of lack that arises out of disappointed expectations can be carefully maintained. Your inner and outer lives can be kept separate. There will be no invasion into your inner world by people offering friendship, who you cannot trust to stay.

I don't let other people get close to me

Some womb twin survivors convince themselves that they do not mind being alone, for that's normal. They convince themselves that they don't need other people. No one can be trusted anyway, so why bother to get close to them, only to be disappointed? If this is your life, long ago you built a great wall around yourself within which you can live without ever being hurt again. You now have a well-maintained, inner space, which will keep you safely away from intimacy for life and defended against hurt - but is it really what you want?

> *From the time I was a small kid, I had the feeling of "being an outsider." Standing outside the circle, watching the others play and a strong feeling of not belonging. I have that feeling in most groups. It doesn't make it easier to be happy to be alive. But in recent years I noticed that I am more sensitive than many of my colleagues and family. I also discovered that I had built a very thick concrete wall around the sensitive part, in order to protect it.*
> *Kristina, USA*

Human beings are social animals and we all need each other. We need our parents, but some young womb twin survivors deliberately alienate them. We need our friends, but some womb twin survivors get either too close and become totally enmeshed, or they push other people away. You may have a real problem with trusting other people to remain faithful. Learning to trust was a primitive affair and began for you in the womb. Because the Beta twins usually do not survive, we will assume that in the womb you were the Alpha twin, who ran the relationship.[f] A twitch of your leg, for instance, got an answering swirl in the amniotic fluid. Your actions may or may not have always elicited a discernible response, but you were capable of learning and therefore able to hope that the response will happen again. If twitching your leg made

---

f.   It is understood that, in some cases, the Beta twin is the sole survivor.

something happen a reasonable number of times, then by a process of conditioning[g] you would continue to twitch until you there was kind of response. The responsiveness in your twin would have become part of your idea of the Way Things Are. This was overturned when your twin died. Your womb script now is *if I reach out, there may be no response, and I will be alone once more.* That is what hurts, so you no longer reach out.

I spend a lot of time talking to myself in a mirror

This statement seems to suggest that womb twin survivors seek out a mirror image of themselves.[h] This may be their lost mirror-image twin. Talking to yourself is generally considered pathological. It is one of the many symptoms of schizophrenia and has also been classified as a symptom of a developmental disorder.[6] Yet for the many womb twin survivors who do talk to themselves, it seems the most natural thing in the world and is an excellent antidote to loneliness. Perhaps for you, your image in the mirror is not necessarily a reflection of yourself but truly your other half, your twin. It can be a comfort to summon up another version of yourself and have a good talk to them. For a young womb twin survivor, the image in the mirror can substitute for an imaginary friend. For an adult, it can still be reassuring to gaze at one's own image and talk to it as if it were another person.

> *I am left-handed and I remember as a child talking to the mirror a lot and playing by myself but it was as if someone else was there. I played alone a lot and I have always been happy to be in my own company because I feel like someone else is there. I am most comfortable alone.*
> Michelle, Ireland

Some womb twin survivors go to great lengths to reconstitute the twin pair. The image in the mirror can give a false sense of two-ness.

> *I always have wanted a twin. I have even gone up to the mirror and taken photos to make it look like there are two of me. Then I used Photoshop to put two of me into a photo. I have even cried at times seeing two of me in the photo.*
> Kat, New Zealand

---

g. For more about foetal conditioning, see page 142

h. For more about mirror-image twins, see page 26

BROKEN RELATIONSHIPS

If you are a womb twin survivor your very first relationship, which you had with your twin, was broken. This may have become a template for all your relationships since then. If so, you may find a pattern in your life. Your womb script may be *my closest and most intimate relationships frequently break down, leaving me feeling sad and alone.*

I have been in an exploitative relationship with another person

If you are a womb twin survivor and you have ever been exploited, this could be a womb script. To keep your Dream alive, you may have a deep emotional need for a style of connection that resembles the one you had with your twin. As a consequence, you will sacrifice anything to keep close relationships alive. Additionally, you may allow intimate relationships to develop that are not good for you. You may choose a friend or partner who uses you and doesn't have empathy with your feelings. You may choose to tolerate selfishness in the other person and thus condemn yourself to a one-way relationship, all taking and no giving. No matter how little empathy or consideration your partner has for your needs, you remain with them. This is the price you are willing to pay to keep the Dream of the Womb alive in your life: you can have a close, intimate relationship but still remain alone and hurting.

I easily get into a love/hate relationship with individuals I want to get close to

The paradox of a love/hate relationship neatly encapsulates the twin-twin relationship in a particular situation. For some reason, a functional intrauterine relationship between twins is impossible, such as when twins develop very differently from each other and one dies as a direct result. The womb script that arises out of this eventuality is, *I hate you but please don't leave me!* Love can turn to hatred very easily if there is a betrayal of trust, and love without trust is impossible for most people. Some womb twin survivors have a particular problem with trusting people to stay. In fact, rather than be abandoned or betrayed themselves, they may pre-empt the possibility by choosing to end the relationship.

I fell out of love with my partner and I was the one who did the leaving, never to trust or love like I had with her ever again. I still love her, but I would never go back. I remember feeling that the end of this relationship felt like a death had occurred. I have no regrets in my decision, as betrayal does not settle well with me.

Rosalind, USA

Some womb twin survivors incite hatred towards themselves, as if they want to be hated. They push people away by choosing to be difficult. They make no effort to maintain the relationship. They exploit others, because they expect others to reach out to them but they reach out to no one. If they meet a womb twin survivor who is willing to be exploited in this way, the relationship may work well for a while, but eventually the one who is exploited will run out of patience. Then love will turn to hate. The final result is that both womb twin survivors are left alone, forsaken and hurting, each lost in their personal Dream of the Womb.

HILARY: HATRED OF HER MOTHER

Hilary has always felt different. Other people seem to be comfortable with life and she craves that. Episodes of depression seem to come from nowhere and she feels intense hatred towards herself. Her parents are very loving but her mother makes Hilary very angry, just by coming into her room. Hilary cannot understand why she hates her mother so much, she just does.

PAINFUL RELATIONSHIPS

The Dream varies according to how long your twin lived. For example, if your womb twin died shortly after the merest spark of life, leaving only an unresponsive presence that lingered on to birth, then your template for relationships would be *things quickly go dead and it never works again.*

I get very intense and involved at the start of a relationship but then I sabotage it somehow

Relationship sabotage precisely reproduces the story of you and your twin in your Dream of the Womb. You and your twin were able to have some awareness of each other sufficient to create some sort of bond between you but the bond was broken by death. In born life when you make an intense connection with someone but sabotage it, you are re-enacting the breaking of that twin bond.

I get involved quickly and intensely in relationships and sabotage them by being "too much" and I wind up feeling ashamed and abandoned and weep with grief over my behavior and aloneness.
Sheila, USA

One way to sabotage a relationship is to get close to someone for a while but then push them away. Another is to be so demanding so that the other person feels "drained dry" and leaves the relationship. This womb script, *I took too much*, is based on being the Alpha twin who got most of the blood supply so that the other twin was unable to survive.

TERESA: A NEED TO BOND WITH MALES

From the age of 11 Teresa has had severe "crushes" on boys. There was one time when there were mutual feelings and they started dating. She then became incredibly emotionally attached and dependent on him. He left her after two months and the devastation was enormous. She cried constantly for weeks. She knows there is "something from her past" causing her to crave intimate bonding with males, and wonders if she once had a twin.

It upsets me if I am unable to reduce the suffering of others

Some womb twin survivors have a mission to heal people in pain and may feel upset if they are unable to help.[i] When the suffering of another person cannot be healed, the distress of the would-be healer seems to be related to empathy and survivor guilt. The rescue mission requires an inordinate degree of self-sacrifice, which for a womb twin survivor is possibly made in reparation, for surviving at the expense of the co-twin.

It upsets me if I am unable to reduce the suffering of others, I think. I take much more care of other people than of me, even if they are my colleagues. I compulsively self-harm, I drive too fast, I forget to eat or drink.
Bernice, Germany

---

i.   For more about the desire to heal the world, see page 191.

234

The desire to relieve suffering in others can become overwhelming. In extreme cases, it is the need of the womb twin survivor to relieve pain in another, rather than the need of the other person to be relieved, that is paramount. This has been called "compulsive caring" which, for the recipient, can feel more like being manipulated than truly cared for.[7]

> *I'll bend over backward to try to help or comfort others, even if it causes me trouble. It doesn't bother me for the most part, even when I'm feeling ridiculously overburdened by my own issues; I'll always take the time out to listen to them and try to help them, even though most of the time I can't help myself.*
> Susanna, Canada

Compulsive caring can be counter-productive. It can lead to unwarranted intrusion into the lives of others and exhaustion to the extent of total "burn out." The compulsion to reduce suffering seems to be driven by a desire to make everything right and restore a lost world where there is no pain and no suffering. That lost world is probably the time long ago in the Dream of the Womb, before it all went wrong and a Special Someone became exhausted, could not cope with life any more, faded away and was gone.

Acting out the Dream in self-sabotage

The next chapter will consider particular kinds of behaviour. This is another non-verbal way in which womb twin survivors try to express what lies in their Dream of the Womb. There are a variety of ways to turn your vague and confusing pre-birth memories into a kind of coded behaviour, which we are gradually beginning to decipher.

21
Self-sabotage

I try things for a while and then, "Halt! This isn't working, this isn't right."
This is the story of my life.
Joan, Australia

This chapter will explore the statements about three kinds of self-sabotage, taken from the Womb Twin research questionnaire. The table below shows what proportion of the selected respondents [a] agreed strongly with each of these statements. [b]

SELF-SABOTAGE - QUESTIONNAIRE RESPONSES	
Hyperactivity	%
I have been searching for something all my life but I don't know what it is	68.4
All my life I have felt restless and unsettled	55.0
I am easily bored	48.7
I know I do not rest enough	44.7
Blocks to healing	
I have strong, inner imaginary life that I use as a coping mechanism	50.4
Sabotaging success	
I want to succeed but I always end up somehow sabotaging my chances of success	44.7

Self-sabotage is so widespread that one could consider it a general human failing or part of the human condition. Viewed objectively however,

---

a. The respondents who were able to provide evidence of their twin.

b. The levels of agreement were 1-5. The term "agreed strongly" refers only to the respondents who checked "1" as the strongest possible agreement with the statement. This explanation applies to all statistics provided for the statements described in this chapter, except where indicated.

in the process of self-sabotage foolish acts are willingly carried out that deliberately dismantle the very foundation of a successful project. These acts are deliberate, conscious and inappropriate choices. They are not instinctual or genetically imprinted. The motive behind these choices is mysterious. If you are a womb twin survivor you will already be aware of how you sabotage your life but you may not be clear about why you do it. Once the idea that self-defeating behaviour is driven by survivor guilt is in place, then it makes perfect sense that you would not feel allowed to succeed, to have riches, good fortune or even personal happiness.

HYPERACTIVITY

Some womb twin survivors take on too much and work themselves to exhaustion. It is as if they are living for two people. They seem to have an extraordinary source of coping energy inside them which demands expression. However, they have a variety of self-defeating ways to waste this precious energy.

I have been searching for something all my life but I don't know what it is

The search for the lost twin can take many forms. It may be a desperate and lonely quest in search of some vague an ineffable Someone or Something. There are womb twin survivors to be found in far-flung places of the world, a long way from home. They only stay a while in any place and soon move on: they have not been home for years. In the vast continent of North America, a certain proportion of people choose to take to the road. They are always on the move while the rest are happy to stay at home. Could this restless group be the womb twin survivors? They may have been inspired by the ever-elusive American Dream but how much is this endless journey an echo of another Dream from long ago before birth? It is a long journey to Somewhere, but it has within it a kind of circularity. Wherever you are, you are still searching, stuck in your Dream of the Womb. Perhaps you are a womb twin survivor who has travelled far from home for reasons you do not quite understand. Perhaps your journeying provides a mode of expression for a deep and painful sense of longing that is never satisfied. You can make your home anywhere but you never belong. You make sure of that by always moving on.

It is a fruitless search, seeking Someone who can never be found. The search may take you into a series of relationships, as you seek out that mysterious, pre-birth twin bond that feels so essential to your well-being. In turn, even after many years, each relationship will prove a disappointment, for it can never replace the intimate bond that is your template for all relationships in your life.

> *I do think I've always been searching for someone to share with at a level that everyone else just falls short of reaching. It's like I've always been looking for that special twin intimacy, but never really find it. I've resigned myself to looking for different things in different people, rather than expecting to find absolutely everything that I need emotionally, in one package. I'm probably overly-open and empathize too easily, share too readily, because I'm always looking for that connection that subconsciously I feel I would have had with my twin.*
> Breda, Australia

Some people feel as if they are searching for themselves. They imagine that they *only partly exist in this world*. Perhaps you are a womb twin survivor and feel this way. If so, you may be in search of *a missing part of yourself*, which is your lost twin. If you do not understand that, you will continue to sabotage your life by never accepting the world and your life as it is.

All my life I have felt restless and unsettled

One way to cope with psychological distress is to avoid thinking about it by being busy. Frenetic activity, constant changes of job, moving house every year and moving from one relationship to another are all signs of being restlessness and unsettled.

> LYNNE: ALWAYS ON THE MOVE
> Lynne, whose twin died in the womb, feels as if she was "cursed" before birth and is constantly depressed. No matter how much she tries to be normal, she says, "This unacknowledged loss is on the tip of my tongue." She lives alone and has created thirty-six different homes for herself in thirty-eight years.

Constant, restless movement is like a journey that always turns in upon itself. As much as you try to avoid the pain, it dogs your footsteps and you never seem to move forward. If you are a womb twin survivor and you have always been restless, then staying in the same place or continuing to do the same thing for a long time may seem somehow wrong. The desire to keep moving may arise out of a deep, inner doubt about your ability to take root and grow.

> *I had five or six jobs before I got married and the longest job I had lasted about six months. Before I got married my relationships didn't last, which made me feel real rejected, but then it was the other person had their own issues at times. I'm quite flirty, I don't want to be but when I get positive attention from someone I like, I like to be around that person. It annoys my husband but I tell him I'm just a friendly person, which I am.*
> Kat, New Zealand

Never finding a place to settle may be in your Dream of the Womb. You might carry a memory of one or more embryos that never managed to implant properly in the womb wall. This could be why you cannot allow yourself to take root and grow. You find it hard to slow down, remain in the same place and stay in the same job for a long time. To be static may seem unthinkable to you at the moment, like a living death, but consider how little you allow yourself to develop. A rolling stone may indeed gather no moss but it is the static stones that are strongest and are chosen to build our greatest monuments. A restlessness of character may be related to trying hard to control events, stop bad things happening to people and keep people happy. It can be related to a vague sense of dread that *a Bad Thing is about to happen*, which is straight out of your Dream of the Womb. The Bad Thing is the death of your twin. Your foetal assumption is, *after a while, the Bad Thing will start to happen* and you live that out as your womb script. Naturally enough, after the initial joys of any new experience, your familiar sense of restlessness begins to increase, along with a vague sense of dread. Yet again, your Dream is realized. You move on, leaving behind an unfinished project, an unrealized dream and possibly also some very disappointed colleagues, who are sad to see you go. Meanwhile, in the far distance is a mysterious, hidden place where everything is fresh and new: that is what keeps you on the move.

I am easily bored

This statement suggests that some womb twin survivors feel as if their life is devoid of meaning and direction. This is certainly true for some. "There ought to be more to life; there is something missing!" they cry. That mysterious, vital spark would bring new energy and life but it is gone. Some womb twin survivors choose not to live a full life but remain frustrated. They use boredom as an excuse for not seizing opportunities in every moment. They are too busy being bored to take part in exciting and creative activities. A boredom study, carried out from 1985 to 1988 using Whitehall civil servants, concluded that those who reported being bored were more likely to die young than those who said they were not bored.[1] The study suggested that finding interest in social and physical activities may alleviate boredom and improve health, thus reducing the risk of being "bored to death." Unfortunately, boredom is a conscious self-sabotaging choice that is unlikely to change, at least until the reasons behind it are understood by the individuals concerned. Some womb twin survivors are not engaged in life at all, as if they have one foot in another world.

> *I have started many careers, jobs and projects only to get bored with them easily and go looking for the next thing to make me feel good. I thought I was the only person in the world that felt a loss like this. I thought there was no one on the planet who could understand this emptiness inside.*
> *Kris, USA*

As we have seen, the strong, inner, imaginary life of the womb twin survivor provides them with a different and possibly more exciting world than ordinary life. Boredom could be described as a petulant reluctance to engage in life. It has nothing whatever to do with what is actually going on, for it is about how interested in life you choose to be. Some womb twin survivors are easily bored at school and complain bitterly that their teacher is "no good." That is because they have chosen not to be interested. They are like butterflies, flitting about from experience to experience, never staying very long and thus missing countless opportunities to fully engage, learn and grow. Just when things might become interesting they move on, thus deliberately sabotaging their personal development. If you are a womb twin survivor and you are easily bored, you do not allow yourself to stay engaged in any activity. You either remain helplessly stuck in a foetal assumption of being *half-alive like a zombie,* or you actively disengage and move on to something else. In your Dream there may have been another brief life that started well but then disengaged and moved on. This is how you remain in a state of arrested development, always moving on and starting afresh, only to find that boredom quickly sets in once the initial excitement has passed: it is your Dream again.

BLOCKS TO HEALING

Some womb twin survivors feel constantly "stuck." They feel unable to move forward in life, as if they are transfixed between two equal and opposite energies. Sometimes they do have a vague sense of a process that must be gone through in order for the self-sabotage to cease. Usually, it is not clear what this process should be.

> *I somehow don't want to let go of my connectedness to my twin, but yet feel that I need to make connection and incorporate this special existence into my life so that my life will then swing into full motion. I feel that I'm stuck in between my old life and the new life of opportunity, abundance and potential that I crave.*
> Greg, USA

Self-sabotage is a perfect vehicle for survivor guilt. In terms of re-enacting the Dream of the Womb, it lets you have a *sad and unfulfilled existence, living half a life.* If you are a womb twin survivor the unclaimed successes of your *half-life* can be set to one side for your twin, like laying an empty place at the dinner table. Anything else would be simply unfair. Choosing to live half a life places a block on the road to your healing and satisfies your secret purpose, which is not to heal.

I have a strong inner imaginary life that I use as a coping mechanism

Keeping the Dream alive takes a great deal of imagination. For instance, creating an imaginary friend is a popular device by means of which sole surviving twins maintain a presence of their lost twin in their lives. If you are a womb twin survivor, you probably had an imaginary friend of your own. We saw in a previous chapter that talking to yourself in a mirror is common among womb twin survivors and this too requires imagination.

I've had a very strong imaginary world of my own since a little kid and it's given me a lot of comfort. Deep down, I have this immense craving for love and unity, but I find it hard to trust people and believe that I'm good enough for them. I'm terrified of the people I love leaving me. I've always used my imagination and various addictions to fill this hole in my life. I've wondered what happened back then to make me this way. I never thought this could at least partly be related to my womb twin.

Anita, Finland

The Womb Twin research project revealed that almost half of the selected respondents had an imaginary friend as a child and also agreed strongly with the statement about having a "strong inner life." The use of imagination in this way does seem to be an excellent coping mechanism. The need for personal support, comfort and companionship drives the imagination of the womb twin survivor to create all kinds of fantasies which can be a major block to healing. For example, womb twin survivors in therapy may try to turn their therapist into their twin.

CAROLINA: FANTASIES ABOUT HER THERAPIST

Carolina, a womb twin survivor on the road to healing, realized she had created an enmeshed relationship with her female therapist. The therapist had noticed that she had been made into a "substitute twin" by her client, which was enabling Carolina to cope with her life alone as a womb twin survivor. This was an unhealthy dependency and not therapeutic in the least, so once this was discovered the therapist brought the sessions to an end, leaving Carolina distraught.

The tendency to create a substitute twin in therapy been noticed for many years and has been described. For example, in the 1950s Wilfred Bion, a psychoanalyst, wrote about this tendency, which he had seen in many of his clients. [3] He described a state of mind that lay somewhere between the conscious and the unconscious, which he claimed was related to events in early life, or the intrauterine state. With access to ultrasound scans and a little more medical knowledge, Bion might have been able to recognise womb twin survivors among his clients. Today we have the benefit of detailed medical knowledge about life before birth and can fully understand why creating a substitute twin may be comforting for a womb twin survivor. By the use of imagination, the lost twin can become incorporated into the reality of born life. In a curious echo of her Dream of the Womb, Janet Frame the New Zealand poet, who was probably a "mirror-image" womb twin survivor [c] entitled the third volume of her autobiography, *The Envoy from Mirror City*.[2] An imaginary inner world is a place to go to avoid problems and difficulties. It is of particular value to hypersensitive womb twin survivors of all ages. Their strong intuitive sense makes them tentative about relationships and unusually aware of the pain of the world, so they escape into fantasy.

Manifestations

The strong inner life of the womb twin survivor can subjectively feel very real. It can include physical manifestations, such as seeing strange lights or experiencing a real sense of the presence of one's lost twin, which may feel like being haunted by a benign ghost. In childhood this sense may be very real and strong. It tends to fade towards adulthood, sometimes leaving a sense of loss in its wake.

> *When I was told about this "twin" I felt, enormously strongly, the presence of "someone" very familiar and very close, almost sitting on my left shoulder. I couldn't shake this feeling for months, and whilst rather strange it was also enormously comforting. Sadly this has mostly gone, although there are occasions when I do feel that this "person" is around.*
>
> Eliz, Ireland

For a womb twin survivor, an interior life of dreams and imagination can be a source of strength in adversity. The capacity to "tune out" of real life in time of trauma can be a great asset. However, in search of those comforting dreams, they may be tempted to remain in bed for a long time, for the sense of the lost twin is nearest when in the state of mind suspended between waking and sleeping.

I know I do not rest enough

Womb twin survivors who do not take enough rest know that they are running themselves into the ground. Not resting enough is associated

---

c.   For more about Janet Frame's twin, see page 122

with low self-esteem. If you feel you have a low value as a person or the job you do is not good enough, then you may try to put that right by working very hard indeed.

NICOLA: TAKING ON TOO MUCH

Nicola seems to attract needy people and gets upset when she cannot heal their hurt instantly. She is an artist, working from home. She moves her work from room to room, so there are materials everywhere. She longs for a tidy house, but clutter just seems to follow her everywhere - it exhausts her just to see it. She is desperate to be liked by everyone and takes on far too much responsibility and charity work. She is a workaholic but never gets anything completely finished. Sometimes she thinks she will die young, as she can't keep up with the demands she sets herself trying to fit a week into every day. There is never enough time for all her ideas and self-imposed tasks. She finds it hard to delegate and feels she should do everything herself. She gets extremely tired. She works seven days a week and her husband feels neglected: she can see why.

If you assume that your achievements are negligible and other people see you negatively, then you will stop caring about anything much, least of all your own well-being. If you secretly carry a foetal assumption that *you have no place in the world and little potential for success*, then you will struggle endlessly to prove yourself. That takes hard work. If you have feel that you many weaknesses and few strengths, a low social status and are hardly able to stand on your own two feet, then you will keep trying, long after you are completely exhausted. There is a driving inner energy that propels you forward. A lifestyle that is perpetually busy means that, even if you are exhausted, you can develop new strengths and capacities. A frenetic life is not an entirely negative thing: it feels like a wonderful creative purpose which can make your life meaningful.

I am an overachiever. I have four academic degrees. I have tried to accomplish enough achievements, both for me and my twin. I recently found out about my twin during a life-saving surgery.
Andrea, USA

244

Extremely hyperactive womb twin survivors however, are at risk of an early death because of their frantic lifestyle. There is another deeper agenda at work in their busy lives, which is to keep their Dream alive. In the Dream of the Womb there are two busy little foetuses. There are bursts of a frantic activity for a while but for one twin this leads to complete collapse and death. Working yourself into burn-out means you take the place of your own lost Beta twin, who did not have enough energy left to survive.

I've always had the feeling that something is missing. I always feel that there is something I should be working on. I'm never fully relaxed, for there is always a long-term task that needs to be done.
Jamie, USA

The mission and purpose of your life is to keep you womb story alive. In order to do that, you are prepared to put your own health at risk.

SABOTAGING SUCCESS

If you are a womb twin survivor there are many ways to assuage the floating feeling of guilt that probably haunts you, and to sabotage your chances of success in your life is an excellent way to do this.

I want to succeed but I always end up somehow sabotaging my chances of success

Self-sabotage may be as simple as holding back, always falling short or not allowing yourself to have a full life. It may be complex and subtle like spending years building a successful business and then allowing it to fail. It may be more obvious, such as endlessly prevaricating about a decision and losing the opportunity. You may be too proud to ask for help, or refuse to exercise self-control and keep yourself from being impulsive. You may become a workaholic, suffer from burn-out and consequently be unable to work at all.

I have recently started seeing a psychotherapist due to my self-destructive tendencies, my on-going addictions to various things; my terrible loneliness even though I have a huge number of friends and the massive feelings of guilt I have about everything. She asked me one day if I had lost a twin. I had read an article about "vanishing" twins and it had made me cry.
Linda, USA

245

MARTIN: SABOTAGING SUCCESS

Martin is constantly building himself up too high with a series of Great Business Ideas that will make him a fortune, only to sabotage each one by not following through the initial excitement to the more mundane business of refining and delivering on the idea. At work, he has a wishful, exaggerated, and unrealistic concept of himself. His work always falls short of his abilities because he rushes it or doesn't finish it properly.

Self-defeating behaviour

Womb twin survivors are prepared to go to great lengths to keep their Dream alive, and to do so some of them regularly engage in self-defeating behaviour. This tendency has baffled psychologists for a long time, but when we consider the lost twin in the Dream of the Womb we may have found a new perspective. From the point of view of womb twin survivors, self-defeating behaviour makes perfect sense and that is what we will explore in the next chapter.

22
Self-defeating behaviour

I never accomplish anything, but only the thought of doing so.
Mark, USA

This chapter will describe in more detail the statements taken from the Womb Twin Research questionnaire that relate to self-defeating behaviour. The table below shows what proportion of the selected respondents [a] agreed strongly with each of these statements. [b]

SELF-DEFEATING BEHAVIOUR - QUESTIONNAIRE RESPONSES	
Holding on, letting go	%
I find it hard to let go of unfinished projects, I am always going to finish them one day	48.9
There is at least one room (including shed or garage) in my home that is completely full of stuff	45.3
Ways to self-harm	
I have a long-term problem with food and eating	47.5
I am addicted to substances or behaviours that are potentially damaging to my health, wealth or well-being	27.9
I compulsively self-harm	11.2

Womb twin survivors have a vast range of self-defeating ways to choose from in order to sabotage their lives, drive their most intimate relationships to destruction, or both. Self-defeating behaviour is so common among people with various personality disorders that a new "Self-defeating Personality Disorder" has been suggested.[1]

---

a. The respondents who were able to provide evidence of their twin.

b. The levels of agreement were 1-5. The term "agreed strongly" refers only to the respondents who checked "1" as the strongest possible agreement with the statement. This explanation applies to all statistics provided for the statements described in this chapter, except where indicated.

For womb twin survivors there is a perfectly normal and reasonable explanation for self-defeating behaviour. It can be seen as a specific re-enactment of a pre-birth tragedy, where a great deal of personal happiness and fulfilment is being deliberately sacrificed, in memory of a lost twin. There are many ways to be self-defeating, each with its own meaning. If you are a womb twin survivor, it may help you to know that there are good reasons why you have chosen one particular kind of self-defeating behaviour over another. A personal study of the particular way you have chosen to sabotage your life will take you straight back to the Dream and give you a clear rendition of what went on in the womb all those years ago. You survived, but your twin did not. That seems to be the crucial issue but there is more to it than that.

HOLDING ON, LETTING GO

Womb twin survivors have a pre-birth experience of holding on and not wanting to let go, which is expressed in specific ways, including the accumulation of possessions and the inability to let go of unfinished projects. These two behaviours go together. The Womb Twin research project revealed that most of the people who strongly agreed to the statement about "stuff" also agreed strongly with the statement about unfinished projects.

I find it hard to let go of unfinished projects, I am always going to finish them one day

This behaviour is concerned with holding on and letting go. If your life and your home is cluttered with projects that have never come to fruition, each unfinished project might be a subtle re-enactment of your Dream of the Womb. The frail body of your lost twin, who died unfinished and faded away, can be in a sense retained by you in each project, which starts with a Grand Plan but never comes to anything. Some womb twin survivors are creative people who start several projects at once and this contributes to the mess and clutter in their homes. Unfinished projects are broken dreams and promises unfulfilled, all of which denies you the satisfaction of a job well done. A constant, imagined reproach emanates from every project lying about in your home or garden waiting to be finished - an excellent resting place for floating feelings of guilt.

248

I can never stay interested in one thing, I seem to get bored very easily. Just in the past month, I started a massive portrait of myself for art class but never got round to finishing it simply because I was bored of it. I've written numerous songs but they all seem to be half-finished and not up to scratch, in my opinion. I'm also writing a book but I've barely finished the first chapter because I feel that it's not going to get me anywhere in life.
Aileen, UK

If you are a womb twin survivor you may hold on to every project you start but leave unfinished. In that way, you are not breaking the promise you made to complete it. If this is your life, then your home is littered with unfinished projects, such as a pile of unread books or a shed filled with potentially useful pieces of wood. Your mind may be filled with unfulfilled dreams such as a new garden design or a major creative project involving recycled waste, which of course must not be thrown away. For you, the original unfulfilled dream is still there, in your Dream of the Womb.

There is at least one room (including a shed or garage) in my home that is completely full of stuff

Some womb twin survivors have a habit of hoarding things. Hoarding is known to be a complex behaviour and generally takes place in the home environment. According to Randy Frost, author of *Stuff*, two behaviours characterize hoarding: acquiring too many possessions and difficulty in getting rid of them. [2] It usually begins in a small way in childhood, with a tendency to collect things. Once the child has money to purchase objects, he or she may buy more than one of the same item, which is known as "double-buying."

Some years ago, I came to the knowledge that I was one of twins, but had been the only one to survive. I have been trying to understand all my life how it is such a seemingly innocuous event could affect me to the extent it has. It does explain some of my behaviors, such as buying two of things that I didn't need.
Nat, USA

The number of hoarders among womb twin survivors (45%) appears to be far above the numbers quoted in research with other groups. One study put the prevalence rate at 4%. [3] However, because this figure

249

was achieved as part of a general study of personality disorders, no real comparison can be made between this and the Womb Twin study.

Five levels of hoarding

A hoarding questionnaire was created in 2003 by the National Study Group on Chronic Disorganization.[4] They set out five levels of the accumulated clutter created by the disorder, each showing increasing disruption in the life of the homeowner. Level One hoarding allows for normal house-keeping and sanitation, whereas Level Two inhibits use of more than two rooms and there is a slight narrowing of household pathways. By the time Level Five is reached, normal sanitation is impossible, because the bathroom and kitchen are unusable and the property has become a public health risk.

> *I always slept with my bed so full of teddies that I could barely fit in! I had a knitted cushion, which I always held. I slept hugging the very edge of my bed.*
> Sophie, UK

Hoarding behaviour can be easily seen. In almost any neighbour-hood one can see a house that is poorly maintained, the windows blocked with piles of stuff and the garden overflowing with items that would normally be kept indoors. There is also the secret hoarding that no one sees: an attic so full that the ceiling joists begun to bow or a garage or shed that cannot be used. Even more secret are the personal storage facilities, where a collection of items can be kept safely, for a monthly fee.

Obsession

Hoarding is usually described as an "Obsessive compulsive disorder."[5] Despite many studies and years of research, the true reasons behind this self-defeating behaviour remain obscure - that is, until we consider womb twin survivors. Many of the most precious hoarded objects once belonged to relatives or friends who have died and are kept in memory of them. Hoarding can be considered as a useful place to settle a floating feeling of shame. The net effect of hoarding, even if it has not gone too far, is an agonising stigma.[6] One way to overcome the stigma is to keep hoarding a secret, which many people do, by using a garage or a shed. When the clutter encroaches on space in the home, however, it becomes visible. Hoarders have willingly adopted a practice that they are ashamed to acknowledge. They have created a home environment that they would prefer not to show to the world. At a level just below that, there are the clutterers, who can still function reasonably normally and can invite people into their homes, but still feel ashamed. Unless their friends are non-judgmental about the state of their house, they will have to do a clean-up job first to make home visits possible.

> *I feel I am extremely selfish, even when I'm trying to give everything away. I feel*
> *a need to share, but hoard in a completely paradoxical manner.*
> Amy, Canada

If your home is cluttered with unfinished projects, they can sap your energy and vitality as you work hard every day to try to find time to finish them all. Of course you fail, because you keep finding more things to do one day. The same applies to unwanted objects you may bring home "in case they come in useful."

Filling space
People who clutter or hoard are compulsively filling their space at home. The space gradually diminishes as time passes. In an extreme case there is hardly any space at all and normal life becomes impossible. People who clutter are hard to live with and many of them live alone as a result. If you are a womb twin survivor who shares a house with others and you fill whole rooms and spaces with clutter and won't let anyone else touch it, here are some questions for you: why would you want to steal space from other people? Why would you want to make yourself unavailable to others by putting a pile of stuff in the way?

Bonded for life to an object
Maybe this is your Dream of the Womb: your Beta womb twin is shrinking in relative size as you grow, until you fill up all the space and take all the nutrients. Your womb twin stops responding and all that is left of the original twin bond is with inert body of your lost twin. So you buy clothes, extra furniture and other items, perhaps a whole houseful. You cannot bear for anything to be lost, for you have lost everything already, before you were born. Perhaps you have been holding on to your stuff because the whole collection has become symbolic of your twin. You cannot bear to let go of any small part of it, for holding on keeps your

Dream alive. This is certainly selfish behaviour but it doesn't feel selfish to you. There has been great expenditure of energy in holding on so carefully, for it all seems to be so precious. The large number of hoarders among the respondents to the Womb twin research questionnaire was unexpected. Before the project began, there did not seem to be any clear connection between accumulating things and the loss of a twin before or around birth. However, the issue of hoarding arose early on in the stories, so it was decided at an early stage to include a statement about it in the questionnaire. The possible connection between hoarding and the Dream of the Womb remains an important area of continuing research.

WAYS TO SELF-HARM

Self-harming behaviour is not simply a lack of self care, it is a deliberate and planned way to inflicting pain and suffering upon oneself. The Womb Twin questionnaire included statements about three styles of self-harm that seemed to be closely connected with being a womb twin survivor.

I have a long-term problem with food and eating

Some respondents to the research questionnaire specified what there problem was with food. The problems ranged from overweight and obesity to allergies, eating disorders and anorexia. It seems in each case that specific food choices are being made so that food can be used symbolically. Eating or starving can be a way to express a vague memory from the womb about a little lost twin, who did not get enough nourishment to survive. To keep the Dream alive, specific food choices may be made, to cause health problems that could bring about a premature death.

My food problems: addiction to sugar. Overeating. When I was younger I ate nothing at all and vomited all the time. I spent some time in hospital at the age of six for an eating disorder. My Mum force-fed me (this is why I vomited.) As a baby I wouldn't eat and was fed the bottle while I slept. My mother had bleeding during her pregnancy with me.
Kalina, Poland

Food addiction
Nature's feedback system works extremely well if you don't deliberately over-ride it. The biofeedback mechanisms that we call "hunger" provide us with a natural appetite for the specific foods our body needs. However,

252

there are some foods that easily override our natural instincts and excite our hunger. This addictive relationship with some food ingredients, such as sugar, provides the food processing industry with millions of willing, if not desperate, consumers.[7]

> *I am definitely an emotional eater. Stress, not enough sleep, sadness - all these things have been known to bring on binges for me. That's why I feel that I self-medicate with food. It seems like an addiction to me.*
> *Jillian, USA*

People who eat out of depression and despair eat themselves into depression and despair. Womb twin survivors are often depressed, as we have seen.[c] Some foods disagree with particular people and are best avoided but food addicts don't avoid these foods: they eat more and more of the wrong kind of food until health problems appear. Choosing to eat too much of the wrong kind of food is a kind of self-harm. Used appropriately, food replenishes worn-out tissues, provides energy for life and bulk to keep the digestive tract healthy. Used inappropriately, food can cause medical problems such as digestive discomfort, obesity and adult onset diabetes. Your difficulty with food may take the form of a mild preoccupation or an utter obsession. Normal, healthy eating may be very difficult for you to maintain. The morbidly obese, who eat themselves to death, are people who know they are eating to die and are not willing to stop. People with anorexia starve themselves and are not willing to eat. These are self-destructive choices and heartbreaking to watch, for this is slow suicide.[8]

I am addicted to substances or behaviours that are potentially damaging to my health, wealth or well-being

Few people will easily admit to their addictions being a subtle version of self-harm. If you are an addict, you are probably aware of the negative consequences of your actions, but if the negative effects are not immediate, it is easy to deny them. It would take courage to admit that you are deliberately and consciously hurting yourself. It is surprising therefore that a third of the respondents were prepared to admit to addictive behaviour. Perhaps the anonymity of the questionnaire enabled

---

c. For more about depression see page 209

them to be honest about their addictions.

VERONICA: DEVELOPING ADDICTIONS

Veronica has no details of her mother's pregnancy, but she was born with *spina bifida*.[d] She was a high-achiever in all areas and excelled at school. As a teenager she starved herself and also binged then purged. At university she says she "went off the rails and hit drugs and alcohol hard." By then she had attempted an overdose twice. Aged 24, having landed a good job, she sat in her friend's house and cut her wrists. She felt desperate and lonely and knew something was very deeply wrong but had no idea what it was or why. She was led to Alcoholics Anonymous and was soon sober and off drugs. She says there is a "gaping hole within her soul." She is considering the possibility that she is a womb twin survivor, which may explain the emptiness inside her.

A study of the womb twin stories gathered during the Womb Twin research project clearly reveals that their addictive behaviour is made by choice. Many of them referred to bad choices, not addiction.

As a teenager, I used many substances and was very interested to try all kinds of drugs. Fortunately I had enough self-control to only "test" the latter but it took me years to give up marijuana. I finally did at 40, when I quit smoking. I had restricted my alcohol use a long time before that. Now in my forties, I have cut out the use of all substances, including cigarettes. I only occasionally drink alcohol, for I am apparently very vulnerable to alcohol. The fear of losing control is bigger than the wish to have fun or party.
Kristin, Belgium

At present, addiction is described and treated as a "disease" from which there is no full recovery without life-long total abstinence.[9] Addiction is seen by some writers as a conscious choice, but the reasons behind that choice remain mysterious.[10] If you are a womb twin survivor and are given to addictive behaviour, your body may have a story to tell. It seems to most addicts that they have no will power at all. But this is only partly true: addiction is best seen as a disorder of the will. The language of addictive behaviour operates in the realm of choice and responsibility.

---

d. For a definition of this term, see Glossary.

Yet addiction does not seem like a choice from the inside, for inwardly you feel helpless, driven and out of control.[11] In your Dream of the Womb, there was your own Beta twin, who did not develop very well. If you have identified too much with that Beta version of yourself, then you will probably feel helpless. That seemingly helpless, Beta energy may be driving your addictions.

> *I hate myself, I always feel sick, and I think about dying every day. I cut myself a lot, and I smoke in hopes that I might die young.*
> *Anonymous, USA*

There are two conflicting energies at work in the addicted individual - one that struggles to control behaviour and the other that remains helplessly addicted. For a womb twin survivor, this is the work of Alpha and Beta energy, operating in opposite directions.

I compulsively self-harm

Self-harm is intentionally injuring oneself, usually using sharp instruments such as a razor blade, but without suicidal intent. Self-harming is known to be practiced mostly by adolescents. The Womb Twin research project shows that self-harm among womb twin survivors is mostly concentrated among young people aged less than 21 years. A study of 1986 military recruits revealed that only 4% had self-harmed.[12] The description of the self-harmers in the 1986 group included some characteristics of womb twin survivors, for they were regarded by the other recruits as having "strange and intense emotions" and "a heightened sensitivity to interpersonal rejection." It was found that over 11% of the respondents to the Womb Twin questionnaire compulsively self-harm so, compared with most military recruits, womb twin survivors are almost three times as likely to practice self-harm.

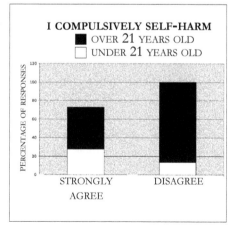

Sensitivity to rejection

Self-harming has been described as being the deviant self-mutilation of the mentally ill and quite different from body mutilation, such as tattooing or ritual wounding, as found in some cultures.[13] The reasons for self-harming may seem mysterious until we consider the emotional pain experienced by some womb twin survivors. They are very sensitive to rejection, as we have already seen in a previous chapter.[e]

> *I feel the suffering of others, particularly those close to me. In relation to self-harm, I haven't actually self-harmed but I get a strong desire to, just in recent months. I feel like cutting my right wrist. My therapist suggests I may be a womb twin survivor and that this indicates I may want to cut the bond with my male twin. I just don't know what to believe. All I know is I have had unbearable anxiety for the last two years, unbearable because I can't connect it to anything in my life. I keep asking, "What is wrong with me?"*
> Leslie, Canada

SHAUNA: A SHARP KNIFE

Shauna, who probably is a womb twin survivor but is unable to find evidence, was a teenager when she started to cut herself. On the same day that her first boyfriend abandoned her for another girl, she used a sharp craft knife to cut her arms and legs. She felt "spaced out" and dissociated from what she was doing to herself. She tried to stop doing it, but every time a relationship broke down she cut herself. She felt as if it were a way to remember a lost love. It felt as if she were a member of a "secret society" of people who are branded for life when a loved one dies or leaves. She is wondering if this "secret society" consists of womb twin survivors.

There may be a rational and intelligent reason why Shauna secretly scars herself in this way. Perhaps this is a physical echo of an emotional wound, a coded message from long ago in the womb when her womb twin brother abandoned her by dying. When her boyfriend abandoned her for another girl, perhaps it was her Dream of the Womb re-enacted. Her seemingly bizarre behaviour may have been triggered by survivor

---

e. For more about sensitivity to rejection see page 224

guilt and the pain of loss. If you are a womb twin survivor and have ever thought of self-harming, the desire to inflict a wound on yourself might be a way to recreate, in your body, the pain that is in your heart. It is probably the pain of a broken relationship, with all the shame and self-blame that may go with it. Self-harm may be the only way to express without words the pain of being a womb twin survivor. It is a pain beyond words, so words cannot possibly express it.

> *I have developed a skin picking disorder, where I pick at my face more than anything, compulsively and irrationally, as a release. I have thought about cutting, to somehow access and release this invisible pain and overwhelming emotion. I find it so hard to connect to the source of this deep longing for connection.*
> Jessie, USA

One day, the story in your Dream of the Womb may finally be made clear. Your deep sense of loss could be understood as genuine and related to a real event. Then at last, having cracked the code of your strange, self-defeating behaviour, you would be able to allow your skin, your body and your life to heal.

Who am I?

As a womb twin survivor you may have spent a great deal of your life wondering who you really are. A poor sense of self can take on many different forms: you may feel like half a person, live the life of two people at once or have several different sides to your character. It is your identity that is at stake and this will be the subject of our next chapter.

257

23

A fragile sense of self

*I've always felt that I don't portray myself to others as who I really am –
there's always something held back, a bitten tongue or a faked reaction.*
Sarah, USA

The table below shows what proportion of the selected respondents[a]
agreed strongly with the statements that suggest a fragile sense of self.[b]

A FRAGILE SENSE OF SELF - QUESTIONNAIRE RESPONSES	
Being half	**%**
All my life I have felt as if something is missing	75.7
I know I am not realising my true potential	69.7
Being alive	
I have a strange, irrational feeling that somehow I don't exist or I'm not really here	36.4
Deep down, I somehow know I experienced death before I was born	36.6
Being two people	
There are two very different sides to my character	55.2
I often feel torn in two between two decisions	51.9
Being your own womb twin	
Deep down, I feel very vulnerable, as if it would not take much to totally annihilate me as an individual	50.2
All my life I have been pretending to be someone else, and I know it's not my authentic self	39.2
All my life I have felt empty inside	48.4
I feel driven by "musts" and "shoulds"	41.1

a.   The respondents who were able to provide evidence of their twin.

b.   The levels of agreement were 1-5. The term "agreed strongly" refers only to the respondents who checked "1" as the strongest possible agreement with the statement. This explanation applies to all statistics provided for the statements described in this chapter, except where indicated.

Womb twin survivors can become so strongly identified with their womb twin that they cannot find their true selves. They may not be sure if they are truly male or female, visible or invisible, of vital importance or of no account whatever. This chapter will explore the various ways in which aspects of the Dream of the Womb can weaken your sense of self.

BEING HALF A PERSON

Some womb twin survivors feel greatly diminished by the loss of their twin. This is largely because they are not yet open to the idea that their pre-birth experience can be a great gift. The following two statements, taken from the Womb Twin research questionnaire, describe some of the ways in which this reduction of self is acted out.

All my life I have felt as if something is missing

A sense of something missing is the commonest characteristic of womb twin survivors and lone twins. It has been known about for many years. The attempt to fill the void, to replace the missing piece in your life, can be a strong driver to success, but the results are not always healthy.

Whatever I do, there is something missing - I have always felt this, as far back as I can remember. Nothing fills the void that I feel. I am beautiful, intelligent, have a prestigious degree, a successful job, have modelled, need ask for nothing - but my feelings of emptiness are all the more because these things do not fill the void. I feel I should appreciate or make the most of things, live life to the full, love what I have. But I cannot help falling into despair.
Carolyn, UK

Womb twin survivors spend all their lives searching for the missing piece in their lives but, to keep the Dream alive, they must make sure it is never found. They remain in therapy for many years to no particular effect, because they require their regular sessions to ease the emptiness inside. If you are a womb twin survivor you will know that the empty space in your life is the place where a special Someone ought to be, but they are no longer there. You probably realise how strong your need is to re-enact the missing piece in your life, by not being your whole self and holding yourself back from reaching your potential.

259

I know I am not realising my true potential

Parents and teachers the world over know the frustration of watching a bright young person fail to reach their potential. This young person may be dreamy and disengaged, or may possess an exaggerated sense of worthlessness that is immune to encouragement and praise.

BARBARA: FEAR OF SUCCESS

Barbara, who now knows she is a womb twin survivor, is the child of two accomplished parents. As a child, she always hid. At the age of five she told her mother she would not go into first grade, she was going into second. The headmistress agreed and so it was. In that class Barbara was the most intelligent but kept quiet about it. When the most popular boy chose her as his girlfriend, she renounced the position by removing all emotional affect from her character. If she wore something to school that got a compliment, she would never wear it again. She shunned all competition, be it academic or social. She did very well in school but expressed little joy about it. She hid her grades to "make sure no one would feel bad." In her prestigious high school, when it came time to apply for college, she made sure to pick colleges that were not competitive, so she could maintain a low profile. In her university studies she became very depressed. The solution she chose was to steer away from her main interests and talents where she might get some attention for talent and pursue subjects she was not good at. She dropped out of music, her greatest passion. One year before realising she once had a twin, she took a risk and started an amateur orchestra for people with instruments in their closets and no place to play. They can enjoy making and performing music in a group. Barbara is now the executive director and conductor. She has finally started reclaiming herself and admits that most of her time so far has not been well used.

If you are a womb twin survivor, it probably feels as if there is no energy available to drive you forward and help you to deliver on your potential. In fact, you have deliberately chosen this path of self-abnegation to keep your Dream alive. If you think back through your life, you may remember times when there were gifts denied and opportunities missed. That is how it is for so many womb twin survivors. They do not fear failure at all, they invite it. Perhaps your greatest fear is that you might succeed. You probably know that you are choosing to hold back in what you could do in life. You may have concocted some excuse that circumstances have worked against you. Deep down, however, you know the truth.

> *My final thesis was so good that my professor suggested I publish it. There wouldn't have been much work to do so and she would have supported me, but somehow I didn't believe that what I wrote could be important or interesting for anyone else, so I never published it and now it's somewhere in our cellar. So are many of my talents. A part of me knows that I would be a good therapist, and another is still unable to go out into the public with what I can do.*
> Petra, Germany

The awareness that one is not living life to the full can creates a sense of unease and prevailing shame. This has been called existential guilt.[1] It is a deliberate denial of your own genetic potential and you look back with regret and remorse to an un-lived life, feeling great guilt at the undone and the unmade. Existential guilt is a useful vehicle for survivor guilt: if you leave your gifts unclaimed and unused this will place you in the sidelines of life, putting you on a level with your little lost Beta twin. Perhaps there is some kind of rough justice in that.

BEING ALIVE

For many womb twin survivors, there are difficult existential issues to contend with. Life and death may be a constant preoccupation for them and a major cause of distress and inner confusion. For some womb twin survivors, simply being alive is a real problem.

I have a strange, irrational feeling that somehow I don't exist or I'm not really here

For some womb twin survivors, feeling ignored or overlooked is quite intolerable because it makes them doubt their own existence. This is hardly surprising if you are a womb twin survivor, because half of you faded away and disappeared not long after conception. If this is your womb story, then probably you have become identified with that

261

fragile, lost half of yourself. Your foetal assumption *I will soon disappear* has set up a womb script of self-doubt, driven by a fear of sinking into nonexistence that comes directly out of your Dream of the Womb. To assuage your self-doubt you need constant reassurance and feedback from other people and the world in general. If you can be seen and other people respond to you, then you can know you are real and in this world. Where the foetal assumption *I probably do not exist* is held by you to be an absolute truth, this will be reflected in your behaviour. In that case, you will choose to act as if you don't exist, in order to guarantee that you are overlooked. In this way you can successfully validate your foetal assumption and keep your Dream alive.

> *I have always felt terribly alone. When I was younger I actually was invisible to many people, i.e. would go out to eat and the waiters would not realize I was at the table. I've tried so many things to feel better, meditation, prayer, therapy, energy work and so much reading! Nothing helped. I also felt as though I was a "fake." I hid my feelings of worthlessness from everyone. I have always wanted so badly to be loved by others and even when they say they love me I don't believe them. I feel as though I've been wearing lead shoes and cannot move because I'll screw it up and someone will get hurt.*
> *Cyndy, USA*

Taken a step further, the foetal assumption *I am invisible* can become *I am not really here.* This can make you doubt your very presence in this world and provokes what has been called "existential anxiety."[1] If you are a womb twin survivor and you experience this kind of doubt and anxiety, it may help you to know that it is precisely because you so badly want to exist that you are afraid of your possible nonexistence.

Another world

A deep sense of "another world" is prevalent among womb twin survivors. Some womb twin survivors can experience a strange feeling of having a foot in another world. If you are a womb twin survivor it probably feels as if you have left part of yourself somewhere else. It is as if you are living some part of your life in the realm of the dead, with one foot in life and the other in death. All these vague feelings, however you happen to make sense of them, add up to the same idea: part of you is missing.

Deep down, I somehow know I experienced death before I was born

A deep conviction that one has experienced death before birth does not mean that one has already died. The foetal assumption, *I have experienced death* arises out of an event that was witnessed rather than experienced personally. However, for some womb twin survivors there is a great confusion between the lost memory of the death of their womb twin and their own death. As we have seen, the general concept of death can be a persistent undercurrent in the lives of many womb twin survivors.

MARGARET: A HELPLESS BYSTANDER

Margaret had a persistent sense of having been the bystander and observer at the death of her twin. She had been the helpless observer while remaining unharmed. This perfectly described her womb experience of being alongside her twin brother who was miscarried, presumably as a result of the puncturing of his amniotic sac with a sharply-pointed object.

A heightened awareness of the various issues surrounding death can result in an increased sensitivity to death in the general sense.

I often think about death and consider my own death but not so much in a melodramatic, suicidal way, but just the possibility of it; the facts of its impending presence.
Sophie, UK

Coupled with survivor guilt, a sensitivity to death may cause a womb twin survivor to assume they caused the death of their womb twin. But this is only a foetal assumption, probably created out of a vague pre-birth impression of a struggle for survival in a marginal situation, where only one was left alive. Once the real situation is fully understood, the misplaced guilt that such ideas may create will soon fade.

BEING TWO PEOPLE

In order to keep both yourself and your womb twin alive in your life, you have to be two people at once. The next two statements describe how womb twin survivors strive to achieve that dual personality.

There are two very different sides to my character

If you are a womb twin survivor, you probably know how you live your life as two separate people. This can be diagnosed as a mental illness. Among the professionals who have no understanding of how womb twin survivors feel, a duality of character seems to defy explanation in terms of normal psychology. In fact, it is a normal and very common trait in the character of the womb twin survivor.

> How do I explain the two personalities that exist in me. My daughter today was reminding me, "Who are you today?" There are definitely two different personalities that expose themselves in my behaviours. I am finally recognizing them. I suffer from depression and have been diagnosed as a schizophrenic. Yes I do feel very strongly that a part of me is missing.
> Kathy, Australia

Perhaps for you, the Dream is very near the surface, as you struggle without success to integrate the two sides of yourself and resolve the constant internal conflict that rages within you. The paradoxical nature of your character probably affects every aspect of your life as you carefully maintain your Dream of the Womb. You feel split in two, so that you can never feel whole or complete. You seek endlessly to prove yourself because you haven't the vaguest clue of who you are. You can't let anyone near you but you for yearn for contact with others. Yet the twins in the Dream of the Womb are never equal, not even MZ twins.[c] When one twin dies and the other lives, it is because there is something badly wrong with one of them. If you think hard about the precise way in which you have divided your character in two, you will become aware of which side of you is the Alpha survivor and which is not.

> I think of myself as dual - bisexual, ambidextrous, bipolar, but as part of the same whole. Less like I'm split, and more like I'm one with a little extra, which I suppose is the case.
> Heather, USA

Being two-sided is hard work. It can be exhausting, self-defeating and extremely uncomfortable. However, if you feel like two people in one, this is not a character flaw but a deliberate and conscious decision.

---

c. Monozygotic twins, created from a single zygote. See page 21

I often feel torn in two between two decisions

Decision-making is a common problem among womb twin survivors. If you are a womb twin survivor, you have a constant and difficult choice to make: either you can live like your Beta twin or you can be your true Alpha self. (If you had other womb mates, there are even more choices.) You truly are two people in one, so your assumed "inability to decide between two choices" would be a reasonable way to live out your duality of character. There are countless ways to be two people in one, each one reflecting the Dream of the Womb. For example, you could be two completely opposite people at different times. If you are an opposite-sex DZ womb twin survivor, you could swing from male-dominated energy to female, as if there are two versions of you. Otherwise, you could have two jobs, two parallel careers, two marriages, two homes, two very different cars or two very different sets of clothing. Clearly, there is great effort involved in keeping yourself and your twin together in born life.

> *I have always felt torn between the two mediums of writing and drawing, such as "When I do one thing, I seem to forget the other," as if there's two of me who can only seem to coexist when I'm drawing yet actually thinking about the sentences that I would put to it if I were narrating a story of sorts. I have always had extreme difficulty making decisions and always have to have a Plan B in the pipeline.*
>
> Eileen, Ireland

The end result of feeling torn between two decisions is always to be held in the same place, stuck between two equal and opposite energies - the powerful Alpha and the helpless Beta. This is a very uncomfortable feeling that has been described as feeling "stuck." It is a common problem among people who seek counselling or psychotherapy. [2] The sensation of feeling stuck is complex. It has within it the helplessness and hopelessness of not being able to move on, in conflict with the frustration of wanting to move on but feeling unable to do so. You may seek professional help and find this effective for a while, but after a while your energy diminishes and you slow to a stop, feeling helpless, frustrated and unable to move. Of course, being stuck is exactly how you feel your life must be, for it keeps both Alpha and Beta energy at work in your life.

BEING YOUR OWN WOMB TWIN

As we have already seen, womb twin survivors easily become identified with their womb twin and this may have happened to you. To identify yourself with someone else is to lose sight of who you truly are. If that person is your missing twin, you may try to be two people at once to keep your twin alive in your life. The following statements reflect how you may have tried to adopt the identity of your womb twin and add it to your own. This practice creates confusion, conflict and distress. We will explore it carefully so it may be fully understood and healed.

Deep down, I feel very vulnerable, as if it would not take much to totally annihilate me as an individual

The fear of annihilation is not the same as the fear of death. After someone dies there is a usually a body and always a memory. To be annihilated is to be totally obliterated and wiped off the face of the earth. In that case, there is no body and no memory - it is as if that person had never existed at all. If you are a womb twin survivor your sense of vulnerability remains at its height, as though your whole self is at constant risk of annihilation. In that case every effort must be made, every day, to maintain yourself as an individual. You must at all times make sure that you are seen, heard, appreciated and loved.

> *The first point of departure from my old self was the realisation that I am not surrounded by enemies. This sounds either trite or obvious, but when one is confined in the prison of denied feelings, expecting at all times to be attacked, then these things are not obvious. The second point of departure was to realize that there were intelligent, reasonable and loving reasons for my way of being, misguided as they might have been. I realize that it is OK to reach out, even though to do so is to exhibit my vulnerability.*
> Tony, UK

Your fear of annihilation could be a vague, pre-birth memory of a twin embryo that died before development was complete. It may be that your twin barely existed before disappearing completely. If you have identified with your virtually nonexistent Beta twin, then your present womb script of *I am being rendered nonexistent* would make perfect sense.

266

All my life I have been pretending to be someone else, and I know it's not my authentic self

We are told that an authentic self is real and whole and carries no elements borrowed or assimilated from anyone else, which means acknowledging and representing one's true self, values, beliefs and behaviours to oneself and others. [3] If you are a womb twin survivor and you are always putting on a false front to the world, then there may be a good reason why you are not acknowledging and living your life as your true self.

> *I am quite a positive confident person outwardly, but I am very sensitive inwardly and get offended very easily. I like to appear confident and happy to make others happy even when I'm not happy.*
> Kat, New Zealand

You may have created a false identity to cover up your inadequacies; you may be too much identified with your chosen profession so that the "real you" is hardly ever visible. You may like to please people so you are perpetually nice and never get angry. You may conceal your true feelings and always say "I don't mind" when really you do. To be "inauthentic" is to project a false self and keep your true self hidden from the world, as if you always wear some kind of mask. There is a natural process whereby one can become identified with a person or social group and even with an imagined concept of how the ideal individual should be. When you identify yourself with a person or group, you are choosing to take on some characteristics of that person, in order to construct an identity for yourself. In the same way, as a womb twin survivor you may have become completely identified with your own fragile, tiny womb twin. This may be so long-established that it feels absolutely authentic for you to run the womb script of *I feel fragile deep inside,* for example, and therefore assume that you are in need of constant emotional support. You have probably felt this way for as long as you can remember and it seems to express your authentic self. The truth is, however, that you have been living the life of your Beta womb twin as if it were your own. This is not your true identity, for the assumption *I am fragile* is in your Dream. You are not fragile, you are the strong Alpha survivor.

267

All my life I have felt empty inside

If you are a womb twin survivor, you may have experienced a sense of inner emptiness. This kind of emptiness inside has been variously described, as a sense of lack[4] or a feeling of meaninglessness.[5] Emptiness inside may be triggered by some external event, such as being left alone, or the death of someone near. For most womb twin survivors it is mostly a sense of being lost, forsaken, yearning and confused.

> *For the last twenty years I have this feeling of not belonging here, that there is something missing, being different, deep-down alone, unsatisfied, paralysed, not knowing who I really am. Mostly I feel as an alien visiting here. I even think now that I am here to be alone, wandering around. Today I still feel "unborn."*
>
> *Nicolas, Belgium*

Inner emptiness has been beautifully described as "an ineluctable trace of nothingness in our being, of death in our life."[6] An inner void inside you may be a womb memory - a sense of having lost something infinitely precious. You probably feel as if the loss of your twin reduced to a fraction of what you might have become, had your twin remained alive. There are a hundred ways to fill inner emptiness. A common one is addiction.[d] Robert Lefever, director of the Promis Clinic in London, has focused his work on what he calls the "spiritual void" that is to be found in all addicts.[7] The Womb Twin hypothesis has an alternative explanation for the spiritual void that drives addictive behaviour: it is the pre-birth loss of your twin who was too weak to be able to survive and remain with you.

I feel driven by "musts" and "shoulds"

If you feel driven you live without agency or autonomy, in a kind of imprisoned, helpless state. You feel unable to think for yourself, make your own choices or make decisions. Everything is done out of duty or a sense of obligation. It is as if you are unable to move unless someone else stimulates you. In any partnership or group you are passive and wide open to influence. You have handed over agency for your life to another person. You have not let yourself live your own life, own your power

---

d. For more about addictive behaviour, see page 252

or use your gifts. This state of mind is normal for many womb twin survivors as they act out the life and character of their weaker Beta twin.

If someone lets me down or disappears, it can send me into a spiral of depression
- a strange empty space within me emerges and I become immobilised and lonely.
I can feel driven for a while, then I seem to lose the momentum, which has caused
problems in my working life.
Carolyn, UK

Carl Rogers (1902-1987) a psychotherapist and writer, created the idea of a self-actualizing tendency,. This is to be found in all human beings and motivates us to develop our genetic potential as far as we can.[8] The self-actualizing tendency is towards becoming your authentic self. It is the You that you could become if you would only allow it. In the words of R.D. Laing, "The ordinary person is a shrivelled, desiccated fragment of what a person can be."[9] Perhaps you have identified just a little bit too much with your lost Beta womb twin. He or she rarely took the initiative and only moved in response to you and probably did not have a well-developed brain as you did. Driven by a foetal assumption, *I am paralysed* and *I am unable to think for myself* you are living out the life of your own Beta twin instead of your own. Womb twin survivors live their lives so caught up in their "unremembered memories" that they feel driven towards certain ways of feeling, thinking and doing. If you are a womb twin survivor you may feel you have no choices in life. But you have chosen never to make any choices of your own and that is how you have kept your beloved Beta twin alive in your life.

Misunderstood

The sadness and tragedy experienced by a womb twin survivor is largely underestimated and misunderstood by the 90% of the population who have not known the death of a twin before birth. If you are a womb twin survivor, you will probably have tried several times to explain to others how you feel about your lost twin. It is not easy. Therefore, we will continue our explorations in a little more detail in the next chapter, when we will consider what womb twin survivors feel about the simple fact of being a twin.

269

24
Being a twin

I don't need any kind of confirmation to be sure that I lost my other half
very soon in life and ever since then I've never really lived.
Divina, Portugal

Even without evidence of your lost twin you still may be a womb twin
survivor: there may be more to learn. This chapter will explore the five
statements from the Womb Twin research questionnaire that are related
to being a twin. The table below shows what proportion of the selected
respondents [a] agreed with each of these statements. [b]

BEING A TWIN	%
I have always had a great interest in twins	73.3
All my life I have had the feeling that I may have once been a twin	62.3
As a child, I had one or more imaginary friends	61.6
Twins in the family	
There are fraternal twins among my blood relations	45.1
There are identical twins among my blood relations	32.7

Some twin-less twins who lost their twins in adulthood find it hard to
believe that the loss of a twin during pregnancy or close to birth can have
a psychological effect on the survivor. Not having known your twin in
born life, it might seem extraordinary to feel grief after such an early loss.
But this is to underestimate the nature of the twin bond that forms in the
womb, long before birth. Adult twins living in an intact twin pair would
naturally focus on the relationship that has built up between them since
birth. Womb twin survivors on the other hand, despite never knowing
their twin in born life, still have a lifelong feeling of being a twin. Because
their twin has died, they too experience a sense of grief and loss.

---

a.   The respondents who were able to provide evidence of their twin.

b.   The respondents were asked for a simple "Yes" or "No" answer

I have always had a great interest in twins

A lifelong interest in twins was predictably very common among the respondents and was the second most popular statement among the respondents who were able to provide evidence of their twin. An interest in twins can be expressed in all kinds of ways. It may be a tendency to scan faces when among people, always noticing twins or people who look similar. It may mean reading books about twins in general and focussing on lost twins in particular. Womb twin survivors seem to take particular interest in anything to do with twinning and published in any medium.

I have absolutely no concrete evidence that I ever had a twin. I just have women's intuition. All my life, ever since I was a child, I have had a bit of an unnatural intense interest in identical twins. I grew up reading the Sweet Valley Twin series, watching Mary Kate and Ashley Olsen, and as I got older, I read and researched everything I could about twins. I am now working on a children's novel about identical twins and a "twin universe."
Ana, Bogota

The fact that many hundreds of people carefully searched the Internet and found the Womb Twin web site, which was little-known at the time, suggests that they were very interested in twins and the death of a twin in particular. Their emotional reaction to the material on the web site was sometimes overwhelming. For these people, their reaction was proof enough that their feelings were related to the prenatal loss of their twin.

I feel a deep sadness and loss and I cry a lot just talking about it, also reading what you have written I felt I was totally relating, as if it was me I was reading about. I felt I could hardly read and had to walk away for a bit and then come back to it and I am also crying as I write this.
Denice, Australia

All my life I have had the feeling that I may have once been a twin

The use of ultrasound has revealed that in many "vanishing" twin pregnancies there are no symptoms at all. If you were conceived before the 1980s when ultrasound scans were more regularly used, and if your mother had no symptoms during her pregnancy with you, then there would be no available evidence of your twin. Until the mid 1990s, the incidence of "vanishing" pregnancies was either unknown or grossly underestimated, so there was nowhere for womb twin survivors to find confirmation of their deep conviction that they once had a twin.

> *When I was in my early teens I became obsessed with the idea of twins and convinced that if I looked hard enough I could find proof of my twin. I had imaginary friends all my life, and still do to this day. I have created a complex world inside my head where I can escape, and be with the twin I always felt I should have had. I did not know about vanishing twin syndrome until very recently. I considered it as a possibility at first, but after doing research I am now nearly certain that I am the survivor of a vanishing twin. Since this discovery I feel like a lifelong question I've had has finally been answered.*
> Sarah, USA

In the absence of any physical evidence, there is no expert, however experienced and highly qualified, who can confirm that you are a womb twin survivor. You will have to rely on your "gut instinct" and your intuition to work out whether or not there was a lost twin in your Dream of the Womb.

> *I feel it deep in every cell of my body that I had a twin in the womb with me. Trust your instincts, is all anyone can say to us who feel this frustration of "no proof." And why does it need to be proven to ourselves or others? When my family is still sceptical, I wish for some kind of physical proof of what I know and feel so profoundly inside me. It's hard to convey this to people who haven't experienced it. I'm sure many of us may have gone through the feeling of this being so right and yet doubting ourselves, and thinking it could all be an invention of our mind. I guess it comes down to accepting our gut feeling.*
> Liza, Germany

It may be that you have been given the idea of being a womb twin survivor recently by a therapist or friend. If you are reading this book to find out whether or not you are a womb twin survivor, there is nothing here that will prove it to you, one way or the other. After all, you are the world's greatest expert on your experience of being yourself. Never let anyone influence you, however persuasive their arguments may be.

I strongly feel, as I have forever felt, that I am a womb twin survivor. The feeling stays with me and most likely will continue to do so to my death. I am happy, yet that void keeps popping into my life, which confuses the hell out of me. A few of the best words that I can think of that can help you in understanding my world are - Lost, yet I'm home. Alone, yet I'm not, yearning for that unknown vacancy, confused as to why I feel this way at times. A confirmation would be a blessing.
Rose, USA

As a child, I had one or more imaginary friends

We have discussed in a previous chapter how womb twin survivors create imaginary friends as a replacement for their twin.[c] The child who creates their own fantasy twin has been generally understood by psychotherapists as feeling lonely because of being forsaken by their family.[1] In the light of the womb twin hypothesis, these cases can be interpreted differently: perhaps these children are womb twin survivors, trying to make sense of their Dream of the Womb.

A fantasy twin?
Among some psychotherapists there is considerable scepticism about pre- and perinatal psychology in general. This is because anyone could build a fantasy about their life before birth and claim that as their personal truth. Sceptical individuals are fond of saying that the feelings associated with being a womb twin survivor are most probably due to some other trauma in born life. Some psychotherapists are very dubious about even mentioning to their clients in therapy the possibility of their being a womb twin survivor. Some have gone further and claim that it cannot be therapeutic, and may be unethical, to replace one fantasy for another.

My therapist suggested to me that I might be a womb twin survivor. It is very surprising to me and I really don't know how to cope with this. It feels like it fits into my life. It feels so familiar.
Guy, Belgium

The idea that a lost twin may be a fantasy can be uncomfortable for womb twin survivors who can produce no evidence of their twin. They lack people to speak to openly about their twin and may become sceptical

---

c.   For more about imaginary friends, see page 240

about their own feelings. In future, as high-quality information about womb twin survivors becomes more available, the prevalent scepticism will no doubt diminish. Sceptical psychotherapists will eventually be reassured that a lifelong sense of having lost a twin in the womb is no fantasy, provided that you are a womb twin survivor. Regardless of these concerns however, the idea that the pre-birth loss of a twin is missed and yearned for by the sole survivor is already gaining ground among therapists of all kinds, particularly among physical therapists, such as kinesiologists.[d]

TWINS IN THE FAMILY

Twinning among blood relatives seems to be very common among womb twin survivors. It has been speculated that there is a "twinning factor" in families, which predisposes them towards multiple births.

My mother's mother miscarried twin boys. My uncle had twin boys. My mother's father had a twin brother. That same grandfather had twin sisters younger than him and his twin. Their father had a twin sister. I am the only twin born to my mother.

Steve, USA

One study suggests that it is probably derived from the paternal line and related to a gene on the Y chromosome.[2] Another study suggests that the tendency may be related to female hormones and therefore passed down the mother's side.[3] Evidently, there is much confusion about what truly causes twinning. The Womb Twin research project showed that womb twin survivors are more likely to have DZ twins in the family than MZ twins.[e] It was also found that a considerable number of

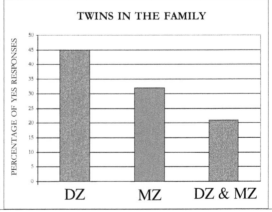

TWINS IN THE FAMILY

d. For more about how kinesiologists diagnose womb twin survivors, see page 164
e. DZ - Dizygotic twins; MZ - Monozygotic twins.

respondents had both DZ and MZ twins in the family, which suggests that the twinning factor is inherited. We have seen how on average world wide, about 10% of singleton births are the result of twin conceptions. Further research is needed in families where twins are conceived but only one baby survives, to see if the tendency to conceive twins also passes down the generations.

The womb twin work

Many hundreds of womb twin survivors have found validation of their situation through the Womb Twin research project and their stories have been a real help and inspiration in creating this book. Over many years, it was gradually discovered that there can be a pathway to healing for womb twin survivors, which has been called the Womb Twin work. At the very beginning of the Womb Twin project, it became clear that simply finding evidence that you are a womb twin survivor, or having your instincts validated if you had no evidence, is not enough. The Womb Twin healing work is still being developed and extended, as more and more therapists of various disciplines have become involved with womb twin survivors and have published their discoveries.[4] There is much more work to be done before the healing path for womb twin survivors is absolutely clear, but the next few chapters will outline what has been learned so far.

PART FIVE

The Womb Twin work

Womb Twin

Amid the flutter of your beating heart
I woke to life and knew you by my side
Together always, from the very start
(But you, but you must go - and I must bide…)
They came with death and and chased you from the womb
And left me in the darkness of despair;
I lived till birth in your reluctant tomb,
With damage that I felt would not repair.
In not forgiving I kept grief alive
But healing came and now, at last, I thrive.

Anonymous

25
Tools for healing

*This is the first time in my life that I don't care
whether I sound foolish or not.*
James, USA

Now that you are aware that you are, or may be, a womb twin survivor, it is time to begin the Womb Twin work. The main task of the work is to gain a better understanding of how your own particular Dream of the Womb has been re-enacted in your life. Every person is created as a self-healing organism, but the natural course of healing can be deliberately blocked. The Womb Twin work is about understanding and removing those blocks, using the available tools. The main tools for healing are trust, truth and intuition.

I saw my counsellor last night and we discussed this further. When she brought it up the previous week, I was fascinated by it and thought it was interesting. But my reaction following it wasn't so much. I felt panicked and couldn't get it out of my mind, especially after visiting the site, completing the questionnaire and reading the e-mails. It felt right in a way, but all my life I've battled with whether I've just made things up. I had a very difficult childhood, yet felt the effects from it I shouldn't be "over-reacting" to. I'm worried that this might be something I lean towards in order to excuse myself from life.
Mandy, UK

TRUST

To start the Womb Twin work, you will need determination. The work is quite difficult in places and you will be fighting with yourself. It is possible to do this work on your own, but daring to trust one other person with this information may be healing in itself. Perhaps you find it difficult to trust other people because of your experiences of being rejected and abandoned by your own womb twin. When you were an embryo learning how to be a person, getting to know your womb twin was an important first lesson in trust. This lesson may have overridden your most basic instincts. It might be the cause of the ambivalence about relationships that lies behind your lack of trust. Ambivalence feels as if is there is one force propelling you forwards to a better life, while another, equal force is dragging you back. You are stuck and you need help.

> *I have abandonment issues, always searching for something or someone, but I do know I was and am loved. Larger than that, is that I have a sense of not belonging even when I know that I really am part of a group. I don't trust people either. So there is always that lack of trust as a barrier to intimacy. My feeling is that I will get hurt by my friend/lover or the person that I love will go away.*
> Mary, Ireland

We need other people. Four hundred years ago, John Donne wrote: "No man is an Island, entire of itself."[1] This holds true today and will always hold true. It would be good to have someone to walk with you as you begin the healing path. If you have always felt that you must do everything by yourself, why not try asking for help? You may be surprised by the results.

Dare to reach out

To build a relationship one needs connection. To make that connection you must reach out to the other person and build your half of it. In the womb you tried reaching out, possibly with little response. That may mean that your foetal assumption is *I am alone, there will be no response from this person.* Perhaps for you there will always be a slight lack of certainty about reaching out to another person, but today you could dare to try and make a connection with someone. When a connection is made, it is a rare thing - something delicate but infinitely precious. This new bridge, this new connection, will need strengthening and nurturing. It must be flexible against the forces that will act against it, light enough to span the abyss and strong enough to carry the shared lives that it links so precariously. If it is well-maintained and nurtured, then this bridge will last a lifetime.

Ask a therapist

Therapists of all disciplines are becoming aware of womb twin survivors among their clients. There is a good chance therefore that you will find someone willing to do the Womb Twin work with you.

280

I know I probably sound like a kid with a hyperactive imagination, but I really feel like this fits. I'd really like to find someone who I can talk to about being a womb twin survivor and figure out if maybe I am one.
Terry, USA

It may be that you are already in therapy but your therapist is unable to help you with this particular aspect of your life. If you need support, it would probably help you to meet other womb twin survivors. If you are very lucky you may find that your therapist is also a womb twin survivor.

Yesterday in therapy my therapist suggested that I am grieving for more than the loss of my own childhood. My grief seems to exist at a much deeper level. I asked him for an example. He told me about his own experience as a twin and his belief that there was a third embryo and how that had affected him and his surviving twin sister. Then I told him about the "feeling" I'd had for the last decade or so about being a surviving twin. I had never told anyone because I have no proof and it sounds a bit insane. Also I explained that I had come to this "sense" independently, or that it had somehow "come to me". Suddenly a lot of psychic puzzle pieces (many of which I have yet to define and cannot yet articulate) seemed to be falling into place.
James, USA

TRUTH

The next tool you will need is to accept the reality of your pre-birth experiences. The prevailing negative public attitude to the Womb Twin hypothesis may be a hindrance, if you are sensitive to public opinion on this issue. However, confirmation has come with every story sent along with the questionnaires and a fresh sense of certainty is growing.

My twin sister was first-born and died five hours after birth. I always had an imaginary "friend" when I was young and I am not sure what age I was told about my sister, but I know I must have been young. And maybe my parents were concerned because I talked to my little "friend" a lot. At times I feel lost and that no one understands how I feel about her. I have been told by some that I couldn't possibly miss her since she didn't survive.
Arlene, USA

The Dream of the Womb is remarkably detailed and precise. Your intuitive ideas about your twin are based on real events, so if you firmly

281

believe what feels true for you, regardless of what people say or whether you have any evidence or not, then a clear picture will begin to emerge of a real memory.

> *I wonder if I was never able to get to the fragile one, to even touch it and try to hold on. I wonder, too, if perhaps I were able to embrace the other but no matter how I tried, couldn't hold on. Or perhaps I held on in ways I didn't want. I sense possibly a desperate reaching. Reaching first for one, while perhaps the other in front of me inadvertently blocks my reach. Then reaching for the other, and perhaps a struggle to keep the second in some position and finally deep, shuddering, infinite grief. A great responsibility to have kept it all together and sense of horrible unfairness at the futility. An inability to accept that I couldn't - and can't - change it, turn it back, make it right.*
> Judith, USA

The various prenatal events that make up the Dream of the Womb can be seen as a spectrum with further gradations in between. The main factor we will consider is the responsiveness of your womb twin, for your twin may or may not have been capable of responding to you

A responsive womb twin

Your womb twin was in complete human form and capable of response. The death of your twin meant the loss of the relationship. Below are some of the variations in your womb story which affected how your relationship with your twin developed and what memory still remains.

Sudden death: Your twin was fully developed and was able to twitch and move. As time passed, a bond was established between you, built on a two-way, reciprocal relationship, which ended abruptly.

Slow death: A bond was established with your fully-developed twin but your twin became sick or didn't thrive. As responses gradually ceased, the bond faded and died along with your twin.

Failure to survive: Your twin's placenta was badly attached to the womb wall, or had overlapped too much with your placenta. It had become impossible for your twin to survive. After good start, your twin responded more and more feebly until there was no response at all.

A tiny body remaining alongside: After the twin bond between you had built up in a reciprocal relationship, your twin slowly died. They would have gradually lost the capacity to respond to you and would have become inert, cold and still. The corpse of your dead twin remained beside you throughout the pregnancy and was delivered with you.

A womb twin incapable of response

You had a womb twin who was abnormally developed, was barely alive at all or who never achieved human form. You had a one-way relationship, which ended at birth.

Unable to respond: Your twin had a fatal abnormality but lived long enough for you to be fully developed and able to attempt to stimulate a response. This relationship was one-sided, with you reaching out and nothing coming back in the way of response. Your deformed twin remained in the womb alongside you for many weeks, only to be miscarried or delivered along with you. An enduring memory remains of something abnormal, unresponsive and inert.

Tentative beginnings: Your embryonic twin developed just enough for the ultrasound scan to pick it up but had disappeared by the next scan a few weeks later. There may have been some tentative beginnings of a relationship but it is unlikely to have been reciprocal.

A vague wraith: Your twin developed abnormally and never made it beyond the embryonic stage. There was no reciprocal relationship. A vague sense remains of a wraith-like figure somewhere near.

A tiny spark of life: Your womb twin was a blighted ovum that sparked briefly into life but never got started, or disintegrated very soon into a chaotic mass of cells.

Two in one: You and your twin were MZ (monozygotic) and shared a placenta. Some of the cells from your MZ twin passed into your own body and you have become two people in one.

Confirmation of your womb twin

Some womb twin survivors do sometimes receive confirmation of their lost twin from experts who know enough to notice the signs. There are two particularly useful methods of doing this.

Regression under hypnosis

This technique involves you being very relaxed, using visualisations or hypnotic induction. Then you are invited to go back in time, year by year, to when you were in your mother's womb. Many womb twin survivors have experienced a real encounter with their womb twin by this method.

> *I had hypnosis to try to discover the core of my issues. I hadn't thought about the vanishing twin situation in a long time and the therapist was unaware. The hypnosis session was based on travelling backwards through my life to find the initial trauma, and it ended up in the womb where I had a strong sense of another, and even what gender they were. The whole experience was so intense and so real that I have no doubts now that I had a twin.*
> Deirdre, UK

Neuro-emotive technique (NET)
If you need confirmation of your womb twin, this is a good way to find it. It seems that this form of applied kinesiology can trigger body memories that are found to be extremely accurate. Also certain questions can be asked of your body about such things as a sense of loss, inner emptiness or an inability to relate. Your bodily reaction to these questions will reveal the true reasons for these feelings. A skilled NET specialist who is aware of womb twin survivors may discover your womb twin before you do.

> *I was in my chiropractors office about five years ago and he was doing some neuro-emotional work on me using applied kinesiology and it came up that an emotion I had held in my body that was causing me problems had to do with love and a female member of my family. He asked if it was my mother, grandmother, aunt, etc. and my arm said no, then he asked sister and it said yes. I told him I did not have a sister. We did it again - same result. Then he said, but you DID have a sister and I instantly burst into tears, knowing deep down it was true. He said he once had a vanishing twin sister too and he knew. It has been the most profound thing to know about.*
> Becky, USA

INTUITION

Never underestimate your own intuition as a tool for healing. It is the ability to take a million tiny pieces of information and to interpret them. The result is a sensation of deep knowledge. Of course, this has as much chance of being wrong as being right, so keep an open mind.

I want to work with some therapist so I'm not alone when I finally find those suppressed feelings. I don't think I could get through the process of dealing with an identical twin by myself. I am not even sure if that's what I am and what I am looking for, maybe it's something else - but what...?
Renie, Germany

Intuition helps us to access the early memories in the Dream of the Womb. The material arises chaotically as vague sensations and feelings that defy explanation or interpretation. You will never get absolute proof of the real nature of your Dream, so you will have to trust your own intuition to make sense of things. It may take a long time, but by the application of relentless logic and the de-construction of every one of your ideas, you can carefully test the validity of everything you believe. In particular you can analyse the way people relate to you and you to them. Gradually, your sense of certainty will increase. You will soon recognize the real relationship you once had with your womb twin.

The defensive wall I have between me and other people was created to protect me from more pain like I experienced when Beth left me. It must have been so painful to be so close to her both emotionally and figuratively and then abruptly be separated forever. In that sense, it is a good thing. It is a conservative thing to do. Actually, it is not risk-taking to tear down the wall. That is because no one can ever replace Beth. So, zero chance of being successful. Who would bet on that? Now, I'm realizing that while this is true and always will be, the strategy is only of limited value. I give my love for her and have good memories of our time together but that is all. It is all one-way traffic. No present or future relationship. Well, that is, if you exclude our meeting up together in Heaven. But that is a long wait. What do I do in the meantime? I read somewhere that this is like seeds being planted. Some grow and some don't. Perhaps this is like that.
Brenda, USA

Finally, you will know the truth in the deepest part of you - that you carry with you always an imprint of your twin, who had a separate story and destiny to yours. You will gradually become acquainted with your womb twin as a real little person by carefully examining your existing feelings, behaviours, relationships and beliefs. Until you have a real understanding of the biological background to your Dream of the Womb it will not be possible to move on in a positive way. It is important to take your time over this first stage, as if you were waiting for a thousand-piece picture puzzle to fall into place by itself. One day you will know that your Dream of the Womb is as clear as you can make it, and it will be time to move on to the next stage of your healing.

No worst

As we walk the healing path, you will find yourself fully acknowledging that something strange has been going on in your life since before you were born. Regardless of what discoveries you make about yourself along the way, there will probably be some kind of pain for you associated with the business of simply being alive. In your Dream of the Womb is the memory of your dying womb twin: this is the source of your pain. That painful memory is the moment once described by Gerard Manley Hopkins as "No worst, there is none."[2] As we move onto the next stage of the Womb Twin work, this painful place in your memory will be referred to as your personal Black Hole. It is the root cause of all the problems in your life and holds the secrets of your healing, so that is where we will go next.

26
The Black Hole

Do you think it is possible for me to ever feel normal? Do you think it is possible that I could learn to accept myself and love myself?
Lena, Belgium

Your Black Hole is the source of the darkness in your life, which is the death of your womb twin. This chapter will explore what feelings are in your Black Hole, how you created it, why you remain in it and how you can begin to find your way out.

The feelings in your Black Hole

The feelings in your Black Hole will take various forms, according to the details of your personal womb story and whether or not your twin was capable of response.

The death of a responsive womb twin

If your womb twin was responsive and then was lost, the pain is in the loss. If this is your story, you have something deep in your mind and soul that is about despair, shame, death, grief and pain. This complex of painful feelings is an integral part of your inner self. However hard you try, it does not heal.

The death of an unresponsive womb twin

If your womb twin remained with you but was unresponsive, the pain in your Black Hole arises out of a frustrated desire for connection. This feels more like resentment than pain. Beneath the resentment lies a terrible sadness, a sense of lack. You have probably adapted to this feeling by deciding that you need nothing and no one.

How you created your own Black Hole

Healing will only begin when you are ready to stop rushing about, looking for different kinds of anaesthetic and using it to forget your inner pain. Only then will you discover that it is self-inflicted and you are the author of your own misfortune. You have built your own Black Hole out of these painful memories and only you can change them.

You have probably blocked your healing growth with a kind of deadening energy. You have been on endless guilt trips, anxious about unfinished business, obligations and possessions. All these projects steal energy and leave you too exhausted and confused to know what to do for the best. You could clear these thoughts out of your head and stand alone and unguarded in the silent, empty space that remains - a terrifying thought. The truth is that you have been deliberately wasting your life energy by actively filling up the painfully empty spaces in your life with negative thoughts.

Why you remain in your Black Hole

Whatever your individual womb story, even with confirmation of your twin and knowing the pain in the Black Hole, you still may feel that the Womb Twin work is not for you. It may be that uncovering your womb story and recognizing that you have been re-enacting it all your life feels threatening in some way. Even with this whole book before you with its message of hope, you may still resist the idea of leaving your Black Hole behind. Living your life in close connection with your twin has always been the most important thing in your life, however hard you may try to deny it. That could be what is keeping you stuck in your Black Hole.

As I grew up I realized that I had cultivated my own double-presence in me as being a bit "my own best-friend." This is never enough to feel completed, but gave me a sincere complicity with my lost still alive in me, through me, by me. Alan, USA

It is possible that you are deeply aware of the fragility of your twin and how easily that tiny life was extinguished. It would be natural if, as the strong survivor, you felt protective of your tiny lost twin and wanted to try very hard to keep him or her alive in your life in any way you could. That would be enough to make you resistant to any change.

Ways to resist change

There are many ways to resist change and we will now explore just a few. The main point to notice is how they all require a great deal of energy to maintain. Each one is an excellent way to uphold your secret agenda, which is to stay just where you are, holding and protecting your little womb twin as if both your lives depended on it.

Avoidance: You can say you are stuck, take it to therapy and spend many expensive sessions getting nowhere. You may allow yourself to make some small progress, in order to give everyone some hope, only to give up after a while and go straight back to where you were.

Rationalisation: You can think of reasonable excuses for why you have not allowed yourself to heal. You may decide that chronic scepticism is the safest option.

Projection: With a certain amount of mental gymnastics you can turn the whole story round. You can claim that your problem is your childhood, your parents or perhaps the uncle who touched you inappropriately. You can insist that it was that car traumatic crash, or the death of your dearest friend, that made you this way.

Displacement: You may decide that it is the other, more vulnerable, womb twin survivors who need healing, not you. You may decide to become a healer yourself, so convinced are you that you do not need any healing at all.

Denial: You may deny your feelings about your womb twin so absolutely that you are completely taken in by your own story. Then you could launch an attack on the Womb Twin project as spurious and potentially damaging.

Identification: You may have a friend or colleague who is resisting healing in the some way. This means that you can resist too, knowing that you have an ally.

Procrastination: You may decide that healing has already happened, can't ever happen at all or will only happen following some unlikely eventuality. This is an excellent way to put things off indefinitely.

Intellectualizing: This is a great favourite. You can turn up to therapy every week and at great expense, argue with your therapist and get absolutely nowhere.

Your resistance to healing, whatever form it takes, is a useful strategy to keep you in your Black hole. We will now consider exactly what kind of place your Black Hole might be and why you are so anxious to stay there.

WHICH BLACK HOLE IS YOURS?

Before you can find your way out, you will need to take a closer look at what is in there. It may not be clear to you yet exactly what your womb story is, but in your Black Hole your feelings are strongest and your senses most acute. In that place, your Dream is at its clearest and most accessible, which is why you have tried for so long to remain there. There seem to be three principle types of Black Hole: a Place of Desolation, a Black Pit and a World Filled with Pain.[a] You might find your own Black Hole somewhere among the following descriptions.

A Place of Desolation

In your Dream of the Womb you are left desolate after the death of your womb twin. The desolation comes from the loss of the close, intimate and empathetic union with your twin. Any similar situation in born life will trigger a feeling of grief and desolation once more. You feel grief if you allow yourself to become really intimate with someone who is unable to give you the high level of intimacy, sharing or empathy that you crave. To keep your sense of loss alive, you repeatedly and unsuccessfully try to replace your twin with a soul-mate. In your Dream you were left alone and forsaken. The desolation arises out of the knowledge that the Someone has gone for ever. You have deep sense of being alone, lost in this dark feeling. You are small, insignificant and shunned by everybody. You are in total isolation. You sabotage your most intimate relationships, because the re-enactment of the Dream is paramount. Nothing, not even your closest relationship in your born life, is more important than that. Co-dependency in marriage is a good example of this kind of sabotage: two womb twin survivors of opposite sexes meet and instantly recognise that they each can fulfil the deeply-felt needs of the other - needs that they hardly know they have. They decide to create a close and intimate relationship and may even pledge themselves to each other for life. After a time, they begin to tear each other apart until they can not tolerate any more. The relationship may be kept going for a decade or two, or ended almost immediately in permanent separation. This is a dance of desolation, straight out of the Dream of the Womb.

---

a. We will continue to use these same three groups in subsequent chapters.

A Pit of Darkness

If this is your personal Black Hole, your whole life has been based on despair. There was hope once, that you vaguely remember in your Dream, but it was soon dashed. You are teetering on the edge of a pit of darkness. It's terrifying, for it seems as if you could easily fall into the abyss. However hard you try to overcome it, and regardless of how much evidence there is to the contrary, the pit of darkness persists in the back of your mind. In your Dream of the Womb, your tiny womb twin was unseen and unnoticed. That is how you feel too. The thought is terrifying, for to be unseen is to be totally extinguished, just like your womb twin. You must prove that you exist so you will not, after all, become your twin - a tiny scrap of a person, dying and disappearing with no chance of a life. You feel a great need to be free and untrammelled, yet paradoxically you have voluntarily created a prison as your place to be.

I am in prison. A mental prison. I have lived in it all my life. As it is, the prison walls only manifested themselves at times of stress, especially emotional stress. Whenever I felt attacked, which could be frequent and after the slightest imagined provocation, I would go into "lock-down mode." Combined with this feeling of attack is an overwhelming feeling of helplessness; of not knowing what to do or which way to go forward. It is a black, hopeless place to be in which all energy is sapped and all hope is gone.
Tony, UK

You willingly endure the pain and torment of trying to be two people at once, in order to heal your primal wound. In your Dream you are being literally torn in two. By being two people at once, you are desperately trying to keep your Dream alive, no matter what the cost.

A World Filled with Pain

If this is your personal Black Hole, you live in a world filled with pain. When in the company of other people, you readily become attuned to their feelings and you have accurate empathy with them. Your hypersensitivity and imagination can undermine your ability to trust in others. You constantly scan their body language. You can sense changes in atmosphere and often answer unspoken questions or carry out unspoken requests. You come in too close to other people, instead of standing clearly in your own space. Because you are so close and empathetic, you quickly become aware of the pain of the people around you. You then adopt this pain as if it were your own. You genuinely believe this will help to heal their pain. It is very hard work, always looking out for problems or difficulties in other people's lives. To cope with this, you need a great deal of time away from people, simply to recover. In those quiet, isolated times, the pain is felt most acutely.

> *I've started being nocturnal again, to avoid people. The only types I ever seem to encounter are neurotics and angry, violent, deceptive, manipulative people, who use me and cause both them and myself misery. I'm tired of living in a society which is apparently grimly determined to destroy itself*
> Peter, USA

Pain is never far away. Life is difficult for you. Disappointed expectations and unfairness are particularly difficult. Rather than let someone down, you will walk that extra mile for them, but be hurt when they won't do the same for you. If you see people being treated unfairly, this enrages you. You deeply resent labels, rules and any other constraints unfairly applied to you, or to others. You are preoccupied with certain social or environmental problems. Above all, you are alone, different, feeling abandoned and somehow far from home. Your life is a painful struggle to find the lost world of your primal past. Driven by a deep sense of mission to restore your Dream of the Womb, you yearn to heal the world and everyone in it.

> *I have been experiencing episodes of rage and self harm since early twenties. I've had an increasing sense that it does stem from pre-birth, and recently felt I was given the insight that I had a womb twin. I have been in caring roles all my working life, although I've recently gotten much better at understanding and setting boundaries, which has helped me begin to separate out what I and others are responsible for. I still have a strong desire to help people heal themselves.*
> Carol, UK

This is a rescue mission through which you too can be saved. You are wounded by the pain of the whole world and that is your Black Hole. If only you could heal the pain of the world, then you would be healed. Whatever your womb story may be, you made a choice long ago to create your own Black Hole and live in it. You can now choose to leave.

Finding a way out of your Black Hole

Now you have rediscovered the loss of your twin in your own Black Hole, the pain can be fully felt and properly attributed. Now you can explore and clarify the way in which these painful feelings from long ago have attached themselves to other losses in your life.

Finding the separate little person
There may be certain characteristics in your nature, such as being histrionic or fragile, which feel alien to your true nature. They feel as if they are *Not You* and you may even describe them as such. You created the *Not Me* out of your Dream of the Womb. You have created the *Not Me* out of a vague imprint in your mind of *Someone being there but gone away*. In the first stage of the Womb Twin work, you began to make your womb twin into a distinct entity in your mind. It may be possible to discover more about the genuine nature of the separate little person who was once there. There may be more real memories or facts about the existence of your womb twin that you can discover, by talking to relatives or consulting medical documents. Your womb twin can be named if they do not have a name already. Giving a name is a very important step, because it marks the fact that your womb twin and yourself were separate little people.

> *A lot of people tend to get my name wrong, and the vast majority of them call me Jennifer. They say that I "just look like a Jennifer." During my freshman and sophomore years in high school I had the same science teacher, and he could not for the life of him remember what my name was. He always called me Jennifer. Some people, I believe, are sensitive to certain things. I've been wondering if perhaps that teacher was getting a sense of a missing twin whenever he looked at me. I think my twin's name was Jennifer.*
> Stephanie, USA

In the end, however stuck you may be, the best route out of the Black Hole is forgiveness. This is because you share something with all womb twin survivors - survivor guilt. Survivor guilt makes the very act of living painful. The good news is that it does not have to be this way forever. It is time you forgave yourself for the way you have been living and that is what we will do next.

293

27
Forgiveness

I am so grateful to you for setting me free. Who knows what's left
but for now I am pleased to say that I have exceeded any healing hopes
I have ever had for myself.
Martina, USA

In this chapter we will explore the issue of forgiveness in the life of the
womb twin survivor, with particular reference to survivor guilt, which
surfaces again and again as a floating feeling of shame.

Pain

Feeling unable to forgive is very painful. Forgiveness can heal that pain,
but somehow you are still holding on to the resentment and bitterness
that causes the pain. You will soon discover how easy it is to forgive other
people and yourself, once you understand fully why you are working so
hard to keep pain alive in your life.

My friend called to tell me that left-handed people may have been "mirror-
image" twins, with one lost in the womb. As soon as I heard it, I felt a great
sense of relief. Maybe I wasn't crazy!
Vania, USA

People hurt one another because they are in some kind of self-inflicted
pain themselves and do not understand why they are hurting. Unless
you are prepared to imagine yourself in the other person's shoes you will
never understand why the other person hurt you. Clearly, forgiveness is
not going to be possible without some understanding and empathy. This
chapter will help you to understand and forgive others and look upon
yourself with a little more mercy.

I have tried many times to alter the destructive patterns that have formulated
what I have become, but to no avail. Basically I have decided that even though
I do not like being here, I will just do my best. But it is not working any more
- neither does prayer for understanding and clarity.
Julie, UK

It has been said that there are two levels of pain - the pain that you experience at this moment and the pain of the past that still lives on in your mind and body.[1] This accumulated pain creates a field of negative energy around you, which is greatly increased by a lack of forgiveness.

Awareness

You are now aware of your Dream of the Womb and the way you are constantly recycling it in your life. With that awareness in place there is no way back to ignorance. Healing will inevitably come into your life whether you seek it or not.

> *I never realized that this was the root of all my behaviors, sabotaging, and detachment. I feel like now that I have discovered the cause of my pain, I can move forward.*
> *Kathy, USA*

However strange the feelings you have had all your life about being a twin, they are true and real. The overwhelming feelings you have often experienced, which appear to be quite disproportionate in the circumstances, have a real basis in lost memories. Fortified by truth and deeper understanding, we will move forward to consider the greatest block of all to forgiveness: survivor guilt.

Survivor guilt

Survivor guilt is simply this: your twin died, you inherited everything that was available but you don't want any of it.

> *My identical twin brother was stillborn. I've always felt loved and prized by my family but I've always felt alone inside and have problems fitting in with society and have a lot of personal issues to work out. I've now come to terms with this, and understood that my twin's passing may be the cause of these problems. I frequently wish that he'd been given the shot at life that I waste and that I'd never earned the gift of a life he never had a chance at.*
> *Bradley, UK*

It is likely that your survivor guilt shows itself most when you do not allow yourself to fulfil your potential. You may keep your gifts hidden, or you may not use them wisely. You may sabotage yourself so that you never know true satisfaction. You may make a good start with various projects but tail off quickly, lose interest and move on. You may have shown great promise as a child, but somehow this has remained unexpressed as you grew older. Despite survivor guilt, you may have managed to be quite successful, but you may still be left with a deep feeling of unease and unrealized potential.

I have had feelings for as long as I can remember to hurt myself - it wasn't so much to kill myself but just to punish me for being alive. I would like to know why I hold myself back from being successful and I'm not using the gifts that I know that I have.

Biddy, Australia

Invented shame

A floating feeling of shame makes a useful place for feelings of survivor guilt to come to rest. You can create a floating feeling of shame by inventing something to be ashamed of and use it to keep you stuck in a treadmill of activities of which you are ashamed. There are countless examples to be found, when we know where to look.

Understanding about womb twin survivors has helped me to see some of the influences in my own life and begin to move on in improved self esteem and the ability to achieve goals rather than self-sabotaging all the time.

Kat, USA

Perfectionism and addiction are excellent ways for survivor guilt to find a means of expression. To be a perfectionist, all you have to do is approach perfectly achievable tasks with an invented, crippling fear of failure. Then you can feel guilty about succeeding, as if success is a failure to fail. You may choose to feel uneasy with success and riches, as if you cannot allow yourself to have them. Then you can set yourself impossible tasks, fail to reach them and feel terribly guilty for letting yourself down.

I have experienced many episodes of severe depression, each one lasting for months. I used to wonder what sins have I committed that I have to go through these punishment time and again. I am a perfectionist and sometimes set rather high expectations of myself so I am doomed to fail in my own eyes.

Gemma, UK

To become an addict is to enter into a major project of invented shame, by means of which you are regularly and willingly precipitated into your

Black Hole. You start by feeling powerless to change, while genuinely believing that your cravings are running your life. At that stage you can be ashamed of your "lack of will power." Then you can feel very ashamed of your bad habits and keep the your addictions secret. After a while, you can let yourself gradually sink into the pit of addiction until everyone notices. They may suggest that you should feel ashamed of yourself. Little do they know that, as the helpless victim of your cravings, you are constantly racked with shame about your behaviour and its consequences. As you get closer to your Black Hole of complete despair, your refusal to admit to any shame about your self-destructive behaviour is yet another thing to be ashamed of.

> *That was always my greatest trial and obstacle - not just accepting help (as I would, once in a while) but asking for it when needing it. It's hard to bend your neck and see the help offered in front of you when you spend so much time looking to the skies crying for help.*
> Edward, USA

Survivor guilt can be healed, provided that you first unravel the knot of your invented shame and rediscover the real, original experience. Then you will be able to understand, accept and forgive your deeply-held feelings of helplessness and emotional need.

WHAT IS THERE TO FORGIVE IN YOUR BLACK HOLE?

We have seen that there are three kinds of Black Hole, a Place of Desolation, a Pit of Darkness and a World Full of Pain. There are also three kinds of resentment that could be healed with forgiveness. The resentment in your personal Black Hole may arise out of being abandoned, living a lie or being unable to relieve suffering. You may find your own story in the three descriptions that follow.

The Desolate Place: Being abandoned

The resentment you feel usually arises out of failed relationships. When relationships don't work, you take the blame and worry that the break -down may have been due to something you did or said. If you sabotaged the relationship, then all the more reason for feeling guilty and ashamed. Are you prepared to believe that after a break-up, a relationship can be mended? There were no second chances in the Dream of the Womb, but here in born life everyone is alive and available for negotiation. There can be no healing without reconciliation, which is the process of letting go of resentment against yourself or other people, leading to a reconstruction of the relationship by means of forgiveness and apology.

> *I had a twin sister. There is no evidence of it. All of a sudden my life has sense, as if I have the missing piece of the puzzle. After several years of therapy I finally was able to talk to my mother and elder sister about my difficulties in life. I was able to overcome a strong pain that I was suffering after having left my partner almost three months before. Something new has begun in my life.*
> Juan, Spain

You may be filled nostalgia for past relationships, as if there once was a time when things were just fine. The search for the perfect soul mate may drive you into codependency, serial monogamy, even promiscuity and adultery. It is not so much a search for a particular person but a specific kind of feeling. It is the way someone makes you feel that is the basis of the attraction. It is vitally important for the success of the relationship that you see your partner for who they truly are and not a substitute for your lost womb twin.

> *I found out when I was a teenager that I was a twin. My twin was stillborn. Recently my girlfriend of six and a half years broke up with me. I never ever felt as down after this. We are trying to work things out now. I've changed a lot since. I'm trying to be a better person. I'd really die if I lost my girlfriend. She's everything to me. At the moment, I feel happy and excited because I think there's real hope. I think things can change for the better.*
> Anthony, UK

Even when an excellent relationship is formed and things go well at first, the lonely tragedy of the lost twin must be played out, to keep recreating the Desolate Place in the Black Hole. Every new partner must be tested to see if they are strong enough to remain, against all odds. You may have put immense pressure on your partner to make them want to leave. Only very strong people could survive such pressure, but that is the whole point. Terrified of abandonment, and by testing your relationships to destruction, you have brought about what you most fear.

298

I feel there are still two parts to me. The driven, outgoing and ambitious business woman and the quiet, dreamy writer, musician and artist. As I got older, I lost touch with the latter and felt that I was living a lie for many years, following the other side, trying to climb up the corporate ladder etc. It's almost as if "HE" (who I name Danny) would have been the ambitious Male, and I'm in truth, the arty female who just loves to write and paint and play guitar. However, I do accept that all of this is part of me and valid and useful! I'm still integrating!

Deborah, UK

Willing apology is a great way to heal broken relationships. An apology given on demand is worthless, so never demand an apology. Just set the tone by apologising for your 50% of the mess and that will leave the way open for the other person to apologise for their 50% of the mess. It is very hard if you apologise for your part in things but the other person just sits there looking aggrieved as if it was all 100% your fault.

This work has helped me realize why I have such difficulty finding and maintaining romantic relationships. I have been looking for that bond that I lost and that bond is only available with a twin. The clarity brings me great affirmation and relief. I know I have a lot of work ahead in therapy, but at least it feels productive and I can stop being so hard on myself in this area.

Vicki, USA

A polite discussion about the fact that two people have been hurt may open things up. Otherwise, just be patient and trust in love to heal things. It is important, once the apology has been made, to forget and move on. This will build for you a new style of connection, which is reconstruction.

The Pit of Darkness: Wearing a mask

If this is your Black Hole you have been trying to live two lives at once. You have been wearing a mask all your life. To keep your Dream alive you have become totally identified with your own Beta twin, the weak and inadequate half of you. Yet all the time the Real You has been the strong Alpha survivor with all the power and capacities of a complete human being. To maintain some kind of balance between these two ways of being, you have pretended to be your Beta twin pretending to be yourself, the Alpha twin. At some level you probably already know this, but perhaps it was not made clear to you before. In a brilliant series of complex, subtle and concurrent manoeuvres that use up a lot of precious energy, you have managed to be two people at once in every moment of your life. It's hard work, so sometimes you give yourself a break from pretending and let your true feelings show. This is how cracks begin to appear in that mask you wear to keep your Dream alive.

A self-inflictor in my youth, I still sometimes deal with tempting thoughts of leaving this reality but have a strong sense of spirit and am only now engaging with who I truly am, having dealt in some small way with my demons.
Jane, Ireland

You have always known, deep down, that your mask is a lie. You also know you need imagination, flexibility and high intelligence to live a lie of this magnitude. If you ever wondered how clever you are, be reassured that it takes brains to live two different lives at once. Out of loyalty to your womb twin, you have tried hard to be two people in one. You have suffered a great deal to manage a lifetime of mental and emotional gymnastics, in order to keep your little Beta twin alive in you. You yearn for that suffering to be acknowledged and the effects to be forgiven, so why not forgive yourself!

I have identified as gay in the past, but I never felt that I belonged in that world or that a gay relationship would really give me what I need. My father was very distant when I was growing up, and I think that is a cause, or that is what I've been trying to find in a gay relationship - of course I've never found that. Maybe the loss of my identical twin brother is also a void I've been trying to fill with a gay relationship. When I "came out" I thought that there would be a world in which I'd be able to fit in and be happy and content. It's been very difficult to accept that coming out isn't the answer either.
Ian, UK

Even if people say they forgive you your transgressions you don't believe them, for in the Pit of Darkness you are afraid that you must be guilty of some "Unforgiveable Act" that defies explanation. A deep consciousness of this mysterious act has created a pool of negativity in your life. The concealment of your shame by denial has paralysed you and the rigidity is maintained by the fear of being discovered. The whole cover-up process acts counter to change and personal progression. But what if this mysterious Unforgiveable Act is the simple fact of your being alive? It is true that you survived and your twin did not, but this was not destruction or murder, it was natural selection. A century ago Charles Darwin recognized that where there is a scarcity of resources the weaker organisms die and the fittest survive.[2] That same competitive situation applies in the womb as much as anywhere else in nature.

I had a NET treatment today. My NET guide started by describing how wonderful the first trimester was for me, that I had an identical twin in the womb and we would caress each other and move and rub against one another and life was wonderful. Then suddenly she started to bump and kick and then she was gone. I felt the loss. During the treatment I worked through the grief. I keep smiling and know now that I was never alone. I didn't "kill" her. Now my personality makes more sense to me, I feel contented or settled in a way I never have before. I can look in the mirror and know who I am.
Linda, USA

A World Full of Pain: Unable to help

If you carry the pain of the world in your Black Hole you cannot forgive the world for being so full of pain and sorrow. Your feelings of shame are caught up in your sense of responsibility towards other people. That is where your survivor guilt surfaces most often. In your desire to heal the whole world by using your gift of empathy, you have probably taken on the painful feelings of others. You have become enmeshed with other people because of your ill-defined personal boundaries. In this way, you have been a sponge to everyone's pain, and you genuinely believe that it helps to be that way. You may think these feelings are yours, but the probability is that you have spent your life burdened with other people's painful feelings. You are far too quick to take on responsibility and spend a lot of time feeling guilty about situations that do not involve you at all.

I have always felt that I was supposed to have a twin. I do feel like I am different from other people, and that I have a great purpose on Earth. I suffered from eating disorders and various other destructive behaviors before I learned to heal myself. Now I am very focused on helping others to heal themselves.
Jen, USA

In a kind of desperate self-sacrifice, you have taken on the pain that the other people close to you could neither handle nor understand. For you, forgiveness would be handing back the pain, placing it where it belongs. It was never yours and may have passed down several generations before it reached you. If you are unable to forgive yourself for failing to heal the World Full of Pain that will be a total block to your healing. Unable to forgive yourself for the sin of being alive, you will be stuck in a perpetual cycle of resentment that will never enable learning and personal development. You probably begrudge others their ability to grow and fume with suppressed rage at your own unrealized potential. As your rage mounts, you can find more and more reasons to be angry and bitter. Resentment keeps you in a perpetual state of pent-up energy, so you can secretly feel that there is much to be aggrieved and angry about but no one seems to understand. You may choose to feel jaundiced by life in general, annoyed by stupid, irritating people or frustrated at the general state of the world. Rage may well express the despair you feel when the World full of Pain refuses to heal, but you know that raging is not the best way to heal the world.

An end to resentment

Whatever may be in your Black Hole, if you forgave yourself the sin of being alive when your twin did not survive, then you would cease altogether to feel resentment. Forgiveness is like being relieved of a heavy load. It brings clarity of mind, lightness of heart and a deep sense of peace. Forgiveness is so good for you that you could make a daily habit of it. In truth, you have nothing in particular to be resentful about, but perpetual resentment is a handy place for the floating feelings of shame in your Dream to come to rest.

> *It was a miracle to find that being a womb twin survivor is, perhaps, the root of all my emotional problems, and that I can start on the long road of healing now that I have a proper explanation.*
> Anna, Canada

Soon, you will be able to find a new way of being your authentic self while building more honest relationships. But first you will have to let go of your womb twin, and that is the next stage of the Womb twin work.

28
Letting go, letting be

I had a twin sister and I lost her somehow. Why did I survive and she didn't?
How do I let go and heal from a loss like this?
Hannah, USA

This chapter will explore the many ways in which holding on to grief and impossible dreams are characteristic of womb twin survivors. We will discover how a carefully-prepared farewell ritual, or some other form of letting go and letting be, could set you free from the painful feelings that lie in your personal Black Hole.

Holding on to grief

Holding on to grief means that it will remain unresolved. Unresolved grief in the lives of womb twin survivors seems to underlie major depression, post-traumatic stress disorder and generalized anxiety. Holding on to grief for your lost womb twin can be resolved by fully expressing it.

Create a focus

One way to let go of grief is to create a focus for it, for where there is no focus, grief cannot fully be expressed. For example, when someone dies and no tangible remains are left, an alternative focus for grief can be created. In the vault of Westminster Abbey in London, England for example, there is the Tomb of the Unknown Soldier. The large engraved stone slab, just inside the main doors, is a focus for the grief of millions of families and friends, who lost a soldier in war but no identifiable remains were ever found. The Tomb of the Unknowns in the Arlington National Cemetery in Washington, USA is there for the same reason. Most of our lost womb twins have no grave, so there is no focus for grief. This makes grieving very difficult.

Becoming aware

Your grieving may have been blocked because you have been unaware until now that you are a womb twin survivor. You may not have realized until now that the loss of a twin could generate such strong feelings.

303

I've heard the story of my twin over and over again while growing up, but never gave it a second thought until recently. Now I am sure that every emotional issue I have relates to my unborn twin. For the first time in my life I grieved for my twin. I can feel his/her presence with me now and it's very comforting.
Kerry, USA

If you have had many deaths in your family, particularly if there have been several deaths in a short time period, you may still be carrying intense grief for them all. When at last you give yourself permission to grieve for your twin, the strength of feeling may take you by surprise.

I'm very emotional now and in the last weeks (in fact years) there is an enormous grief. For a few days, I had a cry that came from so deep that I was completely choked! I cried the whole day and couldn't stop. I have never felt this before.
Gregor, Belgium

The preoccupation with death, which is characteristic of many womb twin survivors, is expressed in many different ways. Some womb twin survivors often think of death, repeatedly risk their lives, attempt to overcome death or work hard to preserve their youth. Once blocked grief can be released by creating a focus and letting the feelings surface, the preoccupation with death diminishes or ceases completely.

Clinging to impossible dreams

Everyone knows that impossible dreams don't work but there are some impossible dreams that are most beguiling to womb twin survivors. Impossible dreams seem to promise some kind of healing for the pain of simply being alive. Dreams can drive habits, addictions and compulsions. Among these are the dream of *I Can be Perfect*, which drives the perfectionist. There is also *Winning a Fortune*, which drives the gambler and speculator. Then there is the idea of a *Safe and Satisfying Place*, which drives people to addiction and compulsive behaviour.

Pain is a constant, which I feed. Then I feel shame about overeating and being fat. Then the shame keeps me away from intimacy because of fear of more pain... and so the cycle continues. This cycle is repeated on so many levels of my life. Not only food, friends, family, but in business and in achieving what I want in my life.
Jack, Australia

Even more seductive is the dream that *There Was Once a Golden Time*, which keeps you immersed in your pre-birth past. Another favourite is *My Lost Twin is Out There Somewhere*, which catapults you into the future in search of a replacement for your twin. By chasing these impossible dreams, you guarantee that none of your possible dreams will ever come true. Of course, that has served your secret purposes until now, for this has been the way to hold back your potential and keep your Dream of the Womb alive. Only by daring to let go of your impossible dreams will you be able to embrace the only possible dream, which is to live a life of healthy realism and reachable goals. Now is the time for these impossible dreams to end.

Dreams and illusions

As you begin to awaken from the Dream of the Womb, you will start to realize that you are no longer able to separate illusion from reality. The feelings are so real in your impossible dreams, that they seem to be true. But we need to question these ideas. For example, you may hear the voice of your twin in your head: is this real or an illusion, born of love and memories?

> *My oldest son has been hearing voices since he was old enough to ask me why someone keeps calling his name.*
> *Greta, USA*

Womb twin survivors often report experiences where they hear their lost twin "speaking" to them. If you have experienced this, it may be driven by a great yearning for contact and dialogue with your lost twin. You have kept your twin alive in your life for a long time. Evidently, this is not doing either of you any good, so truth must now be separated from illusion.

Preparing your ritual of letting go

Healing is letting go of the impossible dream that you can be reunited with your twin. Once that is accomplished, then your possible dreams can come true. We start with making the choice to let go. It will be a deliberate act of choosing. This is to be a heartfelt choice, so it is best not to make it until it can be made definitely. A tentative choice to let go of your twin will not help you at all.

I am much the same, although I did manage to ritually let go of my twin. I always expect these things to have a dramatic "everything is alright now" effect and, given my age and the amount of time I have devoted to finding a way, I am impatient for the light to dawn. I don't want it to be just another step, for I have hoped for them so many times before and time has proved them mostly to be illusions. I felt it to be the path I would tread - now I fear it was just an empty expectation.

Rick, UK

Truth and illusion

On the one hand stands illusion, which is a false perception. You have come to believe that illusion is reality and you are completely taken in by the power of the illusions you have built for yourself. On the other hand stands truth. If you choose to make truth your master, then you will see illusion as a misapprehension. Until now you have been unable to distinguish between the dead and living parts of yourself. Now you can see that the phantom twin you have created is a real memory, not some childish fancy. In the Dream of the Womb there is a ghost of your twin, who once was truly there but is long gone.

Precious memories

The price of awakening from the Dream of the Womb is to face the reality of your original separation from your twin. For a long time, you have been clinging to those dear shreds of memory. The fact is, however, that in letting go of your twin you will not lose any of your precious memories or your sense of connection. It is a strange paradox, but once you have said goodbye to your twin you will feel closer to them than before.

The constant ache/hole in my heart and soul; the constant searching for something or someone; the constant guilt that I feel (for killing my own sister); the pain that never seems to heal; the two sides to my personality; the constant fear of being abandoned or being rejected; why death affects me so badly; my constant battle with mental illness and why I get upset so easily; always trying to make others feel better. This may sound strange but it's like that hole in my life is part of me and, although I hate the depression and the sadness it brings, I don't want it to go away, as it has been with me for 37 years.

Francesca, UK

Letting go is not a moment of real separation but a way to access the memory of a separation event, which happened long ago. You stand to lose nothing by letting go of your twin: rather, you have a huge amount to gain, as we will see.

Planning

Your ritual of farewell will be more profoundly healing, if it is carefully planned. In the planning stages give your intuition full play. Pay special attention to any seemingly irrelevant ideas, as they bubble up from deep inside you. Keep thinking of your ritual and making a note of ideas as they come. In that way the ritual will, in a sense, create itself.

Naming

It will help in creating the ritual and focusing your feelings if you name your twin. Your parents may have had a name already in mind. You may have named your twin for yourself some time ago. As a young child, you may have named your imaginary friend. A name may have already come into your head unbidden, perhaps only a few moments ago. If you are still having a problem finding a name, just wait. Somehow, one will come into your mind. Alternatively, you may choose a name that matches what you imagine to be the characteristics of your twin, such as "Pip" or "Beanie." As your twin's closest relative, you have the right to name your twin, even if your baby twin was stillborn and left un-named by your parents.

A symbol

For the ritual, you will need an object to symbolise your twin. If you wait and let things happen, you may begin to associate some object or substance with your twin. A scarf is particularly good, for you can wear it often and feel warmth and closeness around you. It could be an object you have created, such as a picture or a sculpture. It could be a letter to your twin or a poem. You could create a scrapbook of memories, or tell the story of your twin in the form of a booklet. It could be a precious object, like a ring with sentimental value. It could be an object found in nature, such as a plant, a construction of leaves and sticks or a special stone. Do not start your ritual without it, for it will be the focus for your feelings. Even when you have found it or created it, you will still have to wait for the right moment.

307

Deciding the timing

The correct time to let go of your twin may well prove to be extraordinarily precise. You may realize later that you unconsciously decided on the approximate date of your own conception, the conception of your womb twin or the anniversary of your womb twin's death. If the day when your twin died was your own birthday, because your womb twin was stillborn or died at birth, it may help to carry out the ritual in the evening of the day before your birthday. Then the two dates will not eclipse each other. You will know when the time is right. Don't let anyone, however well-meaning, force you into anything you are not ready for. Also, don't be too wedded to your own plans, for your timing may not, after all, be right. Your dream of the Womb is so deep-seated that it is important to trust your intuition absolutely. Even so, be prepared, for you may have a strange feeling one day that the time is NOW.

> *Yesterday I held a funeral for my twin. The sense of grief was becoming heavier and sharper by the day, to the extent that I couldn't stand feeling that way any longer. I started to plan a funeral for him, but while I was doing it, I suddenly felt I had to do it there and then. As has often happened at such times for me, I managed to find everything I needed at home by dint of a bit of searching, even long lost things turning up at the right moment.*
> *Carol, UK*

Choosing a companion

Other people may be around when you do the ritual or you may do it as part of an organized group activity. You may want to choose a partner, a sibling or other trusted person to accompany you. You may want to include your companion in the ritual activities, but remember to claim space just for yourself.

Choosing your element

One or more of the four elements will be necessary for your ritual as the means to "carry away" your twin. Fire would consume any combustible symbol that you have created, or you could light a candle. Water could carry a floating symbol of your twin, or drown your symbol if it will not float. The air could carry away the symbol if it is light enough to fly. The earth could contain a buried symbol, or nurture a plant or tree.

Ritual space

The setting you choose for your ritual may depend on where you live. Some womb twin survivors are prepared to travel long distances to carry out their ritual.[1] Once you have chosen your space, you can use it in any way you wish, carefully placing certain significant objects in the space, reading a poem, playing certain music or moving around in some way. You will need to claim the ritual space for yourself, taking charge of everything that happens within it.

Being ready

If you are not yet ready, just hold all these ideas in mind for a while. One day, quite suddenly, you will know what to do and it will be time to start.

The womb twin ritual

The nature of womb twin rituals varies greatly. Your ritual may be carefully planned or spontaneous, public or private. It may be simple and may consist only of a short time of painful reflection or prayer, a burning or a burial. On the other hand, it may be elaborate and take several hours, involving many people and various different activities. There is a special ritual for every womb twin survivor and an almost infinite choice of ways to carry it out. Every ritual is perfect, however it is done, so do what your instincts tell you.

An altered state

The womb twin ritual is carried out in a liminal space, in an altered state of consciousness. You are tuning into such a deep part of your soul that you may not realize the meaning of what you are doing until long afterwards. It is important to create plenty of uninterrupted space where the spell will not be broken. The twin symbol will be very important as a vehicle for your feelings. As you let go of your object in your chosen way, you will be acknowledging the reality of your loss. A need may arise for loud laughter, angry outbursts, weeping and even dancing, so be ready for anything!

> *Recently, I did a ritual. I made two fish, a white one and a black one (my starsign is Pisces), representing me and my twin. On the black one, I wrote all the qualities related to my twin (fear, pain, sickness, loneliness) and on the white one my qualities (empathy, joy, caring). First I burned the black fish.*

After one month it still didn't feel right. Suddenly I knew that I had to burn the white fish too. I was still living half a life and still felt as if I needed to be perfect. Then I burned the white one too. That very moment I felt a fire burning inside me, like a warm and comforting glow. This was the right thing to do. The day after my ceremony I started crying and I'm still crying.

Anna, Belgium

LETTING GO OF THE PAIN IN YOUR BLACK HOLE

It may be that a ritual as described above is not the right way for you to let go of your twin. The ways to let go of your twin vary according to your womb story and the Black Hole you have created, so we will consider some alternatives.

Letting go of the Place of Desolation: Welcoming friends

You have been grieving for your twin for the whole of your life, in some way or other. This is the desolate place in your Black Hole. It comes out in all kinds of different ways, such as depression or long periods of unexplained sadness. The lifelong, sad secret of your twin can be brought to light at last: you could make your twin absolutely real. Then, in greeting your twin for the first time and calling him or her by name, you will have established an important personal truth for all time: it doesn't matter what other people say - you know your own heart.

It's only been within the last few years that I've decided to try and memorialize my four womb mates, and claim them as mine. Which is difficult with others trying to shove me into that "singleton" mold I will never fit in to. But I still try and do just that. Admittedly, I have many days where I wish I didn't have womb mates, as it's an awful road to be walking down, being alone and not alone, walking through this life that my womb mates should be sharing with me. And yet I'm the only one left who will keep my womb mates all-too-short memories alive. So I try and do just that.

Irene, USA

You cannot say farewell to your twin if you have never got to know your twin. Do not rush into a ritual of farewell until you fully understand what is in your Dream of the Womb. You may find yourself weeping, uncharacteristically emotional, preoccupied with your twin or unable to function normally. Give it time. Meanwhile, you may find it helpful to try writing "a letter to your twin" describing how it has been for you all these years. The letter could become one of your ritual objects, if the time comes for a ritual. Carol created her own reply from her twin:

"Forgiveness? What of it, my love? I do not need to forgive you for you have not hurt me. You perhaps need to forgive yourself. Walk through the doorway into life and embrace it. You do not even need to live for me at any level, for everything you do will reverberate and I will feel it. Such is the nature of soulship. What is it to forgive? When you go through, you have agreed to step through and at the last moment you let fall behind you everything bad, all the negative emotion, all the bad thoughts and feelings you have had about yourself: blame, anger, sadness, fear, self-denial, sacrifice, punishment, pain, stuckness, torment and anguish. These feelings are no longer necessary, as they serve no purpose now that you have understood you are not to blame. You can step forward in peace and feel light, light, light. Go my love, and live this world."

Once you have allowed your twin to be real and have fully acknowledged your loss, you may find that your attitude changing to other relationships. Fully acknowledging your status as a womb twin survivor can strengthen your resolve to make changes. If you are in a co-dependent, exploitative or abusive relationship, you will find yourself ready to set firmer boundaries and claim more space. You may decide to move on, even if the result is to live alone. If you have been grieving overmuch for other family members, you may find that you are prepared to let them go too, perhaps with a ritual action such as a grave side visit. As the months pass, you will become aware of any relationships that are not working any more. If you are letting a relationship die because you are not putting enough energy into it, then you could re-enliven it by making renewed contact. On the other hand, if the other person is obviously not interested, then it may be time for you to let go of all hopes of a future relationship.

Grief used to be a way of life, now it is healing. In healing I can talk about my experience and live for my sister till we are reunited! It feels like a validation!
Maria, USA

If you have been clinging onto other people for fear of being left alone, then you may find now that you are happier being single – for a while, at least. Now your grief has been properly validated, honoured and fully expressed, you will be stronger, better at standing alone and ready to move on to the next stage of your life.

Letting go of the Pit of Darkness: Letting be

If your Black Hole has within it a sense of having always lived a lie, now is the time for truth. When your Beta twin died, you were left feeling very vulnerable indeed, for you were closely identified with them. Now you know that, whatever else you may be, you are not your Beta womb twin. It is time to let be and accept the truth, that you are the strong survivor. The work will be to integrate the vulnerable Beta and the strong Alpha. It will be like an embrace, a coming together. The process is one of honouring your twin-ship, your status as the sole survivor of a twin pair. To reclaim your status as the Alpha survivor, rather than trying to be both Alpha and Beta at the same time, the death of your Beta twin must be acknowledged as a reality. Then your inauthentic self will be no longer needed. It will be made redundant because you will no longer be keeping your twin alive.

I just don't know how to begin the healing process. Several other twin-less twins have told me I should name my twin and hold a ritual and let my twin go. I think I am scared to death to even name my twin, who I never knew. I am afraid that I will lose even that little part that is holding on, and never to have anything left from my twin.
Chris, USA

To honour your twin-ship, you will need a pair of twin symbols. Because you tend to buy things in sets of two, you may already have a pair. If one is slightly larger then the other, that may be appropriate, particularly if your twin was very much smaller and weaker than you. For instance, Rick found a pebble that had split almost in half, Kay found two gold rings and Jo bought a necklace with two infinity rings hanging together.

Someone saw me today at church and said how lovely my twin necklace was, so I got to tell my story. He was so interested and loving and honoring to me and my story and his wife is a nurse so she knew exactly what I was talking about. It was really validating.
Jo, USA

When you have your twin symbols, you can name one of them for your twin. Then find a suitable place to put them on public display. Don't be shy about displaying your symbols, for this is your chance to honour your twin-ship and your twin. The truth will be evident and public at last.

I am feeling more and more emotionally whole every single day. This completeness and continually increasing confidence within my spirit is amazing and hard to describe but feels very, very real.
Jo, USA

Letting go of the World Filled with Pain: Handing back the pain

If you carry the pain of the world in your Black Hole, you may have already carried out a womb twin farewell ritual but perhaps the pain still remains. In that case, there is more work to be done, for you must now let go of the pain you carry that belongs to others. There are lots of womb twin survivors who routinely gather pain from all around them. Trying to hold and heal the pain of the world is an endless, fruitless mission and may have taken up a lot of your energy so far. Letting go of the pain of others will be easier when you have said your goodbye to your twin and are standing alone, facing life by yourself. In your new-found strength you will be able to see clearly how you have been driven by the dream of *I Can Heal the World*. You now know that this dream is an illusion.

How can I forget about the pain of people around me. Whatever emotional pain they feel, I seem to feel it too. Even if they have forgotten the pain, I haven't. You see their pain is my pain now. But if pain is so hurtful, why not release it? The answer is simple: I'm not allowed to be without pain. Without pain I would be nothing. Pain justifies my existence.
John, USA

It is time to hand the pain back in a daily ritual. The chances are that you have taken on someone else's emotional stuff, so notice the feelings inside you and try identify them as not yours. At some time every day, imagine yourself as usual, being a vessel for the feelings of others. Become aware of how guilty you feel that you can't make the feelings inside you go away. Try and remember who you have been with recently, probably someone who was in pain or in trouble. The chances are that at least some of the pain you feel came from that person. You willingly took on

313

their woundedness, as you have always done. Now imagine cupping your hands, lifting the feeling out of your heart and handing it, with love and respect, back to the owner. Say inside your head: *I know you didn't dump these feelings on me, I am holding them for you because I always want to help. You may hold them now.*

The aftermath

Whatever feelings there may be in your Black Hole, you may carry out a farewell ritual, a public acknowledgment of your twin ship, a ritual of handing back the pain of others or even a combination of all three. Whether you notice it or not, after the letting go and letting be, you will enter into a state of rapid psychic change. If clearing out, throwing away or cleaning activities seem to be the next thing to do, then go with your instincts. This will be part of your healing. If you decide to change something in the way you usually dress or how you do your hair, then go with it. If you want to change your career or take up a new interest, then do it. If you want to go on a diet, give up smoking or start a fitness campaign, then do it. The psychic space is now all yours. Your twin is in the place of the dead and you are here, free to live your own life at last. You now know that the world is not filled with death and dying and you are certainly not alone. Your Black Hole exists only in your Dream of the Womb. You have woken up at last from the Dream and it is time for you to claim your inheritance, Alpha energy.

29
Awakening from the Dream

I don't really know what to think anymore,
as this is completely new territory for me.
Julie, UK

Now that you have let go of your womb twin, you will be entering into a way of being that you have never known before. The Dream is over and it is time to wake up. This may fill you almost at once with unaccustomed joy, energy and confidence. For some womb twin survivors, however, the change is not quite as fast. It may take many years before they feel completely healed. This chapter contains some further guidance that you may find helpful as you begin your journey forward.

There is most definitely some resonating undercurrent that I can't quite put my finger on just yet. I'll have to sit with it a bit and see. Right now I am stringing things together so fast that it will take a while to sort through.
Edward, USA

It may help to imagine that you are making a journey into uncharted territory. We will consider what you might want to bring in your knapsack and the particular kind of energy you will need.

In your knapsack

You will carry your bag every step of the way, so make your bag as light as possible before you start. Along with letting go of your womb twin, you have let go of impossible dreams and resentment, so already your bag is lighter than it has been for a very long time. Yet there are some essential tools that will come in useful for the difficult times and the wonderful times. A sharp knife will be useful to cut the ties with ancestral pain and dead relationships. A trowel will help you to bury your false pride. Above all, you will need lots of energy, but probably not the kind you have used until now. For this new journey you will need a new kind of energy to see you through, Alpha energy.

315

Alpha and Beta

Alpha energy is based in your experience of having survived when your twin died. As a womb twin survivor who has sacrificed everything to keep your Beta twin alive in your Dream of the Womb, you have been using Beta energy. Beta energy often struggles to move at all and is easily drained by activity or stress. On the other hand, Alpha energy is completely effortless and has little to do with your levels of physical energy. It is extremely strong and lifts you up to a different plane of existence. The first surges of Alpha energy can be absolutely exhilarating, but unfortunately they can be short-lived to begin with.

> *Nothing dramatic seemed to have happened, except that I felt more able to handle every day situations. I had more energy available. I felt more empowered and much stronger. I also felt that I am not responsible for other people, I didn't have to help them or please them if I didn't feel like it. I had a greater sense of being a separate entity, with my own boundaries clearly defined. I have a sense of myself as a separate, individual human being. The sense of enmeshment is no longer there.*
> Katrina, UK

Alpha energy is more easily recognised in retrospect. It has a way of coming silently into your life and rendering effortless those tasks that once seemed much too difficult to even begin. You will know you are using Alpha energy when you say to yourself, "Just do it!" and for once you do not hesitate, but just do it.

Self-worth

One of the most astonishing effects of Alpha energy is to increase your self-confidence and sense of self-worth. Once you have awoken from your Dream of the Womb, you will see that you are worth no less than anyone else. And there is no one worth less than you, for we are all of equal worth. Furthermore, low self-esteem is false humility and false humility is only pride. Clearly, that sense of worthlessness is only a foetal assumption that once belonged in your Dream of the Womb.

The love of equal sharing

It is time to lay your burden down and accept that the only way to relate to other people in on a fifty-fifty basis. In other words, the only form

316

of love worth having is the love of equal sharing. This is a relationship of mutual respect, where you love the other person as much as you love yourself. That means that only half of the love goes to them and the rest is for you to keep. That may seem far too selfish at the moment, after so many years of self-sacrifice, but think of this: if the other person wants to give you love as much as you want to give love to him or her, how can fifty-fifty be anything other than completely fair and loving for both of you?

Alpha and Beta energy

There are many ways to recognise Alpha energy rising within you and changing your personality. You will be better able to ask for help and more capable when there is no help to be had. You will be more tolerant of your own failings and more open to learn new skills. You will be more reliable and able to deliver on promises made. You will have stronger opinions, all of your own, but without judging other people.

> *I previously did not know the experience of what it feels like to exist. Until one month ago, I viewed myself through my projections of how I believed others saw me. Now I can look down and see myself sitting here in this chair and realize I exist in this present moment. It may sound weird, but I never had that before.*
> *Amy, USA*

Beta energy is at work in your life when you try to live the Dream and keep alive your weak little Beta twin. Letting go of Beta energy will not happen rapidly or easily, so expect no miracles. Instead, learn to recognise when you are using Beta energy:

- Notice hesitance or indecision and let them go - start to make your own choices.
- Notice resentment at everything and nothing - accept the way things are and watch resentment dissolve away.
- When you feel nervous or anxious, remember your own strength.
- When you want to procrastinate, simply act.
- When you start to create complications, stop and think more clearly.
- When you are feeling weak, remember that you are the Alpha.

317

False Alpha

In the womb, the Alpha twin is more active and lively than the Beta twin. In born life this Alpha quality is expressed as high levels of vitality and purposeful energetic activity. Meanwhile, the Beta is compliant and is able to cope well with not being in control or having what they want. When a Beta womb twin survivor is born, they may choose to become a false Alpha to keep their Dream alive. If you are a Beta twin and try to emulate your lost Alpha twin in this way, you may stretch your capacities to the limit until you become too exhausted to continue. Do remember that your energy is limited, so work within those limits.

Coming into your inheritance

When your womb twin has been allowed to die and has been released, you can live life more fully. The space, the time and energy that your endless search has taken from you is now all yours. You may have spent your life being a false Beta by giving away your Alpha energy. It is a conscious and very powerful act of self-sacrifice, requiring Alpha power to make it.

> *Recently I discovered that I often resist life, simply because I feel responsible for everyone and everything that happens. It is such a burden that I have created in my own mind, that naturally it feels too much to even get out of bed! It was such a relief to discover and let go this image! Previously I always tried to be good, to do things perfectly, etc. (As if I had some survivor guilt.) I never felt I could authentically be me. But now I'm gradually experimenting with stepping outside that and being the me who I want to be. It's very energizing to be myself, rather than constantly holding back.*
> *Alice, USA*

Resistance to healing is a form of self-sabotage but there is Alpha power in that resistance, as we have seen.[a] If you become aware of your own resistance, then you will become conscious of the power that underlies it. That is your Alpha energy and you can now recognise it and own it. You will soon find that Alpha energy always lay beneath your false Beta choices. For instance, now that your twin has gone, you are alone. The false Beta way to be alone is "feel abandoned" but the Alpha way to be alone is to practice autonomy, which is the ability to consciously exercise your right to make active choices. Being passive would be a false Beta choice, but a

---

a. For more on resistance to healing, see page 287

calm acceptance of the status quo would be the Alpha choice. A floating feeling of helpless rage, which leaves you feeling useless, worthless and ineffectual can be turned upside down and recognised as your pent-up Alpha energy seeking an outlet.

Compulsive behaviours

One thing should now be clear: there are blocks on the road ahead but, out of habit, you will put them there. They are repositories of Beta energy that will prevent you from moving forward. You will allow Beta energy to gather into a Black Hole, just as you have done all your life. These blocks are called "compulsive" behaviours but nothing is forcing you. These blocks are your idea and your choice, put in place to keep your Dream alive. Clutter and hoarding is a good example of this.

Compulsive hoarding

You are surrounded with stuff in your Beta space. You feel powerless and unable to have any effect on the large collection of items that surrounds you. If you have a tendency to clutter or hoard, then this is a perfect expression of Beta energy. The end result of hoarding is that you are isolated in the midst of your collection with no room in your life or your home for much else. There is no space left for personal growth, for as all your Alpha energy is diverted into maintaining your piles of cherished possessions. You are literally suffocating in your own stuff.

Rescue yourself with Alpha energy

Hoarding is in your Dream but you are the Dream Master. To keep the Dream alive you decided, for reasons of survivor guilt, to delegate your Alpha power to some inanimate objects. Alpha energy is effortless, so you are never short of energy for bringing things into the house. If you take a dispassionate look at it all, you may be quite surprised how many possessions you do have, for it has required no effort to collect it.

> *I literally have created a wall between me and society with my clutter. The wall, very conveniently, stops me from having to deal with more pain and reminds me of the good times. I have a love / hate relationship with clutter. My emotional energy is drained when I look at it but yet I can't seem to live without it. I've realized on a conscious level that I need to move on, yet can't seem to get past that point and actually toss a significant amount of stuff.*
> Brenda, USA

319

It is very difficult when a large number of your possessions are packed into bags or boxes or littered all over the floor, so that you can hardly move. The presence of so many things can precipitate you into your Black Hole. There you sit, at once exhausted and overwhelmed by the enormity of the task you have set yourself. It may help you in that situation to understand that hoarding is a reflection of your Dream of the Womb, and that every item you collect is a potential focus of Beta energy.

MARTINA AND HER CLUTTER

Martina's fraternal twin (who was a surviving identical twin herself) died just after birth. Martina has since come to realize that she too had an identical twin, lost very early in the pregnancy, which makes her a womb quadruplet survivor. Martina cluttered her home with personal treasures and her own artwork. Most of her collection of clutter was in her bedroom and was concealed behind a large, translucent, blue curtain. She did not like making her bed, for that was like, "putting a lid on a coffin, too sterile, like hospital." Martina was in an incubator for months because she and her twin were born nearly three months early. Her twin sister was barely acknowledged, because the doctors had no idea there were to be twins. Martina being the stronger one, was given the only incubator. As her Alpha energy rises, she is gaining a sense of mastery over her behaviour. The familiar, exhausting Beta feeling of compulsion is beginning to diminish. For example she finds that when the sink is full of dishes, she is overwhelmed by them and gets momentarily lost in her Beta space. She uses her Alpha energy to get the dishes washed. She has noticed her tendency to leave food in her fridge for a long time, and this too has a meaning. Dirty glass dishes, some with rotting food inside, represent her twin, whose body was "donated to science." She has been keeping her twin's memory alive in a glass jar like, "a specimen." She leaves clothes littered around and particularly keeps clothes in her own bed. She can imagine clothes as "the places that people once occupied." She sees the bags she leaves around her home as empty amniotic sacs. For her, the main thing is "filling up the empty space, the place in my life where my womb quads would have been."

Clearing the space

It is time to clear space and release your Alpha energy. Bury the corpse, clear out the rubbish and chase the ghost into the light of day. Let it all be gone so you can claim your psychic space. Consider what ought to be in that space in your life, which you have never allowed yourself to own. It has been a dead place in your heart, with all the joy and fulfilment sucked out of it. If you open your heart and make space, the joy can rush in. As you move forward in your life, swept up in a glorious surge of Alpha energy, never forget that your brain was fashioned by your pre-birth experiences into patterns which will tend to persist. To illustrate this tendency, we will take a brief look at the three kinds of personal Black Hole and see how they have been healed.[b]

Ending desolation

You will now use your Alpha energy to claim your own personal space and set firm boundaries. If you remember always to keep your distance from other people, then your Alpha energy will be concentrated in the small area of operation that is truly yours. In your private space is all your freedom and power, so do be careful to keep it contained. Do not let it leach away in a desperate quest for companionship. Your relationships will be stronger and healthier as a result. Surrounded by friends, it will then be possible for you to find tiny fragments of your lost twin in each of them. One will give you companionship, another laughter and so on. No one person can replace your twin. Instead, you will find that you can have many brothers or sisters. When you put all these fragments together, it will ease the emptiness inside.

Out of the pit

The biggest block to your progress will be a sense of being "held captive" in your Beta space, where you feel too weak and vulnerable to escape. You are so used to being both Alpha and Beta at exactly the same time, that you have forgotten how to use Alpha energy without always injecting some Beta energy into it somehow. When you feel overwhelmed, remember that you have slipped into your Beta space. There is a simple and highly effective way to get back into your Alpha space: recognise the truth, that

---

b.   The three Black Holes are fully described in Chapter 26

you have never left your Alpha space. Being a false Beta has always been a choice and the capacity to choose is an Alpha quality in itself. Next time you wake up in your Beta space, remember that you chose to invite Beta energy into your life. You had a rational, loving and intelligent reason for the choice you made, but it was based on a misunderstanding. Alpha energy will give you the strength to begin relating to people in a new way: equally. For far too long you have allowed other people, duties and bad habits to steal your energy. Now you will share. If you take space belonging to another person, they will complain and claim it back. If someone takes your space, you will negotiate your rights using Alpha energy: you will complain and claim it all back.

Handing back the pain

If you have always wanted to heal the pain of the world, first you will have to heal yourself. With your new-found Alpha energy all kinds of things that seemed impossible become possible. Alpha energy will help you to see that your life journey is made of steps along the road. If you bring your Alpha energy into every small step, the results will be astonishing. You will soon recognise that Alpha energy is not to be used to overpower or persuade others: it is made for sharing. By sharing your power you will become a force to be reckoned with. You will be able to express yourself more freely. If any one hurts you, you will find it easy to complain. If there is loss in your life, you will grieve appropriately and then move on. Alpha energy is effortless, intelligent and calm. Agitation, struggle and thoughtlessness are an expression of Beta energy and are exhausting. As soon as you stop trying too hard, calm down and start thinking clearly: the Alpha energy will flood in. This kind of energy is as much about letting be and allowing as it is about getting things done. If something is a real struggle and beyond your capacities, delegate the task or ask for help. Soon, you will quietly accept the present situation in your life with all its limitations. You will allow yourself to settle down, wherever you are. You will begin to want what you get and love what you have. You will break new ground, make new friends and revive old friendships. You will gladly do whatever work has to be done. Even your mission to heal the world and everyone in it may be achievable after all, if you are clear about which group you are trying to heal and enliven.

Time for personal growth

It is time now for you, an awakened womb twin survivor, to grow into the person you were created to become. This kind of growth is not about getting larger. It is being stripped absolutely bare of pride, impossible dreams and additional burdens: all that has to go. Once you are sufficiently stripped down, all your Alpha energy will be set free. Gradually this new energy will become more dependable and you will slip into your Beta space less and less often. Then you will be able to practice intelligent thinking, calm in spirit, in every situation. You will find yourself bolder and readier to trust in your capacity to cope. You may decide as to let go of more and more as time passes. Letting go is a wonderful feeling of cleansing and renewal, but do not let go of too much, for this might weaken your Alpha energy, which needs to be well-fed.

Restoration

Along with growth comes restoration. Broken family ties can be mended and neglected tasks can be revisited. Gradually and imperceptibly, you will be strengthened, as you become more firmly rooted in this world. With good care of your body, sufficient rest and good nutrition, you will become healthier. Given enough time and space to recover your energies, you will be amazed at how much you can achieve. With a calm but determined spirit, you will stop wasting energy on useless regretting.

Being yourself

You will quickly discover that, regardless of your other talents, your greatest gift is your capacity to be completely yourself. Alpha energy will allow your whole personality to shine out and make a difference in the world. Now is the time to hand over your gifts to the world, and your principal gift is yourself: it is time for your light to shine.

323

30
The Healer : a dialogue

The Healer said, *You can be healed.*

I said, *Thank you very much, that's very kind of you.*

But inside I knew that the healer didn't understand how much it hurt me just to be alive. So I was nice to her, because it was kind of her to care so much. I knew she didn't understand how it was for me and I did not want to hurt her by saying that the whole thing was a waste of time, that it was not what I wanted, that I just wanted her to get off my back.

Many other healers came. They tried to be polite and loving, but I knew they were thinking I was a bad person. They said I must change, so I tried, I really did. I tried to be nice and be friendly. I did everything I was told to do. I completed all the healing tasks they set me - or at least I tried but they did not know how hard it was for me to do them.

Again they looked at me as if I was stupid because I was so slow. I could not make up my mind how to do things. I didn't know where to start. There was such a mess in my life and I was so afraid! I didn't know what to tackle first. They kept suggesting schedules of work and gave me ideas about how to get my life on track. None of them were any good for me. I couldn't do them.

It's so obvious, all this stuff. It makes me annoyed but I'm trying to be nice. It's patronising of them even to make all suggestions, like I am some kind of idiot. I'm not stupid. I know that all these so-called good ideas would work but I also know that I won't do it. I really don't want to. I just want them to stop getting at me all the time.

Am I not good enough, just as I am? Am I so bad? Why am I always judged and found wanting? It hurts me so much when they say these things about me. It makes me angry. No one cares about me enough to notice how hard this is for me.

When is someone going to see that I don't want to change into another kind of person? How can I possibly do that? This is me, and that's that. They want me to change and I can't.

When I say that, they begin to accuse me and tell me that my behaviour is unacceptable, that it's all my fault and I am a bad person. I don't need them to rub it in. I know. I am worthless, useless, unable to take charge of my life, unable to do anything much that has any meaning at all, except this. So I will do this - it's what I do. It's me, being me.

This is my truth, the meaning of my life. They are asking me to throw away my identity! Well, they can wish. I will not throw it away and become some other person and live some other life. This is my way of being. I will hold on to this because it is all I have. There is nothing else. Without this I may as well be dead. Without this I would no longer exist. In fact, this is keeping me alive - this thing I do, this thing I must do, this thing I must never stop doing.

To stop doing this would be a betrayal of all I hold dear. It would mean a kind of spiritual death. It would mean guilt and pain and terror. So don't try to heal me! Please do not try, I don't want it, it hurts too much even to think about.

Love me enough to leave me alone and accept me just as I am. Please do not ask me to change. Just love me as I am. Leave me alone here, for this is the only life I know. I can't do it any other way.

Then the Healer said, *I know how much it hurts you to simply be alive. I know how guilty you feel at being alive. I believe that the thing you most fear is the truth.*

I was angry and I said, *I am the only one who knows the truth about me, so don't think you know what my truth is like!*

The Healer spoke gently and said, *I mean the truth of your intrinsic goodness and wholeness, given to you at conception.*

I felt sorrowful as I said, *That was a long time ago. Maybe I was that once, but no more.*

The Healer was silent then, for everything had been said that must be said.

I waited a long time but there were no more healing words. There was only the memory of what the Healer had said. I struggled with that truth, that I was created good.

325

I wanted it to be true but I knew in my heart it could not possibly be true. I struggled for many dark nights and many lonely days.

Then I came to a river. I said to myself, *I could wash myself clean of all the things I have done to myself and be healed!* So I washed myself carefully and I was clean - but I was not healed.

Then I walked through fire and the badness was burnt out of me and there was great pain - but I was not healed.

Then I came to a mirror, and I saw myself in truth. I felt pity and regret at my un-lived life and I wept. Through those tears I felt the healing begin. I stood up and knew once again my original wholeness and perfection.

I was able then to let go of the person I had been pretending to be all my life and become myself.

Appendices

Appendix A
Signs and indications of a possible twin or multiple pregnancy

The mother's pregnancy
Mother abnormally large around the waist in the first three months
First trimester bleeding
Complete miscarriage but pregnancy continued
Suspected miscarriage but pregnancy continued
Attempted abortion but pregnancy continued
Doctor or nurse suspected twin pregnancy
Another person suspected twins
Mother experienced blunt trauma in an accident or assault when pregnant
Mother experienced infection during pregnancy
Mother experienced severe trauma during pregnancy
Mother experienced starvation through illness famine or hyperemesis
Mother took hyper-ovulation drug (eg. Clomid)
More that one embryo transplanted after IVF
Ultrasound evidence of second sac

Features of labour and delivery
Birth was traumatic
Breech birth
Small for dates
Placenta unusually large

Physical evidence of the lost twin after delivery
Additional sacs or cords found
Fetus papyaceous
Marks or lesions on the placenta
Twin stillborn or dies close to birth

In body of survivor
Dermoid cyst
Teratoma
Foetus in foetu
Sexual organs of opposite sex
Secondary sexual characteristics of opposite sex
Cerebral palsy in the survivor

Birth defects in survivor
Split organs
Congenital abnormality
Left handed

Other associations with twinning
Ambidextrous
Chimerism
Mosaicism

Appendix B
Data Analysis of Womb Twin Survey

UNIVERSITY OF HERTFORDSHIRE
STATISTICAL SERVICES AND CONSULTANCY UNIT
[http://go.herts.ac.uk/sscu]
Lindsey Kevan, Neil Spencer. 4th September 2009

Abstract

The Statistical Services and Consultancy Unit (SSCU), which is part of the Business School at the University of Hertfordshire, were contracted to carry out the following services:

1. Data management.
2. A full analysis of the "effects" against "q64stuff" to identify potential relationships.
3. Analysis to identify the commonest psychological effects for "A" (the strongest possible agreement) responses for those respondents for whom evidence of a womb twin exists.
4. To identify any differences in "effects" amongst fraternal and identical survivors.

Methodology
The data analysis was carried out using SPSS by a member of the SSCU.

2. A full analysis of the "effects" against "q64stuff" to identify potential relationships.

To accomplish this a binary logistic regression using a forward selection method (Wald) was carried out on the dependent variable "q64stuff" against the "effects" (q19-77). From the binary logistic regression, the variables "q30vulnerable", "q33addicted", "q61unfunished" and "q69unwell" are included in a model for "q64stuff". Table 1 in the appendix shows the development of the model. This leads us to conclude that there is a significant relationship between "q64stuff" and these four variables.

Table 1: output from the binary logistic regression

	B	S.E.	Wald	df	Sig.	Exp.(B)
Step 1[a] a61 unfinished	1.353	.309	19.138	1	.000	3.869
Constant	-.788	.204	14.959	1	.000	.455
Step 2[b] q30 vulnerable	1.082	.319	11.549	1	.001	2.952
a61 unfinished	1.296	.320	16.435	1	.001	3.653
Constant	-1.345	.277	23.624	1	.000	.260
Constant	-1.621	.300	29.189	1	.000	.198
a. Variable(s) entered on Step 1: q61 unfinished.						
b. Variable(s) entered on Step 2: q30 vulnerable.						
c. Variable(s) entered on Step 3: q33 addicted.						
d. Variable(s) entered on Step 4: q69 unwell.						

329

	B	S.E.	Wald	df	Sig.	Exp.(B)
Step 3[c] q30 vulnerable	.907	.328	7.625	1	.006	2.477
q33 addicted	.920	.360	6.506	1	.011	2.508
q61 unfinished	1.271	.326	15.196	1	.000	3.563
Constant	-1.510	.290	27.130	1	.000	.221
Step 4[d] q30 vulnerable	.843	.332	6.436	1	.011	2.324
q33 addicted	.864	.365	5.602	1	.018	2.374
q61 unfinished	1.179	.332	12.613	1	.000	3.251
q69 unwell	.737	.371	3.951	1	.047	2.089
Constant	-1.621	.300	29.189	1	.000	.198
a. Variable(s) entered on Step 1: q61 unfinished.						
b. Variable(s) entered on Step 2: q30 vulnerable.						
c. Variable(s) entered on Step 3: q33 addicted.						
d. Variable(s) entered on Step 4: q69 unwell.						

3. Analysis to identify the commonest psychological effects for "A" responses for those respondents for whom evidence of a womb twin exists. *(See Appendix A for details)*

To accomplish this, a table was created that shows for each "effect", the proportion of these selected respondents who gave an "A" response. Table 2 shows each "effect" in ascending order of the proportion of the selected respondents who gave an "A" response.

Table 2: of the commonest psychological effects

	Statement	Count	Table N%
q53	dyslexia	19	7.4%
q27	male with female	21	8.1%
q76	harm	26	11.2
q75	guilt being alive	46	18.5
q51	paranoid	58	22.5
q33	addicted	68	27.9
q43	mirror	71	28.4
q63	privileged	71	27.2
q54	upset	75	29.8
q69	unwell	77	30.1
q23	alone in dark	78	33.6

q46	perfectionist	80	31.6
q50	not close	82	32.0
q26	female with male	84	31.9
q45	psychic	87	35.5
q48	exploitative	87	34.0
q56	guilty	89	35.9
q28	unable to cope	91	36.8
q62	feel not there	94	36.4
q65	lack energy	96	36.8
q60	death before born	96	36.6
q22	suicide	98	40.0
q34	inauthentic	98	39.2
q32	death and dying	100	38.5
q52	musts and shoulds	102	41.0
q37	love-hate relationship	103	40.1
q38	reduce suffering	110	42.0
q20	problem with food	112	45.7
q47	hard to forgive	112	43.8
q19	depression	115	48.7
q70	maintain privacy	115	46.9
q77	sabotage success	115	44.7
q64	stuff	116	45.3
q39	difficulty falling asleep	117	45.3
q40	not rest enough	119	44.7
q44	disappointment	120	48.4
q25	intense then sabotage	120	47.8
q49	empty inside	124	48.4
q71	empathy & intuition	124	48.1
q59	inner life	128	50.4
q61	let go unfinished	128	48.9
q31	bored easily	128	48.7
q67	lack self esteem	129	51.8
q29	greive deeply	129	49.6
q74	heal the world	130	49.6

q30	feel vulnerable	131	50.2
q68	torn in two	136	51.9
q35	pain of others	136	51.7
q72	restless and unsettled	142	55.0
q41	two sides to character	143	55.2
q73	deep pain wont heal	143	54.8
q57	unsatisfied	145	56.0
q66	anger	153	59.3
q36	alone	163	62.2
q21	fear abandonment	165	64.2
q24	searching	175	68.4
q55	different from others	176	67.4
q58	not realising potential	182	69.7
q21	rejection	188	72.9
q42	missing	193	75.7

4. To identify any differences in "effects" amongst DZ and MZ womb twin survivors

To accomplish this a Mann-Whitney U test was carried for each "effect" to see if there was a difference between responses given by these two groups.

Table 3 Test statistics

		Mann-Whitney U	Wilcoxon W	Z	Asymp.Sig.(2-tailed)
q29	grief	689.500	1770.500	-2.193	.028
q30	vulnerable	667.000	1796.000	-2.189	.029
q75	guilt alive	657.000	1785.000	-2.191	.028

Table 3 shows the results from the three Mann-Whitney U tests that show a significant difference between the two groups (fraternal and identical) at the 5% level of significance. However, when using a 5% level of significance, there is a one in twenty chance of obtaining a p-value less than 5% so we would expect a number of the tests to give p-values of less than 5% even if no real difference existed. We should thus treat with caution the fact that there are "effects" in Table 3 shown as being significantly different.

332

References

Chapter 1: The Making of You

1. Karr, T. L., (2007) Fruit flies and the sperm proteome. *Human Molecular Genetics*, Vol.16, Special edition No. 2, pp.124-33
2. Pillitteri, A., (2009) *Maternal and Child Health Nursing: Care of the Childbearing and Child Rearing.* Lippincott Williams & Wilkins, p.93
3. Piotrowska, K., F. Wianny, et al., (2001) Blastomeres arising from the first cleavage division have distinguishable fates in normal mouse development. *Development*, Vol.128, No.19, pp. 3739-3748
4. Eyal-Giladi, H., (1997) Establishment of the axis in chordates: facts and speculations. *Development*, Vol.124, No.12, pp.2285-9
5. Horton, H. L. & P. Levitt, (1988) A unique membrane protein is expressed on early developing limbic system axons and cortical targets. *Journal of Neuroscience*, Vol. 8, No.12, pp.4653-61
6. Rockwell, P.E., (1970) Letter. *Albany Times-Union*, March 1
7. Piontelli, A., (2002) *Twins: From Fetus To Child.* Routledge, p.29

Chapter 2: How Twins are Made

1. Hedricks, C., et al., (1987) Peak coital rate coincides with onset of luteinizing hormone surge. *Fertility and Sterility.* Vol. 48, No.2, pp. 234-8
2. Dunson, D. B., C. R. Weinberg, et al., (2001) Modelling multiple ovulation, fertilization, and embryo loss in human fertility studies. *Biostatistics*, Vol. 2, No. 2, pp.131-45
3. Tuppen GD, C. Fairs, et al., (2002) Spontaneous superfetation diagnosed in the first trimester with successful outcome. *Ultrasound in Obstetrics and Gynecology* Vol.14, No. 3, pp. 219-221
4. Elliot, D. & F. End, (1995) Twins-with two fathers: a fertility clinic's startling error. *Newsweek,* July 3rd, p.38
5. Bortolus, R., V. Zanardo, et al., (2001) Epidemiology of identical twin pregnancy (article in Italian.) *La Pediatria Medica e Chirurgica*, Vol. 23, Nos, 3-4, pp. 153-8
6. Hall, J.G., (2003) Twinning. *Lancet*, Vol. 362, No. 9385, pp. 735–743
7. Piontelli, A., (2002) *Twins: From Fetus To Child.* Routledge, p.19
8. Derom, C., Derom R, et al., (1987) Increased monozygotic twinning rate after ovulation induction. *The Lancet*, Vol. 1, No, 8544, pp.1236-8
9. Aston, K.I., (2008) Monozygotic twinning associated with assisted reproductive technologies: a review. *Reproduction*, No.136, pp. 377-386
10. Schachter M. et al., (2001) Monozygotic twinning after assisted reproductive techniques: a phenomenon independent of micromanipulation. *Human Reproduction*, Vol. 16, No. 6
11. Hall, J.G., (2003) *op. cit.* p.737
12. Hall, J.G., (2003) *ibid*
13. Hall, J.G., (2003) *ibid*
14. Hunter, K., C. Bunker, et al., (1964) *Duet for a Lifetime.* Michael Joseph.
15. Kothari, M.L., Mehta, L.A.,(1985) Non-identicality of monozygous twins. *Journal of Postgraduate Medicine*, Vol. 31, no.1. pp.1-4

16. Scott, J.M & M.A Ferguson-Smith, (1973) Heterokaryotypic monozygotic twins and the acardiac monster. *Journal of Obstetrics and Gynaecology of the British Commonwealth*, Vol. 80, No.1, pp.52-59

17. Hall, J.G., (2003) *ibid*. p.738

18. Springer, S.P. & G. Deutsch, (1998) *Left Brain, Right Brain: Perspectives from Cognitive Neuroscience*. W.H. Freeman & Co.

19. Machin, G.A., (1996) Some causes of genotypic and phenotypic discordance in monozygotic twin pairs. *American Journal of Medical Genetics*. Vol. 61, No. 3, pp. 216-228

20. Bruder, C. E., A. Piotrowski, et al., (2008),Phenotypically concordant and discordant monozygotic twins display different DNA copy-number-variation profiles. *American Journal of Human Genetics*, Vol. 82, No.3, pp.763-771

21. Shibata D., (2009) Inferring human stem cell behaviour from epigenetic drift. *Journal of Pathology*, Vol. 217, No.2, pp.199-205

22. Edwards, J. H., T. Dent, et al., (1966) Monozygotic twins of different sex. *Journal of Medical Genetics*, Vol. 3, No.2, pp.117-23

23. Kothari, M.L., (1985) *op. cit.*

24. Keith, L. G. & J. J. Oleszczuk, (2002) Triplet births in the United States. An epidemic of high-risk pregnancies. *Journal of Reproductive Medicine*, Vol. 47, No. 4, pp. 259-65

25. Imaizumi, Y., (2003) A comparative study of zygotic twinning and triplet rates in eight countries, 1972-1999. *Journal of Biosocial Science*, Vol. 35, No. 2, pp. 287-302

26. Keith, L.G (Ed.) & I. Blickstein (Ed.), (2002)*Triplet Pregnancies and Their Consequences*. Taylor & Francis

27. Keith, L.G (Ed.) & I. Blickstein (Ed.), (2002) *ibid*. p.13

28. Noble, E. et al., (2003) *Having Twins And More: A Parent's Guide to Multiple Pregnancy, Birth, and Early Childhood*. Houghton Mifflin Harcourt p. 340

29. Piontelli, A., (2002) *Twins: From Fetus To Child*. Routledge, p.128

Chapter 3: When a Twin Dies Close to Birth

1. Stevenson A., (2010) *Half Baked: The Story of My Nerves, My Newborn, and How We Both Learned to Breathe*. Running Press

2. Sandbank A., (1998) *Twins and the Family*. TAMBA (Twins and Multiple Births Association) Guildford, England.

3. Progrebin A., (2009) *One and the Same*. Doubleday

4. Piontelli A., (2008) *Twins In The World: The Legends They Inspire and the Lives They Lead*. Palgrave Macmillan

5. Roberts, S.C., (1987) Vaccination And Cot Deaths In Perspective. *Archives of Disease in Childhood*, Vol. 62, No.7, pp. 754-759

6. Pharoah P., (2007) Sudden Infant Death Syndrome in Twins and Singletons. *Twin Research and Human Genetics, Supplement: Abstracts From the 12th International Congress on Twin Studies, Belgium, 8–10 June*

7. Fellman, J. & A. W. Eriksson, (2007) Estimation of the stillbirth rate in twin pairs according to zygosity. *Twin Research and Human Genetics*, Vol.10, No.3, pp. 508-13

8. Ghai,V. & D.Vidyasagar, (1988) Morbidity and mortality factors in twins. An epidemiologic approach. *Clinical Perinatology*, Vol.15, No.1, pp.123-140

9. Henderson, J.L., (1945) The definition of prematurity :a proposed minimal weight standard for viable premature infants. *BJOG. An International Journal of Obstetrics & Gynaecology*, Vol. 52, No.1, pp. 29-35

10. Engle, W.A., (2006) A recommendation for the definition of "late preterm" (near-term) and the birth weight–gestational age classification system. *Seminars in Perinatalology*, Vol. 30, No.1, pp.2-7

11. Forman, V., (2009) *This Lovely Life*. Mariner Books

12. Fogel B., H. Nitowsky, P. Gruenwald, (1965) Discordant abnormalities in monozygotic twins. *The Journal of Paediatrics*, Vol. 66, No. 1, pp. 64-72

13. Ohkuchi A, H. Minakami et al., (2002) Intrauterine death of one twin, with rescue of the other, in twin-twin transfusion syndrome. *Ultrasound in Obstetrics & Gynecology*, Vol. 19, No.3, p.293

14. Senat M.V., J.P. Bernard et al., (2002) Management of single fetal death in twin-to-twin transfusion syndrome: a role for fetal blood sampling. *Ultrasound in Obstetrics & Gynecology*, Vol. 20, No. 4, pp. 360-3

15. Tarkan L., (2008) Lowering Odds of Multiple Births. *New York Times*, Feb 19th

16. Umstead, M.P. & M.J. Gronow, (2003) Multiple pregnancy: a modern epidemic? *The Medical Journal of Australia*, Vol.178, No.12, pp. 613-615

17. Hatkar, P.A. & A.G. Bhide, (1999) Perinatal outcome of twins in relation to chorionicity. *Journal of Postgraduate Medicine*, Vol.45, No.2, pp. 33-7

18. Ménézo, Y., (1999) Birth weight and sex ratio after transfer at the blastocyst stage in humans. *Fertility and Sterility*, Vol. 72, No. 2, pp. 221-224

19. Loos, R., C. Derom, R. Eeckels, et al., (2001) Length of gestation and birthweight in dizygotic twins. *The Lancet*, Vol. 358, No. 9281, pp. 560-561

20. Progrebin A., (2009) *op. cit.*

Chapter 4: The Death of a Twin in the Second Trimester

1. Nishida, H. & I. Sakuma, (2009) Limit of viability in Japan: ethical consideration. *Journal of Perinatal Medicine*, Vol. 37, No. 5, pp. 457-60

2. Olga, B. & J. Olsen, (2001) Sex Ratio and Twinning in Women With Hyperemesis or Pre-eclampsia. *Epidemiology*, Vol.12, No.6, pp.747-749

3. Ghulmiyyah, L., Wehbe, S. et al. (2004) Successful obstetrical management of 110-day intertwin delivery interval without cerclage: counseling and conservative management approach to extreme asynchronous twin. *Pregnancy and Childbirth*, Vol. 4, No. 23

4. Ong, S.S., Zamora, J. et al., (2006) Prognosis for the co-twin following single-twin death: a systematic review. *British Journal of Obstetricts and Gynaecology*, Vol.113, No.9, pp.992-8

5. Ville, Y. et al., (1995) Preliminary experience with endoscopic laser surgery for severe twin-twin transfusion syndrome. *New England Journal of Medicine*, Vol. 332, No. 4, pp. 224-7

6. De Lia, J.E. et al., (1995) Fetoscopic laser ablation of placental vessels in severe previable twin-twin transfusion syndrome. *American Journal of Obstetrics and Gynecology*, Vol.172, No 4, Part 1, pp.1202-8

7. Salomon, L.J. et al., (2010) Long-term developmental follow-up of infants who participated in a randomized clinical trial of amniocentesis *vs* laser photocoagulation for the treatment of twin-to-twin transfusion syndrome. *American Journal of Obstetrics and Gynecology*. Vol. 203, No. 5, pp. 444. e1-7

8. Urig, M.A. et al., (1988) Twin-twin transfusion syndrome. The surgical removal of one twin as a treatment option. *Fetal Therapy*, Vol. 3, No. 4, pp.185-8

9. Zankl, A.& E. Boltshauser, (2004) Natural history of twin disruption sequence. *American Journal of Medical Genetics*, Part A, Vol.127a, No. 2, pp.133-138

10. Szymonowicz, W. et al., (1986) The surviving monozygotic twin. *Archives of Diseases in Childhood*, Vol. 61, No. 5, pp. 454-8

11. Enbom, J. A., (1985) Twin pregnancy with intrauterine death of one twin. *American Journal of Obstetrics & Gynecology*, Vol.152, No. 4, pp. 424-9

12. Kilby, M. D. et al., (1994) Outcome of twin pregnancies complicated by a single intrauterine death: a comparison with viable twin pregnancies. *Obstetrics and Gynecology*, Vol. 84, No. 1, pp.107-9

13. Woo, H. H. et al., (2000) Single foetal death in twin pregnancies: review of the maternal and neonatal outcomes and management. *Hong Kong Medical Journal*, Vol. 6, No. 3, pp.293-300

14. Malinowski, W., R. Koktysz, P. Stawerski, (2005) The case of monochorionic twin gestation complicated by intrauterine demise of one fetus in the first trimester. *Twin Research and Human Genetics*, Vol. 8, No.3, p.262-6

15. Kobayashi, K. et al. (2005) Fetal growth restriction associated with measles virus infection during pregnancy. *Journal of Perinatal Medicine*, Vol. 33, No.1, pp. 67-8

16. Lazzarotto T. et al, (2003) Congenital cytomegalovirus infection in twin pregnancies: viral load in the amniotic fluid and pregnancy outcome. *Pediatrics*, Vol. 112. No. 2, pp.153-7

17. Willerman, L. & J. A. Churchill, (1967) Intelligence and birth weight in identical twins. *Child Development*, Vol.38, No. 3, pp.623-9

18. O'Neill, Y. V., (1974) Michele Savonarola and the *fera* or blighted twin phenomenon. *Medical History*, Vol. 18, No.3, pp. 222-39

19. Redwine, F. O. & R. E. Petres, (1984) Selective birth in a case of twins discordant for Tay Sachs disease. *Acta Geneticae Medicae et Gemellologica* (Roma), Vol. 33, No.1, pp. 35-8

20. Aberg, A. et al., (1978) Cardiac puncture of fetus with Hurler's disease avoiding abortion of unaffected co-twin. *The Lancet* ,Vol. 2, pp. 990-991

21. Maymon, R. et al., (1995) First trimester embryo reduction: a medical solution to an iatrogenic problem. *Human Reproduction*, Vol.10, No.3, pp. 668-73

22. Frederiksen, M. H. et al. (2009) [Foetal reduction--a retrospective survey]. *Ugeskrift for Laeger*, Vol.171, No.39, p. 2825-9

23. Evans, M.I. et al., (2004) Do reduced multiples do better? *Best Practice & Research Clinical Obstetrics & Gynaecology*, Vol. 18, No. 4, pp. 601-612

24. Sentilhes, L. et al., (2008)[Multifetal pregnancy reduction: indications, technical aspects and psychological impact]. *Presse Medicale*, Vol.37, No.2, pp. 295-306

25. Bryan, E., (2002) Loss in higher multiple pregnancy and multifetal pregnancy reduction, *Twin Research and Human Genetics*, Vol.5, No.3, pp.169-74

26. Dimitriou, G. et al. (2004) Cerebral palsy in triplet pregnancies with and without iatrogenic reduction. *European Journal Of Pediatrics,* Vol. 163, No. 8, pp. 449-451

Chapter 5: The Death of a Twin in the First Trimester

1. Kurjak, A. & V. Latin, (1979) Ultrasound diagnosis of fetal abnormalities in multiple pregnancy. *Acta Obstetricia et Gynecologica Scandinavica*, Vol.58, No.2, pp. 153-61

2. Arck, P. C. et al. (2001) Stress and immune mediators in miscarriage. *Human Reproduction*, Vol.16, No.7, pp.1505-11

3. Craig, M., (2001) Stress and Recurrent Miscarriage. *Stress: The International Journal on the Biology of Stress*, Vol. 4, No. 3, pp.205-213

4. Yang, J. et al., (2004) Vaginal bleeding during pregnancy and preterm birth. *American Journal of Epidemiology*, Vol.160, No.2, pp.118-25

5. Harville, E.W. et al. (2003) Vaginal bleeding in very early pregnancy, *Human Reproduction*, Vol.18, No.9, pp.1944-1947

6. Saidi, M. H., (1988) First-trimester bleeding and the vanishing twin. A report of three cases, *The Journal of Reproductive Medicine*, Vol. 33, No 10, pp.831-4

7. Finberg, H. J. & J. C. Birnholz, (1979) Ultrasound observations in multiple gestation with first trimester bleeding: the blighted twin, *Radiology*, Vol. 132, No.1, pp.137-42

8. Staff reporter, (2001) Anger of woman who gave birth after abortion. *Daily Telegraph*, 23rd November

9. Inion, I. et al. (1998) An unexpected triplet heterotopic pregnancy after replacement of two embryos. *Human Reproduction*, Vol. 13, No.7, pp.1999-2001

10. Small, M.F., (1998) Love with the proper stranger. *Natural History*, September

11. Small, M.F., (1998) *ibid.*

12. Pharoah, P. O., (2002) Neurological outcome in twins. *Seminars in Neonatology*, Vol.7, No. 3, pp. 223-30

13. Glinianaia, S. V. et al., (2002) Fetal or infant death in twin pregnancy: neuro-developmental consequence for the survivor. *Archives of Disease in Childhood, Fetal & Neonatal Edition*, Vol. 86, No. 1, pp.9-15

14. Pharoah, P. O., (2000) Consequences of in-utero death in a twin pregnancy. *The Lancet*, Vol. 355, No. 9215, pp. 1597-602

15. Pharoah, P. O. and Y. Dundar, (2009) Monozygotic twinning, cerebral palsy and congenital anomalies. *Human Reproduction Update*, Vol.15, No. 6, pp. 639-48

Chapter 6: When Twins Unite

1. Toufexis, A. et al. (1994) The Brief Life of Angela Lakeberg. *Time Magazine*, 27 Jun

2. Dyer, C. (2000) Conjoined twins separated after long legal battle. *British Medical Journal*, Vol. 321. No. 7270, p.1175

3. Harris, J. (2001) Human Beings, Persons and Conjoined Twins: An Ethical Analysis of the Judgment in Re. A. *Medical Law Review*, No. 9, pp.221-236

4. Bashir, M.,(2003) Living With the Miracle of Gracie. *The Sunday Times*, 3 Aug

5. Chatterjee, S. K. et al., (2009) Ischiopagus tetrapus conjoined twins: 22 years after separation. *Journal of the Indian Association of Pediatric Surgeons*, Vol.14, No.1, pp.36-8

6. Wallis, C. & J.M.R Doman, (1996) The Most Intimate Bond. *Time Magazine*, 25 March

7. Boulot, P. et al., (1992) Conjoined twins associated with a normal singleton: very early diagnosis and successful selective termination. *Journal of Perinatal Medicine*, Vol.20, No.2, p.135-7

8. Fitzpatrick, C., (2000) Psychosocial Study of a Surviving Conjoined Twin. *Clinical Child Psychology and Psychiatry*, Vol. 5, No.4, pp. 513-519

9. Chou, S. Y. et al. (2001) Sacral parasite conjoined twin. *Obstetrics and Gynecology*, Vol. 98, No. 5, pp.938-40

10. Wang, T. M. et al. (1982) Craniopagus parasiticus: a case report of a parasitic head protruding from the right side of the face. *British Journal of Plastic Surgery*, Vol. 35, No. 3, pp. 304-311

11. Hirayama, Y. et al. (2007) Sacral parasite with histopathological features of an unequally conjoined twin. *Pediatric Surgery International*, Vol. 23, No.7, pp.715-20

12. Wark, P., (2003) The boy with a twin inside. *The Times*, 5 Dec

13. Boyce, M. J. et al.,(1972) Fetus in fetu: serological assessment of monozygotic origin by automated analysis. *Journal of Clinical Pathology*, No. 25, pp.793-798

14. Nagar, A. et al. (2002) Foetus in foetu. *Journal of Postgraduate Medicine*, No.48, p.133

15. Higgins, K. R. & B. D. Coley, (2006) Fetus in fetu and fetaform teratoma in two neonates: an embryologic spectrum? *Journal of Ultrasound Medicine* Vol. 25, No. 2, pp. 259-63

16. Basu, A. et al., (2006) Fetus in fetu or differentiated teratomas? *Indian Journal of Pathology and Microbiology*, Vol.49, No. 4, pp. 563-5

17. Ihara, T. et al., (1984) Histologic grade and karyotype of immature teratoma of the ovary. *Cancer*, Vol. 54, No.12, pp. 2988-94.

18. Kazez, A. et al. (2002) Sacrococcygeal heart: a very rare differentiation in teratoma. *European Journal of Pediatric Surgery*, Vol.12, No.4, pp.278-80

19. Malan, V. et al., (2006) Chimera and other fertilization errors. *Clinical Genetics*, No.70, pp 363–373

20. Pearson, H., (2002) Dual identities. *Nature*, Vol.417, No. 6884, p.10-1

21. Ainsworth, C., (2003) The stranger within. *New Scientist*, No 2421, p.34

22. Bird, G. W., (1982) Another Example of Hæmopoietic (Twin) Chimærism in a Subject Unaware of Being a Twin. *Journal of Immunogenetics*, Vol.9, No.317, p.322

23. Schoenle E. et al., (1983) 46,XX/46,XY chimerism in a phenotypically normal man. *Human Genetics*, Vol.64, No.1, pp.86-9

24. Strain, L. et al., (1998)A true hermaphrodite chimera resulting from embryo amalgamation after in vitro fertilization. *New England Journal of Medicine*, Vol.338, No.3, pp.166-169

25. Verp, M.S, Harrison, H.H., Ober, C., el al (1992), Chimerism as the etiology of a 46,XX/46,XY fertile true hermaphrodite. *Fertility and Sterility*, Vol.57, No.2, pp. 346-9

26. McBeth, J., (2005) Woman with two wombs tells of joy after giving birth to twins. *The Scotsman*, 31 Oct.

Chapter 7 : Womb Companions

1. Varma, T.R., (1980) Double uterus with twin pregnancy in the left and singleton in the right horns: a case report. *Journal of Obstetrics & Gynaecology*, Vol.1, No.1, pp.36-37

2. Mold, J. E. et al. (2008). Maternal alloantigens promote the development of tolerogenic fetal regulatory T cells in utero. *Science*, Vol. 322, No. 5907, pp.1562-5

3. Burlingham, W.J., (2009) A lesson in tolerance - maternal instruction to fetal cells. *New England Journal of Medicine*, Vol. 360, No.13, pp.1355-7

4. Heifetz, S.A., (1996) The umbilical cord: obstetrically important lesion. *Clinical Obstetrics & Gynaecology*, No.39, pp.571-87

5. Boyd, P.A,, (1984) Quantitative structure of the normal human placenta from 10 weeks of gestation to term. *Early Human Development*, Vol.9, No.4, pp.297-307

6. Aherne W., & Dunnill, M.S., (1966) Morphometry of the human placenta. *British Medical Bulletin*, Vol. 22, No.1, pp.5-8

7. Winer-Muram, H.T. (1983) Uterine myomas in pregnancy. *Canadian Medical Association Journal.* No.128, pp.949-950

Chapter 8: Vanishing Twins Revealed

1. Anderson, W. F., (1957) Blighted Twin: Report of Three Cases. *Canadian Medical Association Journal*, Vol.76, No. 3, pp. 216–218

2. Quenby, S. et al., (2002) Recurrent miscarriage: a defect in nature's quality control? *Human Reproduction*, Vol. 17, No. 8, pp. 1959-1963

3. Whitehouse, D.B., (1955) Mono-amniotic twins with one blighted; case report. *Journal of Obstetrics and Gynaecology of the British Empire.* Vol. 62, No. 4, pp. 610-1

4. Melnick, R.N. & Godsick, W.H., (1958) Blighted twin diagnosed by x-ray. *New York State Journal of Medicine*, Vol.58, No.10, pp.1743-4

5. Moore, R.M. et al. (1990) Use of diagnostic ultrasound, X-ray examinations, and electronic fetal monitoring in perinatal medicine. *Journal of Perinatology*, Vol.10, No.4, pp.361-5

6. Peres, M.R.,(2007) *Focal Encyclopaedia of Photography : Digital Imaging, Theory and Applications.* Focal Press, p. 279

7. Nilsson, L., (1966) *A Child is Born: The Drama of Life Before Birth*, Delacorte Press

8. Levi, S.J., (1976) Ultrasonic assessment of the high rate of human multiple pregnancy in the first trimester. *Clinical Ultrasound*, Vol.4, No.1, p.5

9. Kurjak, A., & Latin, V., (1979) Ultrasound diagnosis of fetal abnormalities in multiple pregnancy. *Acta Obstetricia et Gynecologica Scandinavica*, Vol.58, No.2, pp.153-61

10. Bernard, K.G., & Cooperberg, P.L., (1985) Sonographic differentiation between blighted ovum and early viable pregnancy. *American Journal of Roentgenology*, Vol.144, No. 3, pp.597-602

11. Finberg, H.J. & J.C. Birnholz, (1979) Ultrasound observations in multiple gestation with first trimester bleeding: the blighted twin. *Radiology*, Vol.132, No.1, pp.137-42

12. Hanna, J.H. & J.M. Hill, (1984) Single intrauterine fetal demise in multiple gestation. *Obstetrics and Gynecology*, Vol.63, No.1, pp.126-30

13. Wright, L., (1997) *Twins: Genes, Environment and the Mystery of Identity.* Weidenfield and Nicholson

14. Landy, H.J. et al., (1982) The Vanishing Twin. *Acta Geneticae Medicae et Gemellologia (Roma)*, Vol. 31, No. 3-4, p.179-94

15. International Planned Parenthood Federation, (1983) The Vanishing Twin. *Research in Reproduction*, Vol.15, No.4, pp.1-2

16. Maly, Z. & Burnog, T., (1986) The disappearing twin, a new phenomenon in ultrasonic diagnosis in pregnancy. [Article in Czech.] *Ceskoslovenska Gynekologie*, Vol.51, No.3, pp.147-9

17. Daw, E.G., (1992) Fetus vanescens, fetus compressus and fetus papyraceus. *Journal of Obstetrics & Gynaecology*, Vol.12, No. 6, pp.375-376

18. Landy, H.J., & Keith, L.G., (1998) The vanishing twin: a review. *Human Reproduction Update*, Vol.4, No.2, pp.177-183

19. Ainsworth, C., (2001) And then there was one. *New Scientist*, No. 2313, October

20. Davis, C., (2007) *Where Did It Go?* Chapter in Hayton, A. (Ed.), *Untwinned: Perspectives on The Death Of a Twin Before Birth*. Wren Publications

21. Landy, H.J. et al.,(1986) The "vanishing twin": ultrasonographic assessment of fetal disappearance in the first trimester. *American Journal of Obstetrics and Gynecology*, Vol.155, No.1, pp.14-9

22. Boklage, C.E., (1995) *The Frequency And Survivability Of Natural Twin Conceptions*. Chapter in Keith, L.G., Papiernik, E., et al. (Eds) *Multiple Pregnancy: Epidemiology, Gestation and Perinatal Outcome*. Parthenon

23. Imaizumi, Y., (2003) A comparative study of zygotic twinning and triplet rates in eight countries, 1972-1999. *Journal of Biosocial Science*, Vol. 35, No. 2, pp.287-302

24. Akinboro, A., Azeez, M.A. et al., (2008) Frequency of twinning in southwest Nigeria. *Indian Journal of Human Genetics*, Vol.14, No. 2, pp.41-7

25. Pector, E.A., (2007) *Twin Traditions Worldwide For Life Death And Mourning*, Chapter 2 in A. Hayton (Ed.) *Untwinned: Perspectives on The Death of a Twin Before Birth*, Wren Publications

26. Imaizumi, Y., (2003) *op. cit*

27. Galton, F., (1883) *Inquiries into Human Faculty and its Development*. Macmillan

28. Hur, Y-M, J.S. Kwon, (2005) Changes in Twinning Rates in South Korea: 1981–2002. *Twin Research and Human Genetics*, Vol.8, No.1, pp. 76-79

29. Keith, L. G. and J. J. Oleszczuk (2002) Triplet births in the united states. An epidemic of high-risk pregnancies. *Journal of Reproductive Medicine*, Vol.47, No.4, pp. 259-65

30. Gibson, F.L. et al. (2002) Children conceived through ICSI and IVF at 5 years of age: behavioural adjustment, parenting stress and attitudes: a comparative study. *Fertility and Sterility*, Vol.78, pp. 28-29

31. De Pascalis, L. et al. (2008) Psychological vulnerability of singleton children after the "vanishing" of a co-twin following assisted reproduction. *Twin Research and Human Genetics* Vol.11, No.1, p.93-8

32. Blickstein, I. (2004) Do multiple gestations raise the risk of cerebral palsy? *Clinical Perinatology*, Vol.31, No.3, p.395-408

33. Pharaoh, P.O., & Cooke, R.W., (1997) A hypothesis for the aetiology of spastic cerebral palsy - the vanishing twin. *Developmental Medicine and Child Neurology*, No.39, p.292–296

34. Hvidtjorn, D. et al (2006) Cerebral palsy among children born after in vitro fertilization: the role of preterm delivery - a population-based, cohort study. *Pediatrics*. Vol. 118, No. 2, pp.475-82

35. Bruck, I., Antoniuk. S.A., et al., (2001) Epilepsy in children with cerebral palsy. *Arquives de Neuropsiquiatrie*, Vol.59, No.1, p.35-39

36. Pharoah, P.O., (2007) Prevalence and pathogenesis of congenital anomalies in cerebral palsy. *Archives of Disease in Childhood. Fetal and Neonatal Edition*, Vol. 92, No.6, pp. F.489-93

37. Pharoah, P.O. & Y. Dundar, (2009) Monozygotic twinning, cerebral palsy and congenital anomalies. *Human Reproduction Update*, Vol. 15, No. 6, pp. 639-48

38. Taylor, C.L. et al., (2009) The risk of cerebral palsy in survivors of multiple pregnancies with cofetal loss or death. *American Journal of Obstetrics and Gynecology*, Vol. 201, No 1, pp. 41

39. Clua, E. et al., (2010) Analysis of factors associated with multiple pregnancy in an oocyte donation programme. *Reproductive Biomedicine Online*, Vol. 21, No. 5, pp.694-9

40. Brodtkorb, E. & G. Myhr, (2001) Short communication: Is monochorionic twinning a risk factor for focal cortical dysgenesis? *Acta Neurologica Scandinavica*, Vol.102, No.1, pp.53-59

Chapter 9: Clues to a Vanishing Twin Pregnancy

1. Staff reporter, (1999) What's in a yam? Clues to fertility, a student discovers. *Yale Medical Bulletin*, Summer, pp. 9-10

2. Bortolus, R., V. Zanardo, et al., (2001) [Epidemiology of identical twin pregnancy], *Pediatria Medica e Chirurgica*, Vol. 23, No. 3-4, pp.153-8

3. Hecht, B.R., Magoon, M,W., (1998) Can the epidemic of iatrogenic multiples be conquered? *Clinical Obstetrics and Gynecology*, Vol. 41, No 1, pp. 127-137

4. Laurance, J. (2009) Seeing double: the village in deepest Kerala where twins have taken over. *The Independent* , May 12

5. People's Daily Online, (2010) 98 sets of twins born in same village in 54 years. *Peoples Daily web site [english.people.com.cn]*, retrieved January 2011

6. Stevenson, R. E. & J. G. Hall, (2005)*Human Malformations And Related Anomalies*. Oxford University Press, p.1385

7. Boklage, C.E., (1990) Survival probability of human conceptions from fertilization to term. *International Journal of Fertility*, No. 35, pp.75 -94

8. Bortolus, R., V. Zanardo, et al., (2001) *op. cit.*

9. Friedman, B.E., Rosen, M.P. et al., (2005) The effect of a vanishing twin on perinatal outcomes. *Fertility and Sterility*, Vol. 84, Supp.1, pp. S1-S2

10. Glick, M.M. & E.L. Dick, (1999) Case Reports: Molar pregnancy presenting with hyperemesis gravidarum. *Journal of the American Osteopathic Association*, Vol. 99, No. 3, pp.162-162

11. Basso, O., Olsen, J., (2001) Sex ratio and twinning in women with hyperemesis or pre-eclampsia. *Epidemiology*, Vol. 12, No.6, pp.747-749

12. Paauw, J.D. et al. (2005) Hyperemesis gravidarum and fetal outcome. *Journal of Parenteral and Enteral Nutrition*, Vol. 29. No.2, pp. 93-6

13. Chasen, S.T., Perni, S.C., et al. (2006) Does a "vanishing twin" affect first-trimester biochemistry in Down syndrome risk assessment ? *American Journal of Obstetrics and Gynecology*, Vol. 195, No.1, pp. 236-9

14. Bingham, P. & Lilford, R.J. (1987) Management of the selected term breech presentation!! Assessment of the risks of selected vaginal delivery versus cesarean section for all cases. *Obstetrics and Gynecology*, Vol. 69, No 6, pp. 965-78

15. Friedman, B.E., M.P. Rosen, et al., (2005) *op. cit*

16. Pinborg, A., Lidegaard, O., et al. (2005) Consequences of vanishing twins in IVF/ ICSI pregnancies. *Human Reproduction*, Vol. 20, No.10, pp. 2821-9

Chapter 10 : Bodily evidence of a womb twin

1. Milham, S., (1966) Symmetrical conjoined twins: an analysis of the birth records of twenty-two sets. *The Journal of Pediatrics*, Vol. 69, No. 4, pp. 643-647

2. Zeitlin, J. et al., (2002) Fetal sex and preterm birth: are males at greater risk? *Human Reproduction* Vol.17, No.10, pp. 2762-8

3. Kraemer, S., (2000) The fragile male. *British Medical Journal*, Vol. 321, No.7276, pp.1609-12

4. Jongbloet, P.H., (2004) "Conception origin" versus "fetal origins" hypothesis and stroke. *Stroke*, Vol. 35, p.e1

5. Loos, R. et al., (2001) Length of gestation and birth weight in dizygotic twins. *The Lancet*, Vol. 358, No. 9281, pp. 560-561

6. Fellman, J. & A. W. Eriksson (2007) Estimation of the stillbirth rate in twin pairs according to zygosity. *Twin Research and Human Genetics*, Vol 10, No. 3, pp.508-13

7. Boklage, C.E., (1985) Interactions between opposite-sex dizygotic fetuses and the assumptions of Weinberg difference method epidemiology. *American Journal of Human Genetics*, Vol. 37, No. 3, p. 591-605

8. Lambalk, C.B., (2007) Freemartins: history, biology and possible clinical relevance. *Abstracts From the 12th International Congress on Twin Studies, Belgium*, 8–10 June 2007, *Twin Research and Human Genetics Supplement*, p.38

9. Miller, E.M., (1994) Prenatal sex hormone transfer: a reason to study opposite-sex twins. *Personality and Individual Differences*, Vol. 17, No. 4, pp. 511-529

10. Van Anders, S.M, et al., (2006) Finger-length ratios show evidence of prenatal hormone-transfer between opposite-sex twins. *Hormones and Behavior*, Vol 49, No.3, pp. 315-319

11. Manning, J. T. et al., (1998) The ratio of 2nd to 4th digit length: a predictor of sperm numbers and concentrations of testosterone, luteinizing hormone and oestrogen. *Human Reproduction*, Vol. 13, No.11, pp. 3000-4

12. Manning, J.T., (2002) *Digit Ratio: A Pointer to Fertility, Behavior, and Health* (A volume in the *Rutgers Series in Human Evolution*, Ed. Robert Trivers.) Rutgers University Press

13. Malas, M.A. et al., (2006) Fetal development of the hand, digits and digit ratio (2D-4D). *Early Human Development*, Vol. 82, No.7 pp.469-75.

14. Manning, J.T., (2002) *op cit.*

15. Medland, S.E. et al., (2008) No effects of prenatal hormone transfer on digit ratio in a large sample of same- and opposite-sex dizygotic twins. *Personality and Individual Differences*, Vol. 44, No.5, pp. 1225–1234

16. Cattrall, F. R. et al., (2005) Anatomical evidence for in utero androgen exposure in women with polycystic ovary syndrome. *Fertility and Sterility*, Vol. 84, No. 6, pp.1689-92

17. Markkula, R. et al., (2009) Clustering of symptoms associated with fibromyalgia in a Finnish twin cohort. *European Journal of Pain*, Vol.13, p.7, pp. 744-50

18. Gupta, A. & A.J Silman, (2004) Psychological stress and fibromyalgia: a review of the evidence suggesting a neuro-endocrine link. *Arthritis Research and Therapy*, Vol. 6, No.3, pp. 98-106

19. Seyle, H.,(1950) *The Physiology And Pathology Of Exposure To Stress*. Oxford

20. Kelly, M.C.,(1998) *Fibromyalgia, Fatigue And You*. Kelmed Publications

21. Carter-Saltzman, L. et al. (1976) Left-handedness in twins: incidence and patterns of performance in an adolescent sample, *Behavior Genetics*, Vol.6, No.2, pp.189-203

22. Runner, M.N, (2005) New evidence for monozygotic twins in the mouse: Twinning initiated in the late blastocyst can account for mirror image asymmetries. *The Anatomical Record*, Vol. 209, No.3, p.399

23. Sommer, I. E. et al. (2002) Language lateralization in monozygotic twin pairs concordant and discordant for handedness. *Brain*, Vol.125, Part 12, pp. 2710-8

24. Boklage, C.E., (1977) Schizophrenia, brain asymmetry development, and twinning: cellular relationship with etiological and possibly prognostic implications. *Biological Psychiatry*, Vol.12, No.1, p.19-35

25. King, M., (2000) *Wrestling With the Angel: A Life of Janet Frame*. Counterpoint, p.400

26. Carter-Saltzman, L. et al., (1976) Left-handedness in twins: incidence and patterns of performance in an adolescent sample. *Behavior Genetics*, Vol. 6, No.2. pp.189-203

27. Curtis, H., & L.F. Petrinovich, (1977) Left-handedness. *Psychological Bulletin*, Vol. 84, No. 3, pp. 385-404

28. Richardson, A.J., (1994) Dyslexia, handedness and syndromes of psychosis-proneness. *International Journal of Psychophysiology*, Vol.18, No.3, pp. 251-263

Chapter 11: The Grief of a Lone Twin

1. Hayton, A., (2009) Attachment issues associated with the loss of a co-twin before birth. *Attachment: New Directions in Psychotherapy and Relational Psychoanalysis*, Vol. 3, No. 2, pp. 144-156

2. Tancredy, C.M. & R.C. Fraley, (2006) The nature of adult twin relationships: an attachment-theoretical perspective. *Journal of Personal & Social Psychology*, Vol. 90, No. 1, pp.78-93

3. Piontelli, A., (2002) *Twins: From Fetus to Child*. Routledge, p.90

4. Woodward, J., (1998) *The Lone Twin*. Free Association Books, p.125

5. Thorpe, K. & Gardner, K., (2006) Twins and their friendships: differences between monozygotic, dizygotic same-sex and dizygotic mixed-sex pairs. *Twin Research and Human Genetics*, Vol. 9, No.1, pp. 155-164

6. Segal, N.L., (2000) *Entwined lives: twins and what they tell us about human behavior*. Plume

7. Wallace, M., (1996) *The Silent Twins*. Vintage

8. Staff reporter, (1993) Jennifer Gibbons, 29, 'Silent Twin' of a Study. *New York Times*, March 12

9. Schave, B & J. Ciriello, (1983) *Identity and Intimacy In Twins*. Praeger

10. Piontelli, A., (2002) *op.cit.* p.140

11. Case, B.J., (1991) *We Are Twins, But Who Am I?* Tibbutt Publishing

12. Macdonald, A.M., (2002) Bereavement in twin relationships: an exploration of themes from a study of twinship. *Twin Research*, Vol. 5, No. 3, pp. 218-226

13. Segal, N.L., & Ream, S.L., (1998) Decrease in grief intensity for deceased twin and non-twin relatives: an evolutionary perspective. *Personality and Individual Differences*, No.25, pp. 317-325

14. Segal N. & S. Blozis, (2002) Psychobiological and evolutionary perspectives on coping and health characteristics following loss: a twin study. *Twin Research*, Vol. 5, No. 3, pp. 175-187

15. Woodward, J., (1988) The Bereaved Twin. *Acta Geneticae Medicae et Gemellologia (Roma)* Vol. 37, No. 2, pp.173-80

16. Woodward, J., (1998) *The Lone Twin: Understanding Twin Bereavement and Loss.* Free Association Books, p.45

17. The Lone Twin Network, P.O. Box 5653, Birmingham, B29 7JY [www.lonetwinnetwork.org.uk]

18. Twinless Twins Support Group International, P.O. Box 980481, Ypsilanti, MI 48198, USA [www.twinlesstwins.org]

19. Dawn, C.M., (2007) *The Surviving Twin: Psychological, Emotional, And Spiritual Impacts Of Having Experienced A Death Before Or At Birth.* Chapter in Hayton, A. (Ed) *Untwinned: Perspectives on The Death of a Twin Before Birth.* Wren Publications

20. Bowlby, J., (1979) *The Making and Breaking of Affectional Bonds.* Routledge

21. Bryan, E.M., (1995) The death of a twin. *Palliative Medicine.* Vol.9, No. 3, pp.187-9

22. Woodward, J., (1998) *op.cit.* p.101

23. Hopkins, J., (2007) *Elvis.* Plexus

Chapter 12: A Womb Twin Remembered

1. Verny, T. R. & J. Kelly, (1981)*The Secret Life Of The Unborn Child.* Summit. p. 12

2. Valman, H.B. & J.F. Pearson, (1980) What the foetus feels. *British Medical Journal*, Vol. 280, No. 6209, p.233-4

3. Birnholz, J.C. & B.R. Benacerraf, (1983) The development of human foetal hearing. *Science*, Vol. 222, p. 4623, p. 516-8

4. Chamberlain, D. B., (2007) *Babies Are Conscious.* Chapter in Hayton, A. (Ed.) *Untwinned: Perspectives On The Death Of A Twin Before Birth.* Wren Publications

5. Chamberlain, D. B., (2007) *op.cit.* p.132

6. Piontelli, A. et al., (1999) Differences and similarities in the intra–uterine behaviour of monozygotic and dizygotic twins. *Twin Research*, Vol. 2, No.4, pp. 264-273

7. Chamberlain, D. B., (2007) *op.cit.* p.136

8. Chamberlain, D. B., (2007) *op.cit.* p.131

9. Wade, J., (1996) *Changes Of Mind - A Holonomic Theory Of The Evolution Of Consciousness.* State University of New York Press, p.25

10. Hepper, P. G., (1997) Fetal habituation: another Pandora's box? *Developmental Medicine and Child Neurology*, Vol.39, No.4, p.274-8

11. James, D., (2010) Foetal learning: a critical review. *Infant & Child Development*, No.19: p.45–54

12. Manrique, B. et al. (1998) A controlled experiment in prenatal enrichment with 684 families in Caracas, Venezuela: Results to age six. *Journal of Prenatal and Perinatal Psychology and Health*, Vol.12, Nos. 3-4, p.209-234

13. Van de Carr, R., & Lehrer, M., (1996) *While You Are Expecting: Your Own Prenatal Classroom*. Humanics Trade

14. Hepper, P.G. & S. Shahidullah, (1993) Newborn and foetal response to maternal voice. *Journal of Reproduction and Infant Psychology*, No.1, p.147-153

15. Arabin, B., R. Bos, et al. (1996) The onset of inter-human contacts: longitudinal ultrasound observations in early twin pregnancies. *Ultrasound in Obstetrics and Gynecology*, Vol. 8, No. 3, p.166-73

16. Liley, A.W., (1972) The foetus as a personality. *Australian and New Zealand Journal of Psychiatry*, Vol. 6, p.99

17. Piontelli, A., (2002) *Twins : From Foetus To Child*. Routledge, p.23

Chapter 13: My child is a Womb Twin Survivor

1. Dawn, C.M., (2003) *The Surviving Twin: Exploring The Psychological, Emotional And Spiritual Impacts Of Having Experienced A Death Before Or At Birth*. PHD Thesis, Santa Barbara Institute, California USA, p.153

2. Piontelli, A., (2002) *Twins: From Fetus to Child*. Routledge, p.6

3. The Center for Loss in Multiple Birth (CLIMB), P.O. Box 91377, Anchorage, AK 99509, USA

4. Progrebin A., (2009) *One and the Same*. Doubleday, p. 186

5. Kollantai, J., (2002) The context and long-term impacts of multiple birth loss: A peer support network perspective. *Twin Research*, Vol.5, No. 3, p.165–168

6. Stillbirth and Neonatal Death charity (SANDS) 28 Portland Place, London, W1B 1LY, England

7. Twins and Multiple Birth Association, (TAMBA) 2 The Willows, Gardner Road, Guildford, GU1 4PG, England

8. Dr. Elizabeth Pector's web site for parents of multiple birth is [www.synspectrum.com/articles.html]

9. Pector, E., (2004) How bereaved multiple birth parents cope with hospitalization, homecoming, disposition for deceased, and attachment to survivors. *Journal of Perinatology*, Vol. 24, No.11, p.714-22

10. Sandbank, A., (1988) *Twins and the Family*. TAMBA, p.170

11. Hayton, A., (1998) *Not Out of Mind*. Arthur James/Wren Publications

12. Hayton, A., (1995) *Lucy's Baby Brother*. Eddlestone Press/Wren Publications

13. Bourne, S. & E. Lewis, (1991) Perinatal bereavement. *British Medical Journal* Vol. 302, p.167-8

14. Briscoe, L. & C. Street, (2003) Vanished twin: an exploration of women's experiences. *Birth*, Vol.30, No.1, p.47

15. Conway, K. & G. Russell, (2000) Couples' grief and experience of support in the aftermath of miscarriage. *British Journal of Medical Psychology*, Vol.73, No.4, pp. 531-545

16. Beutel, M. et al. (1995) Grief and depression after miscarriage: their separation, antecedents, and course. *Psychosomatic Medicine*, Vol. 57, No. 6, pp. 517-526

17. Broen, A.N. et al. (2004) Psychological impact on women of miscarriage versus induced abortion: a 2-year follow-up study. *Psychosomatic Medicine*, No.66, p.265-271
18. Schulz, L., (2003) *The Survivor.* Pleasant Word Publishing, p.64
19. Dawn, C.M., (2003) *op.cit*, p. 153
20. Pinheiro, C. & Maria da Luz Alves da Silva, (2009) *Me and My Twin.* Wren Publications
21. Aron, E., (2002) *The Highly Sensitive Child: Helping Our Children When The World Overwhelms Them.* Broadway, p.4

Chapter 14: A Womb Twin Discovered

1. Stuttaford, T., (1996) Ghost of the missing twin. *The Times*, Aug.8, p.14
2. Babcock, B., (2009) *My Twin Vanished, Did Yours?* Tate Publishing, p. 32
3. Babcock, B., (2009) *ibid.* p.107
4. Janov, A., (2000) *The Biology of Love*, Prometheus Books
5. The Association of Pre- and Perinatal Psychology and Health (APPPAH) P.O. Box 1398, Forestville, CA 95436, USA [www.birthpsychology.com]
6. James, J., (2007) *The Vanishing Twin Syndrome, And The Traumatic Reality From This Loss,* Chapter in Hayton, A. (Ed.) *Untwinned: Perspectives on the Death of a Twin Before Birth.* Wren Publications
7. Chamberlain, D., (1999) Transpersonal Adventures in Prenatal and Perinatal Hypnotherapy, *Journal of Prenatal and Perinatal Psychology and Health*, Vol.14, No 2, p.90
8. Chamberlain, D., (1999) *ibid.* p.93
9. Austermann, A., (2006) *The Surviving Twin Syndrome.* Konigsweg-Verlag, p.184
10. Cogley, J., (2005) *Wood You Believe, Volume One: The Unfolding Self. Healing & Self-Awareness Exploring Spirituality And Psychology Through Handcrafted Wood Symbols.* AuthorHouse
11. Myers, D., (2000) *Intuition: its Powers and Perils.* Yale University Press
12. Bishop, D.V.M. & S.J. Bishop, (1998) Twin language: a risk factor for language impairment? *Journal of Speech, Language, and Hearing Research*, February, pp.150-160

Chapter 15: The Lost Twin in the Dream of the Womb

1. Ruiz, D.M., (1997) *The Four Agreements.* Amber-Allen Publishing, p.49
2. Freud, S., (1977) *Inhibitions, symptoms and anxiety. Standard edition.* W.W. Norton & Co., p.138
3. Rank, O., (1929) *The Trauma of Birth.* Kegan Paul & Co.
4. Nandor, F., (1949) *The Search for the Beloved: A Clinical Investigation of the Trauma of Birth and Prenatal Condition.* University Books
5. Ployé, P.M., (1973) Does prenatal mental life exist? *International Journal of Psycho-Analysis*, No. 54, pp. 241-246
6. Laing, R.D., (1970) *Sanity, Madness and the Family: Families of Schizophrenics.* Pelican Books
7. Laing, R.D., (1976) *The Facts of Life.* Pantheon Books, p.36

8. Lake, F., (1981) *Tight Corners In Pastoral Counselling*. Darton, Longman and Todd.
9. Janov, A.,(1973) *The Primal Scream*. Abacus
10. Janov, A. (2000) *The Biology of Love*. Prometheus Books, p.17
11. Arthur Janov's forthcoming book has the working title of *Life Before Birth*
12. Leboyer, F., (1975) *Birth Without Violence*. Knopf
13. Grof, S., (1985) *Beyond The Brain: Birth, Death, And Transcendence In Psychotherapy*. State University of New York
14. Spensley, J., (2008) *Graham Farrant, 1933-1993, Healing Life of Many Births*, online article. [primal-page.com/gfobit.htm] Retrieved Sept 2010
15. Farrant, G., (1988) Cellular Consciousness and Conception. *Pre- and Perinatal Psychology News*, Vol.2, No.2
16. The Association for Prenatal and Perinatal Psychology and Health (APPPAH), P.O. Box 1398, Forestville, CA, 95436, USA
17. Verney, T.R., (Ed.) (1986) *Pre- And Perinatal Psychology: An Introduction*. Human Sciences Press
18. From the APPPAH web site [www.birthpsychology.com] retrieved June 2010
19. Arabin, B., R. Bos, et al. (1996) The onset of inter-human contacts: longitudinal ultrasound observations in early twin pregnancies. *Ultrasound in Obstetrics and Gynecology*, Vol. 8, No.3, p.166-73
20. Woodward, J., (1998) *The Lone Twin : A Study In Bereavement And Loss*. Free Association Books, p.1.
21. Woodward, J., (1988) The Bereaved Twin. *Acta Geneticae Medicae et Gemellologia (Roma)* Vol.37, No.2, pp.173-80
22. Bowlby, J., (1969) *Attachment and Loss, Vol. 1: Attachment*. The Hogarth Press
23. Noble, E., (1993) *Primal Connections*. Simon & Schuster
24. Pector, E., *Raising Survivors Of Multiple Birth Loss*. Document from Dr Pector's own website [www.synspectrum.com/survivors3.doc] Retrieved Sept 2010

Chapter 16: The Womb Twin Research Project

1. Pozzebon, M., (2004) *Conducting and Evaluating Critical Interpretive Research: Examining Criteria as a Key Component in Building a Research Tradition*. Chapter in *Information Systems Research*, Springer

Chapter 17: An Unusual Person

1. Aron. E., (1999) *The Highly Sensitive Person: How To Survive And Thrive When The World Overwhelms You*. Thorsens

Chapter 18: Signs of Psychological Distress

1. Weissman, M. et al. (1999). Prevalence of suicide ideation and suicide attempts in nine countries. *Psychological Medicine*, Vol. 29, No.1, p. 9-17
2. Roedding, J.,(1991) Birth trauma and suicide. A study of the relationship between near death experience and later suicidal behaviour. *Pre and Perinatal Psychology Journal*, Vol. 6, No. 2, Winter.

3. Ward, S.A., (2007) *Suicide And Pre-And Perinatal Psychotherapy*, Chapter in A.Hayton, (Ed.) *Untwinned: Perspectives On The Death Of A Twin Before Birth*. Wren Publications

4. Grof, S.,(1986) *Beyond the Brain: Birth, Death, and Transendence in Psychotherapy*. State University of New York Press

5. Ombelet, W. et al. (2006) Perinatal outcome of 12,021 singleton and 3108 twin births after non-IVF-assisted reproduction: a cohort study. *Human Reproduction*, Vol. 21, No. 4, p.1025-32

6. Tomassini, C. et al. (2003) Risk of suicide in twins: 51 year follow-up study. *British Medical Journal.* Vol. 327, No. 7411, p. 373-4

7. Stroebe, M. et al. (2005) The broken heart: suicidal ideation in bereavement. *American Journal of Psychiatry*, Vol. 162, No.11, p. 2178-80

8. Feldmar, A., (1979). *The Embryology Of Consciousness: What Is A Normal Pregnancy?* Chapter in D. Mall & W. Watts (Eds.), *The Psychological Aspects of Abortion*. University Publications of America., p. 15-24

9. Ward, S.A., (2007) *op. cit.*

10. McCall, W.V. et al. (2010) Insomnia severity is an indicator of suicidal ideation during a depression clinical trial. *Sleep Medicine*, May 15th

11. Laing, R.D., (1967) *The Politics of Experience*. Routledge & Kegan Paul, p.113

Chapter 19: Difficult Feelings

1. Segal N.L. et al., (2002) Monozygotic and Dizygotic Twins' Retrospective and Current Bereavement-related Behaviors: An Evolutionary Perspective. *Twin Research*, Vol. 5, No.3, p.188-195

2. Maier, S.F. & M.E. Seligman,(1976) Learned helplessness: theory and evidence. *Journal of Experimental Psychology: General*, Vol.105 No.1, pp. 3-46

3. Freud, S., (1920, 1954) *Beyond the pleasure principle*. In *Complete Psychological Works*, *Standard Ed.* Vol 3. Translated and edited by J.Strachey. Hogarth Press

Chapter 20 : A Problem With Relationships

1. Tancredy, C.M. & Fraley, R.C., (2006) The nature of adult twin relationships: an attachment-theoretical perspective. *Journal of Personality and Social Psychology*, Vol. 90, No. 1, 78-93

2. Bowlby, J.,(2005) *The Making And Breaking Of Affectional Bonds*. Routlege

3. Hayton, A., (2009) Attachment Issues Associated with the Loss of a Co-twin Before Birth. *Attachment: New Directions in Psychotherapy and Relational Psychoanalysis*, Vol. 3, No. 2 p.144-156

4. Fraley, R. C. & Davis, K. E., (1997) Attachment formation and transfer in young adults' close friendships and romantic relationships. *Personal Relationships*, No. 4, pp.131–144

5. Gunderson, J.G., (1996) The borderline patient's intolerance of aloneness: insecure attachments and therapist availability. *American Journal of Psychiatry*, No.153, pp.752-758

6. Sverd, J. et al. (2003) Pervasive developmental disorders among children and adolescents attending psychiatric day treatment. *Psychiatric Services* No.54, pp.1519-1525

7. Hughes, J., (1980) Manipulation: a negative element in care. *Journal of Advanced Nursing*, Vol.5, No., pp.21-9

Chapter 21: Self-sabotage

1. Britton, A., M.J.Shipley, (2010) Bored To Death? *International Journal Of Epidemiology*. Vol.39, No 2, p. 370-371
2. Frame, J.,(2004) *Janet Frame An Autobiography: To the Is-Land; An Angel at my Table; The Envoy from Mirror City*. Vintage
3. López-Corvo, R.E., (2003) *The Dictionary Of The Work Of W.R. Bion*. Karnac books, p.143

Chapter 22: Self-defeating Behaviour

1. Cruz, J. et al. (2000) *Self-Defeating Personality Disorder Reconsidered*. Journal of Personality Disorders, Vol. 14, No.1, p.64-71
2. Frost, R.,(2010) *Stuff: Compulsive Hoarding and the Meaning of Things*. Houghton Mifflin Harcourt
3. Samuels, J. F., O. J. Bienvenu, et al. (2008) Prevalence and correlates of hoarding behavior in a community-based sample. *Behavioral Research and Therapy*, Vol. 46, No.7, p.836-44
4. National Study Group on Chronic Disorganization (NSGCD) 1693 S. Hanley Rd. St. Louis, MO, 63144, USA [www.nsgcd.org]
5. Tolin, D.F., R.O.Frost, G.Steketee, (2007) *Buried in Treasures: Help for Compulsive Acquiring, Saving, and Hoarding*. Oxford University Press, USA
6. Frost, R.,(2010) *op. cit.*
7. Hayton A., (2000) *Food And You: Stage One, An Introduction To The Four Zero Experience*. Wren Publications
8. Hayton, A (2008) The possible prenatal origins of morbid obesity. *Journal of Prenatal & Perinatal Psychology & Health*, Vol.23, No. 2, pp.79-89
9. Lefever, R.,(2000) *Kick the Habit*. Carlton Books
10. Heyman, G.M.,(2009) *Addiction: A Disorder of Choice*. Harvard University Press
11. Schaler, J.A.,(2002) *Addiction is a Choice*. Open Court Publishing
12. Klonsky, E. D. et al. (2003). Deliberate self-harm in a nonclinical population: prevalence and psychological correlates. *American Journal of Psychiatry*, Vol.160, No.8, p.1501-8
13. Favazza, A.R., (1996) *Bodies under siege: self-mutilation and body modification in culture and psychiatry*. The Johns Hopkins University Press

Chapter 23: A Fragile Sense of Self

1. Yalom, I., (1980) *Existential Psychotherapy*. Basic Books, p. 277
2. Fernandes, F.,(2007) *Working With The Concept Of Stuckness*. Chapter in W. Dryden (Ed.) *Key Issues For Counselling In Action*. Sage Publications, p.160
3. Snyder, C. R. & S. J. Lopez, (2006) *Positive Psychology : The Scientific And Practical Explorations Of Human Strengths*. Sage Publications. p.241

4. Loy, D. (1998) Lack and transcendence: the problem of death and life in psychotherapy, existentialism, and Buddhism. *Philosophy East and West*, Vol. 48, No. 4
5. Frankl, V., (2006) *Man's Search for Meaning*. Beacon Press
6. Loy, D. R., (1992) Avoiding The Void: The Lack of Self in Psychotherapy and Buddhism. *The Journal of Transpersonal Psychology*, Vol. 24, No. 2 pp.151-180
7. Lefever R.,(2000) *Kick the Habit*. Carlton Books
8. Rogers, C.R.,(1951) *Client-centred Therapy*. Constable, p.489
9. Laing, R., (1967) *The Politics of Experience*, Routledge & Kegan Paul p.22

Chapter 24: Being a Twin

1. Burlingham, D.T. (1945) The fantasy of having a twin. *Psychoanalytic Study of the Child*, No.1, p. 205-210
2. St Clair, J.B., (2002) Paternally derived twinning: a two-century examination of records of one scottish name. *Twin Research*, Vol.5. No.4, p. 294-307
3. Chenevix-Trench, G., S. Healey, N.G. Martin (1993) Reproductive hormone genes in mothers of spontaneous dizygotic twins: an association study. *Human Genetics*, Vol. 91, No. 2, p.118-120
4. Austermann, A., (2006) *The Surviving Twin Syndrome*. Konigweg-Verlag

Chapter 25 : Tools for Healing

1. Donne, J., (1839) *Meditation Xvii. Nunc Lento Sonitu Dicunt, Morieris*. From Henry Alford, (Ed.) *The works of John Donne*. Vol 3. John W. Parker, p. 574
2. Hopkins, G.M., (1918) *No Worst, There Is None. Pitched Past Pitch Of Grief*, in *Poems of Gerard Manley Hopkins*. Humphrey Milford

Chapter 27: Forgiveness

1. Eckhart Tolle, E., (1999) *The Power of Now*. Hodder and Stoughton, p.29
2. Darwin, C., (1859) *On the Origin of Species*. John Murray

Chapter 28: Letting go, letting be

1. "Nicholas", (2008) *Last Rites*, Chapter in *A Silent Cry: Womb Twin Survivors Tell Their Stories*. Wren Publications, p.181

Glossary

Amniotic fluid	The fluid surrounding a foetus within the amnion
Amniotic sac	The sac in which the foetus develops, also known as the bag of waters
ART	Assisted reproductive technology. Includes IVF, use of fertility drugs, artificial insemination, GIFT, ICSI
Asphyxiation	Death by lack of air
Blastocyst	An embryo that has developed for five to six days after fertilization
Blastomere	A cell produced by division of the egg after fertilization
Caesarean delivery	Surgical procedure in which one or more incisions are made through a mother's abdomen to deliver one or more babies
Capacitation	Preparation of a spermatozoon to enable penetration of the ovum
Capillaries	The smallest kind of blood vessels, one cell thick
Cervical cerclage	The cervix is stitched closed in to prevent a miscarriage
Chimera	An organism containing cells from of two or more genetically-distinct sources
Chromosome	A string of DNA molecules in a thread-like structure
Cortical dysgenesis	Abnormal development of the cerebral cortex
Cytomegalovirus (CMV)	A common virus that is part of the herpes group of viruses, which can also cause cold sores or genital warts
Dizygotic	Formed from two zygotes
DNA	Deoxyribonucleic acid, a self-replicating material present in nearly all living organisms as the main constituent of chromosomes. It is the carrier of genetic information
Ectopic pregnancy	When an embryo begins to develop outside the womb, usually in the fallopian tube
Epigenetic drift	The process of change in the genetic composition of a pair or small group due to chance or random events rather than by natural selection, resulting in changes in genes frequencies over time
Epigenetics	The study of changes in gene function brought about by environmental influences
Cerebral palsy	A group of neurological disorders caused by damage to the brain during the pregnancy
Foetus papyraceous	A twin foetus that died after 12 weeks of development and has been pressed flat against the uterine wall by the growth of the living foetus
Foetal pole	A thickening on the margin of the yolk sac, visible at six weeks of pregnancy

FSH	Follicle stimulating hormone, which stimulated the production of eggs
Gamete	Cells with half the usual number of chromosomes which fuse during fertilization to create a zygote
GIFT	Eggs and sperm are placed directly into the fallopian tubes, where fertilization will hopefully occur
HCG	Human chorionic gonadotropin
Hydatidiform mole	A rare mass or growth that forms inside the uterus at the beginning of a pregnancy.
Hyperovulation drugs	Fertility drugs causing hyperovulation (stimulated release of multiple eggs by the mother)
ICSI	The injection of a single sperm directly into an egg outside the body. The embryo is placed into the uterus.
Immune system	A network of cells, tissues and organs that work together to defend the body against attacks by "foreign" invaders
Implantation	An event that occurs early in pregnancy in which the embryo adheres to the wall of uterus
Intrauterine	Inside the womb
IVF	Harvesting and fertilization of ova outside the body and placement of the embryos into the uterus
Luteinizing Hormone	A hormone that stimulates ovulation and the production of testosterone in the male
Menstrual cycle	Menstrual cycles are counted from the first day of menstrual bleeding in a woman. The cycle is usually around 28 days
Mitochondria	An organelle found in large numbers in most cells. Facilitates respiration and energy production.
Mo-mo twins	Monozygotic monoamniotic twins, created from one zygote and sharing a placenta and amniotic sac.
Monoamniotic	Sharing an amniotic sac
Monozygotic	Formed from one zygote
Morula	Embryo at an early stage of embryonic development, consisting of a ball of blastomeres
Mosaic	An individual with cells of two genetically different types
MRI scan	A form of medical imaging that measures the response of the atomic nuclei of body tissues to high-frequency radio waves when placed in a strong magnetic field
Multiple birth	A pregnancy when more than one baby is conceived and survives until birth
Neural tube	The brain and spinal cord in its earliest stages

Oestrogen	A group of steroid hormones that maintain female sexual characteristics
Oocyte	A female germ cell in the process of development
Ovulation	When one or more eggs are released from the ovaries
Ovum	The egg, the female gamete
Petrie dish	A flat glass dish with a lid
Placenta	A flattened circular organ in the uterus which nourishes the foetus through the umbilical cord
Polycystic ovary syndrome	A condition in which the ovaries do not work properly because of the presence of several cysts.
Radiographer	Someone who operates an ultrasound machine to make ultrasound scans
Resorbed	The absorption into the circulation of cells or tissue
Singleton	A baby conceived and born alone
Sonogram	A visual image produced from an ultrasound examination also known as an ultrasound scan
Spermatozoon	The male sex cell by which the ovum is fertilized
Stillbirth	The birth of an infant that has died in the womb or is born without breathing
Stricture	Abnormal narrowing of a tube or duct in the body
Superfetation	The occurrence of a second conception during pregnancy, giving rise to embryos of different ages in the uterus
Testosterone	A steroid hormone that stimulates development of male secondary sexual characteristics
Trophoblast	A layer of tissue on the outside of the developing embryo which forms the major part of the placenta
Ultrasound scan	A visual image produced from an ultrasound examination also known as a sonogram
Vagina	The muscular tube leading from the external genitals to the cervix
Vaginal bleeding	Bleeding from the vagina
Womb script	A series of prenatal experiences that are repeated in coded form in born life
Womb twin survivor	The sole survivor of a twin or multiple conception
Zona pellucida	The clear zone that can be seen surrounding the morula
Zygote	A large cell created from the fusion of two gametes
Yolk sac	A sac where blood is formed and which provides nutrition to the developing embryo in the first four or five weeks.

Lightning Source UK Ltd.
Milton Keynes UK
UKHW02f2017190618

324487UK00016B/410/P